POST
ANESTHESIA
CARE
NURSING

POST ANESTHESIA CARE NURSING

KIM LITWACK, PhD, RN

**Associate Professor, College of Nursing,
Rush University;
Unit Leader, Post Anesthesia Recovery,
Rush-Presbyterian-St Luke's Medical Center
Chicago, Illinois**

with 50 illustrations

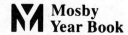

**Mosby
Year Book**

St. Louis   Baltimore   Boston   Chicago   London   Philadelphia   Sydney   Toronto

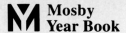
**Mosby
Year Book**

Editor: Nancy L. Coon
Developmental editor: Suzanne Seeley
Project manager: Patricia Gayle May
Production editor: Sheila Walker
Designer: Laura Steube

Printed in the United States of America

Mosby-Year Book, Inc.
11830 Westline Industrial Drive, St. Louis, Missouri 63146

Library of Congress Cataloging-in-Publication Data

Litwack, Kim.
    Post anesthesia care nursing/Kim Litwack.
        p.   cm.
    Includes bibliographical references.
    Includes index.
    ISBN 0-8016-6081-5
    1. Postoperative care.   2. Surgical nursing.   I. Title.
    [DNLM: 1. Postoperative Care.   2. Postoperative Period—nurses'
instruction.   3. Surgical Nursing.   WY   161 L782p]
RD51.L58   1990
617.919—dc20
DNLM/DLC
for Library of Congress   90-6517
                                                                            CIP

C/RRD/RRD   9   8   7   6   5   4   3   2   1

To Danny with love

PREFACE

To practice in the post anesthesia care unit (PACU), a nurse must be able to integrate physiologic, medical, surgical, and anesthesia information to set appropriate patient care priorities. PACU nursing demands the integration of unique knowledge and skills to optimize the status of each patient.

Professional specialization demands specialized knowledge. Unfortunately, existing references for the emerging specialty of PACU nursing are either written by physicians, with little emphasis on nursing care or nursing issues, or by nurses, with little emphasis on techniques, technologies, or drugs, and their effects. *Post Anesthesia Care Nursing* has been written to provide this needed body of information.

Post Anesthesia Care Nursing is written for the practicing PACU nurse by a practicing PACU nurse. It is drawn from experience, science, research, and practice. The text will also prove useful to nurses preparing for CPAN certification, to PACU unit managers, advanced students in collegiate schools of nursing, intensive care unit nurses who receive patients directly from the operating room, operating room nurses who are directly involved with intraoperative and postoperative care and recovery of surgical patients, and clinical specialists with responsibility for the PACU. The emphasis of the text is on understanding *why* we do what we do.

FEATURES OF THE TEXT

Chapter 1 examines the past, present, and future influences on PACU nursing and PACU care. Chapter 2 relates the importance of preoperative assessment to PACU care. Chapters 3 and 4 focus on anesthetic agents and techniques, emphasizing the nursing implications required to provide optimum care for the postanesthetic patient. Chapter 5 provides a systematic discussion of postanesthetic and postoperative assessment. Chapter 6 focuses on hemodynamic monitoring, an increasingly essential technology in the PACU. Chapters 7 and 8 address common postanesthetic problems and emergencies, identifying patients at risk and recognition and treatment of problems. Chapter 9 examines the needs of special patient populations. Chapter 10 examines quality assurance issues specific to the PACU. Chapter 11 examines the legal issues specific to the PACU and PACU nursing.

The text features chapter objectives and chapter-specific references. Each chapter includes review questions (and answers) designed to assist the PACU nurse in further study. The review questions may also be used as a pretest before reading the chapter, or in preparation for the CPAN certification examination.

ACKNOWLEDGMENTS

Although this text is the written word of one author, I wish to acknowledge the following individuals for their assistance in critiquing chapters for content: Drs. David Rothenberg, Sam Parnass, Floyd Heller, Kate Kierney, Peter Murphy, and Timothy Lubenow; Richard Schillo, Deb Levin, Cynthia Motton, and Tim Buell. A special thank you goes to Donna Ritacco for her expert typing of the manuscript, and to Nancy Coon, Nursing Editor, Suzanne Seeley, Developmental Editor, and Sheila Walker, Senior Production Editor at Mosby-Year Book. My work was enhanced by all of their efforts.

Kim Litwack

TABLE OF CONTENTS_____

CHAPTER 1

It has been said that to understand where we are going, we have to know where we have been. In the area of post anesthesia care, it is important to have an understanding of the history of the post anesthesia care unit (PACU), post anesthesia care nursing, and the development of the professional organization for post anesthesia care nurses.

POST ANESTHESIA CARE NURSING

Chapter Objectives

After reading this chapter, the reader should be able to:

1. Identify factors that contributed to the development of the post anesthesia recovery unit.
2. Identify the purpose of the post anesthesia care unit (PACU).
3. Discuss future trends that are likely to influence the PACU.
4. Discuss the role of the PACU nurse as specialist.
5. Discuss the role of the PACU nurse as generalist.
6. Identify the purpose of the American Society of Post Anesthesia Nurses (ASPAN).

POST ANESTHESIA CARE UNITS: PAST, PRESENT, AND FUTURE

Prior to the 1940s, documentation of the existence of post anesthesia recovery rooms is somewhat vague and controversial. Some texts cite the Mayo Clinic in Rochester, Minnesota (1942) as having had the first post anesthesia rooms.[6] However, references have been found citing the existence of recovery rooms in 1904 (Boston City Hospital), 1923 (Johns Hopkins Hospital), 1932 (Cook County Hospital, Chicago), and 1938 (New Britain General Hospital, Connecticut). It is difficult to confirm or validate the existence of the first post anesthesia care unit (PACU) in the United States.[3] It is possible, however, to identify factors that contributed to making the existence of PACUs desirable.

In the 1940's, the Anesthesia Study Commission of the Philadelphia Medical Society published a report of a study reviewing cases of patient deaths that occurred within 24 hours of the induction of anesthesia.[11] The Commission evaluated each case, with the goal of determining the cause of death, and, more important, whether the fatality appeared to be preventable or nonpreventable. A total of 306 postoperative fatalities were studied.

The most common factors contributing to postoperative death were identified, in order of occurrence, as inadequate management, poor oxygenation, and excessive dose of anesthetic agent. Other contributing factors included error in judgment, poor choice of anesthesia, inadequate supervision, error in technique, problems with sedation, intraoperative respiratory obstruction, and laryngospasm.

It is interesting to note, that of the 306 fatalities reported, 144, or 47%, were classified as preventable. That is, it was believed by a majority of members of the Commission that, if some factor of management pertaining to anesthesia had been instituted differently, the fatality would probably not have occurred.

In an effort to reduce the morbidity and mortality associated with anesthesia, the Commission called for the presence and maintenance of post anesthesia rooms. The post anesthesia rooms were to be staffed by specially trained nurses, under the direction of Anesthesia Departments, with provisions made for the presence of resuscitation equipment.

In 1951, using the Anesthesia Study Commission data as evidence, Lowenthal and Russell went on to detail the requirements for a successful recovery unit and the advantages of a recovery room.[9]

The requirements for a successful recovery unit were identified as follows: supervision, personnel, equipment, space, location, and availability. The authors called for a unit that would be supervised by anesthesiologists with surgeons available, staffed by nurses oriented to the unique needs of the post anesthesia patient, and supplied with oxygen, suction, airways, medications, and intravenous fluids. The unit was to accommodate two litters for each active operating room and was to be located on the same floor as the operating rooms. The unit should, ideally, be open for use 24 hours a day.

The advantages of a recovery unit were identified as (1) centralization of patients, equipment, and personnel, (2) increased patient safety, and (3) economy of resources. The authors also cited the advantage of protection afforded the physician and the hospital against liability. The recovery unit was seen as a means to save lives and as a way to reduce the morbidity and mortality associated with anesthesia and surgery.

Whether it is referred to as *postop, postop recovery (POR), postoperative ward (POW), recovery room (RR), post anesthesia recovery (PAR), post anesthesia recovery unit (PARU), post anesthesia recovery area (PARA), or post anesthesia care unit (PACU),* the goal of the unit is to provide optimal patient care for the postanesthetic and postsurgical patient.[3]

It is interesting to note that the initial PACU was a combination postanesthetic and postsurgical unit, or what today would be considered a combination of a PACU and surgical intensive care unit. Over time, the trend was to separate the care of the postsurgical patient into immediate care (post anesthesia) and ongoing care (postsurgical). The PACU became separate from the surgical intensive care unit.

As we move into the 1990s, the trend is once again toward combining the two units. This time, the move toward consolidation is the result of an increasing demand for intensive care beds. It has been speculated that the hospitals of the future will be for intensive care and ambulatory patients only.

More and more surgery is being performed on an outpatient basis, including types of surgery traditionally associated with inpatient hospitalizations (cholecystectomies, mastectomies, tonsillectomies). With the increase in technology, surgical equipment, medications, and resources, the remaining inpatients require much care and attention (high acuity). The intensive care units have become life support units, with patients requiring ventilator support, polypharmacy, and technologies for organ function (ventricular assistance devices, dialysis, transplantation). Patients who traditionally have spent the night in the intensive care unit for careful monitoring, including thoracic and vascular surgery patients, are now returning to general surgical units on the day of surgery, greatly increasing the acuity level and staffing needs of the surgical floors.

In addition, the demand for intensive care beds is increasing as the general population increases in age. With increasing age comes the chronic health care problems of cardiac disease, vascular disease, pulmonary disease, and orthopedic degeneration (see Chapter 9). These medical problems are rarely curable; they require continual management of symptoms.

Turnover of staff in the intensive care units is high, partly because of the high-acuity and chronic nature of the diseases of the patients in these units. It is a challenge to recruit and retain staff. Lack of adequate staffing may force bed closures.

As intensive care beds become filled, with no cessation of the surgical schedule, the overflow of patients is being cared for in the PACU. Now, in addition to providing acute postanesthetic and postoperative care to the surgical patient, the PACU is becoming a unit for extended care and extended recovery of surgical patients.

In addition to providing care for postsurgical patients, the PACU is becoming a special procedures unit. PACUs are being used for electroconvulsive therapy (ECT), elective cardioversions, blood donations, and endoscopies, as pain centers for epidural injections, and as holding areas for preoperative patient preparation. PACU, in many instances, seems to stand for Put All you Can in the Unit.

Although the PACU may prove to be the ideal unit for many special procedures—because of the availability of personnel, resources, and space and the potential to maximize patient safety—use of the PACU for more than postanesthetic and postoperative care of surgical patients may cause many problems. These problems include staffing, space, safety, and, from a management perspective, morale issues.

Most PACUs plan staffing requirements based on patient census and acuity. It is difficult to plan for times when the intensive care unit is full and patients are required to remain in the PACU overnight. As a result, most PACUs have, by necessity, developed an on-call system to provide nursing care at times of unpredictable patient admissions. Although availability of an on-call nurse meets the immediate need of night or weekend coverage, the nurse is then faced with the problem of having to work a regularly scheduled day after being awake all night.

Space may become an issue. The ideal PACU has at least one and a half spaces for every operating room. If most of the patients on the operating schedule are short-procedure outpatients, two PACU spaces per operating room are recommended. Unfortunately, if these spaces become occupied by nonsurgical patients, it is difficult to provide service to the day's surgical patients.

Safety may become compromised if patients are discharged from the PACU prematurely to make space for the next patient from the operating room to be admitted. However, it is the rare PACU nurse who has not at some time pulled a patient into the hall or off to the side to await discharge, a technologic assistance device (analgesia pump), or a clean room. Thus the six bed PACU becomes a seven or eight bed unit. Although the physical space may be adequate to handle seven or eight patients, several of these patients may find themselves without direct access to cardiac monitors, oxygen, or suction devices. Liability and the potential for patient injury become significant risks.

Morale of staff and management has become an increasing problem. The nurses begin to perceive the PACU as a "dumping ground" and to believe that every other unit in the hospital except the PACU can "say no." The PACU is perceived by those external to the unit as a place of unlimited resources and personnel. PACU nurses may feel a lack of support from hospital and nursing management as the unit is asked to do more, often without additional staff, resources, or equipment. Additional responsibilities will be met with less resistance if the increased workload is a planned event, one that is supported by management, both verbally and with resources.

The PACU of the future is likely to continue to be a unit of high-acuity patients. The demand will be for highly specialized nurses. Technologic advances will become standard, increasing monitoring capabilities. New drugs and surgical advances will continue to be developed and incorporated into care.

The subspecialty of ambulatory surgery will place additional demands on the PACU. Some hospitals have already begun to feel the outcome of providing care in a more invasive and intensive manner. The trend is increasingly toward home care and 23-hour observation units. Families are playing an increasing role in postoperative care.

PACU NURSES: PAST, PRESENT, AND FUTURE

When the Anesthesia Study Commission called for the existence of post anesthesia units, it was recognized that the nurses who were to work in these units would require specialized training, targeted toward the management of postoperative emergencies and toward meeting the needs of the postanesthetic and postsurgical patient.[9,11] Postoperative emergencies included obstructed airway, decreased gas exchange, cardiovascular depression, and aspiration. Meeting patient needs called for the nurses to provide care and monitoring in the areas of airway and respiratory activity, heart rate and blood pressure, temperature, comfort, intravenous fluids, surgical drains, catheters and urinary output.[4] It is interesting to note that despite the advances in science, technology, surgery, and anesthesia, postoperative emergencies and postoperative patient needs have not changed in over 50 years!

The PACU nurse today must possess highly specific knowledge and skills along with a broad base of general knowledge and skills. The PACU nurse must have expertise specific to the needs of the post anesthesia patient. This includes knowledge of anesthetic agents and techniques (Chapters 3 and 4), postoperative priorities and assessment (Chapter 5), and postoperative problems and emergencies (Chapters 7 and 8). The PACU nurse must possess skills in airway management, basic and advanced life support measures, and postsurgical care.

As a generalist, the PACU nurse cares for pediatric, adult, and geriatric patients, as well as ambulatory (low-acuity) and intensive care (high-acuity) patients. The PACU nurse provides care to patients after all surgical procedures and is, therefore, expected to be familiar with all surgical specialties. Because surgical patients often have chronic medical problems, the PACU nurse is expected to have a working knowledge of such disorders, including cardiac, pulmonary, endocrine, and renal disorders. If the PACU provides care to patients after delivery or for electroconvulsive therapy, the PACU nurse will be expected to have knowledge of obstetric and psychiatric patients. Now that PACUs are providing ambulatory care services, the PACU nurse is expected to have knowledge of community health issues, including knowledge of community resources.

The PACU nurse institutes many nursing actions independently, using the nursing process. The PACU nurse works collaboratively with anesthesiologists and surgeons, residents, and nurse anesthetists. The PACU nurse coordinates the provision of respiratory, ECG, laboratory, and blood services. The goal is to help the patient become ready for discharge to an intensive care, general surgical, or medical unit or to home. The role of the PACU nurse as patient care coordinator is schematically depicted in Fig. 1-1.

The PACU nurse of the future will continue to practice as a post anesthesia specialist and a postoperative generalist. The increasing patient acuity will require nurses to possess strong physiology backgrounds, with increasing emphasis on the "why" of practice,

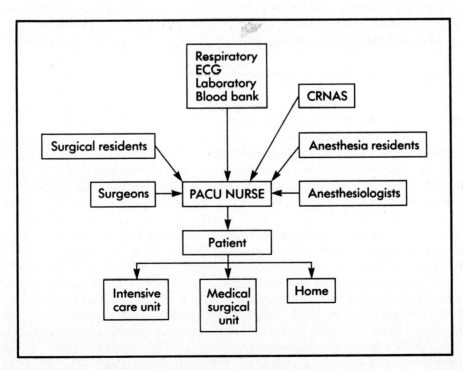

FIG. 1-1. The PACU nurse as patient care coordinator.

not just the "how to." Nurses will be required to master the critical care skills of hemo-dynamic monitoring, respiratory care, and vasoactive pharmacology. Technologic advances in cardiac and respiratory monitoring will be standard for patients. Nurses will increasingly integrate computers into their care and management of patients.

Not only will the PACU nurse need "high tech" post anesthesia care skills, he or she will also have to be "high touch," providing care to patients on a more extended basis. The PACU nurse will increasingly incorporate the family into the care of the postsurgical patient. The families of intensive care and ambulatory surgical patients will need information and comfort.

To practice in the PACU, today or in the future, the PACU nurse will truly be *Pro*active, *A*ssertive, *C*onscientious, and *U*nderstanding. Post anesthesia nursing demands it. Patients deserve it.

AMERICAN SOCIETY OF POST ANESTHESIA NURSES: PAST, PRESENT, AND FUTURE

In 1979 the American Society of Anesthesiologists (ASA) Committee on Anesthesia Care Teams extended an invitation to nursing leaders of recovery room associations across the country to join with them to discuss the formation of a national organization of recovery room nurses.[3]

Seven PACU nursing representatives from Florida, Connecticut, Oklahoma, Illinois, Alabama, New Jersey, and the Northwest joined with six anesthesiologists to form a national organization with the goals of education, communication, and establishment of an identity for recovery room nurses. Membership and funding issues were also discussed. A Steering Committee was created to work out the details of forming a new association, including those concerning officers, bylaws, and subcommittees.

In May of 1980, officers were elected, bylaws were drafted, and a board of directors was appointed. Committee chairmen and members for the Executive Committee, Nominating Committee, Finance Committee, Bylaws Committee, and Publications Committee were chosen. The aspen leaf was selected as the organization's logo.

At the next meeting, held in October 1980, the bylaws were approved, the Articles of Incorporation were signed, and the organization known as the American Society of Post Anesthesia Nurses (ASPAN) became an official organization of and for Recovery Room nurses.[3]

Since that time, the strength of the association has continued to increase. Membership is drawn from state associations, which now exist in almost every state and region. The Society publishes its own journal, *The Journal of Post Anesthesia Nursing*, bimonthly. The Society newsletter, *Breathline,* is also printed bimonthly, in alternate months from the Journal. In 1986, certification in post anesthesia nursing became an option. The examination, currently offered twice a year, provides post anesthesia nurses the opportunity, if successful, to become CPANs: certified post anesthesia nurses. Certification is maintained through continued clinical practice in post anesthesia care and through continuing education. Certification is renewed every 3 years.

The original purposes of the organization—education, communication, and professional identity—have been retained and expanded. The current purposes of the American Society of Post Anesthesia Nurses are identified in the box below.[2]

Future plans for ASPAN are drawn from its mission statement and 5-year strategic plan. Activities, programs, and strategies are directed toward maintenance and fulfillment of the Society's mission. The current mission statement is presented in the box on p. 8.[1]

Information about ASPAN may be obtained from the national office; information about certification may be obtained from the Professional Examination Service. The addresses of both are listed below:

AMERICAN SOCIETY OF POST ANESTHESIA NURSES
11512 Allecingie Parkway
Richmond, Virginia 23235
Phone: (804) 379-5513
FAX: (804) 379-1386

PROFESSIONAL EXAMINATION SERVICES
ABPANC
475 Riverside Drive
New York City, New York 10115
Phone: (212) 870-3161

PURPOSE OF ASPAN

The purposes for which the Society is organized are exclusively educational, scientific and charitable in nature and include the following:

A. To associate and affiliate into one organization of all licensed nurses who are engaged, or otherwise especially interested, in the care of patients in the immediate preanesthesia and post anesthesia period.
B. To provide education with respect to pre and post anesthesia patient care through conferences, courses, symposia, and the publication of articles, bulletins and periodicals that will maintain and upgrade standards of post anesthesia patient care and promote the professional growth of licensed nurses who are engaged, or otherwise especially interested, in the care of patients in the immediate pre and post anesthesia period.
C. To study, discuss and exchange professional knowledge, expertise and ideas on pre and post anesthesia patient care and to facilitate cooperation between post anesthesia nurses and physicians and other medical personnel concerned with care of the patient in the immediate pre and post anesthesia period.
D. To encourage specialization and research in pre and post anesthesia nursing.
E. To promote public awareness and understanding of the care of pre and post anesthesia patients.
F. To cooperate with universities, government agencies or any other organizations in matters affecting the purposes of the Society.

ASPAN: MISSION STATEMENT

1. To increase recognition of the value and importance of all phases of post anesthesia nursing, particularly among
   a. Consumers
   b. Hospital administrators
   c. Medical staff
   d. Nursing specialties
2. To maintain and upgrade standards in all phases of post anesthesia patient care and to promote the professional growth of nurses interested in the care of patients in the post anesthesia period.
3. To assist members of the Society to understand and succeed in the changing health care industry.
4. To promote a positive and professional image for the members and for the association itself.

Reprinted with permission, American Society of Post Anesthesia Nurses; Richmond, Va.

SUMMARY

The specialty of post anesthesia care has been and continues to be based on the goal of providing optimal care to the postanesthetic and postsurgical patient. The motto of the American Society of Anesthesiologists is "vigilance." The goal of post anesthesia care is patient safety.

REFERENCES

1. American Society of Post Anesthesia Nurses: Restructuring of long range planning committee, strategic plan development, unpublished document, 1987, The Society.
2. American Society of Post Anesthesia Nurses: Standards of practice, Richmond, Va, 1986, The Society.
3. American Society of Post Anesthesia Nurses: Historical record of ASPAN, Richmond, Va, 1982, The Society.
4. Atkinson R, Rushman G, and Lee J: A synopsis of anaesthesia, ed 8, John Wright & Sons, Bristol, 1977.
5. Davidson H: A practice of anaesthesia, ed 4, Philadelphia, 1978, WB Saunders Co.
6. Dripps R, Eckenhoff J, and Vandam L: Introduction to anesthesia: the principles of safe practice, ed 7, Philadelphia, 1988, WB Saunders Co.
7. Jolly C and Lee J: Post-operative observation ward, Anaesthesia 12(1):49-56, 1957.
8. Kalisch P and Kalisch B: The advance of American nursing, Boston, 1978, Little, Brown & Co, Inc.
9. Lowenthal P and Russell A: Recovery room: life saving and economical, Anesthesiology 12(4):470-476, 1951.
10. Pask E: Committee on deaths associated with anaesthesia, Anaesthesia 10(1):4-8, 1955.
11. Ruth H, Haugen F, and Grove D: Anesthesia study commission, JAMA 135(14):881-884, 1947.

Review Questions

1. *In the 1940s the Anesthesia Study Commission of the Philadelphia Medical Society investi-gated postoperative deaths to identify* _____.
   a. The responsible individual
   b. Rationale for lawsuits
   c. Cause and preventability
   d. Hospitals that should be closed for being unsafe

2. *The most common cause of postoperative death was found to be* _____.
   a. Inadequate management
   b. Excessive anesthesia
   c. Errors in supervision
   d. Laryngospasm

3. *The ultimate purpose of the PACU is to* _____.
   a. Prevent postoperative death
   b. Provide optimal care for the postanesthetic and postsurgical patient
   c. Centralize resources
   d. Prevent liability associated with surgical care

4. *Use of the PACU as a special procedures unit is designed to* _____.
   a. Demoralize PACU nursing staff
   b. Minimize staff "down-time"
   c. Generate increased revenue
   d. Maximize patient safety

5. *The practice of PACU nursing requires* _____.
   a. No specialized training or orientation
   b. Graduate level specialization
   c. That all care delivered be supervised by an anesthesiologist
   d. Specialty knowledge and a generalist orientation

6. *The PACU nurse's practice may be* _____.
   a. Totally independent and self-initiated
   b. Collaborative only
   c. Independent and collaborative
   d. The outcome of only medical orders

7. *The original goals (established in 1980) of ASPAN were* _____.
   a. Education, communication, professional identity
   b. Education, practice, research
   c. Education, science, and charity
   d. Practice, community, and collaboration

8. *The current purposes (1990) of ASPAN are* _____.
   a. Practice-based and research-supported
   b. Educational, scientific, and charitable in nature
   c. Guided by education, technology, and service
   d. Organizational, commercial, and representational in nature

9. *Successful completion of the post anesthesia certification examination allows a nurse to carry the title* _____.
   a. CPON: Certified Postoperative Nurse
   b. CRRN: Certified Recovery Room Nurse
   c. CPAN: Certified Post Anesthesia Nurse
   d. PANS: Post Anesthesia Nurse Specialist
10. *Certification must be renewed every 3 years by* _____.
   a. Letters of reference
   b. Continued post anesthesia practice
   c. Nomination
   d. Continuing education credit

Answers

10. b and d   5. d
9. c   4. d
8. b   3. b
7. a   2. a
6. c   1. c

CHAPTER 2

Patients scheduled for surgery bring with them a history of medical problems and prior surgeries, a family history of disease or illness, and a personal history or indication for surgery. It is important for the anesthesia care team to be aware of this patient history in preparing for and administering anesthesia. The nurse in the post anesthesia care unit (PACU) will use the patient history in planning for and instituting post anesthesia care.

It is the goal of this chapter to describe the purpose and components of the preanesthetic assessment, to identify specific patient situations that may have an impact on intraoperative and post anesthesia care, and to discuss the concept of risk assessment and the factors that must be considered when selecting the ideal anesthetic.

RELATIONSHIP BETWEEN PREOPERATIVE STATUS AND POST ANESTHESIA CARE

Chapter Objectives

After reading this chapter, the reader should be able to:

1. Identify the purpose of the preanesthetic visit.
2. Identify and discuss the components of the preanesthetic assessment.
3. Identify and discuss specific patient situations that may influence intraoperative or post anesthesia care.
4. Explain the determination of a physical status rating.
5. Discuss variables that may influence anesthetic options.

PREANESTHESIA VISIT

Just as the surgeon sees the patient to confirm the diagnosis or indication for surgery before scheduling surgery, the anesthesiologist should also see the patient preoperatively to obtain data from which to plan the patient's anesthetic course. Ideally, each time an anesthetic is administered, it should be the best anesthetic for that particular patient at that moment in time.

The preanesthetic visit is designed to reduce intraoperative and postoperative morbidity and mortality. The patient's preoperative status can be improved, and intraoperative management can be anticipated and planned. The information gathered during this visit allows the anesthesiologist the opportunity to anticipate postoperative problems and to alert the PACU nurse to areas requiring extra concern or attention. By visiting the patient before surgery, cancellations and delays in scheduling can also be minimized.

Chart audit

Before visiting the patient, the anesthesiologist should first carefully perform a chart audit. The patient's chart, both current and historical, is a rich source of data and a potential time-saver in data collection. The patient's chart should contain data from admission, including patient demographic information such as sex, age, height, weight, vital signs, and admitting diagnosis. Admission data, current laboratory data, x-ray reports, and/or ECGs should be found in the chart.

The anesthesiologist should review the documented history and physical examination information provided by the surgeon or surgical service (residents). By doing so, the anesthesiologist may identify areas of concern, which can be further explored during the actual patient interview.

Finally, the chart audit may provide an account of previous anesthetics. By reviewing previous anesthetic records, the anesthesiologist can identify which anesthetic agents and techniques have been used and with what outcome. Notes concerning intraoperative or postoperative problems should be carefully investigated. If the previous anesthetic record documents the need for fiberoptic intubation, the anesthesiologist can further explore the cause of the difficulty in accessing the airway. If the previous anesthetic record documents a problem with an adverse reaction to a medication, the anesthesiologist can alter techniques accordingly.

After reviewing the chart, the anesthesiologist should then plan to meet with the patient.[36]

Patient interview

Another purpose of the preanesthetic visit is to promote the development of a relationship between the patient and the anesthesiologist. The formation of a professional relationship before surgery helps to promote trust and decrease anxiety. The anesthesiologist will be one more familiar face seen on the day of surgery.

Because the preanesthetic visit is usually the first meeting between the patient and the anesthesiologist, it should take place when both parties are capable of committing time and attention to the meeting. Ideally, the anesthesiologist will not be between cases and therefore rushed and pressed for time. The patient should not have visitors, be in the middle of a meal, or be imminently on the way to the x-ray department. The meeting should occur in a place where patient privacy can be maintained, such as in the patient's room or in a separate preadmission testing area. With the increase in ambulatory surgery, this interview may occur the morning of surgery.

The primary purposes of the patient interview are to obtain patient information, to provide information about the operating room and anesthesia, and to obtain consent for anesthesia or for a specific technique. The interview is also a time for the anesthesiologist to assess the patient's emotional state and readiness for surgery. The anesthesiologist can explore the patient's expectations about surgery and anesthesia and can reinforce or clarify these expectations as indicated. The anesthesiologist can also determine the patient's level of knowledge about anesthesia and surgery, again clarifying misconceptions and reinforcing understanding.

Patient history

The patient history is one of the best measures of patient status. The focus of the patient history should be targeted and specific and designed to assist the anesthesiologist in planning the anesthetic and in anticipating problem areas. The components of the patient history are summarized in the box below.

Initially, the anesthesiologist should explore the patient's understanding of the need for surgery and specific patient complaints that may have caused the patient to seek medical attention. The patient scheduled for a valve replacement who indicates preadmission symptoms of dyspnea, angina at rest, and the need to sleep upright will alert the anesthesiologist to potential problems with cardiopulmonary function. The patient scheduled for a total hip arthroplasty who indicates preadmission problems with mobility and pain will alert the anesthesiologist to potential problems with musculoskeletal function.

The anesthesiologist should also inquire about previous anesthetics. This will provide the anesthesiologist with a surgical history of the patient, including the age of the patient at the time of exposure to anesthetics. If the patient's last experience with surgery was a herniorraphy in infancy, knowledge about surgery and memories of the anesthetic will probably be nonexistent. However, if the surgery occurred in the recent past, the patient may remember vivid details about both the surgery and the anesthetic.

In inquiring about previous anesthetics, the anesthesiologist should also ask about the incidence or occurrence of postoperative problems. The patient may report having had an allergic reaction to a medication, may remember problems with delayed awakening, may have been paralyzed on awakening, may have experienced a postdural puncture headache after a spinal anesthetic, or may also recall problems with nausea and vomiting, pain, or myalgias.

Problems related to surgery may include reports of hemorrhage requiring transfusion, inability to wean from a ventilator, or venous stasis causing postoperative pulmonary embolism.

It is also important for the anesthesiologist to inquire about the patient's family health history, including any adverse reactions or problems with anesthesia. Anesthesiologists were first made aware of a phenomenon, later to be known as malignant hyperthermia, when a young man in Australia reported that 10 of his family members died while undergoing anesthesia. The genetic predisposition to malignant hyperthermia is now well documented. There is also a family predisposition to pseudocholinesterase de-

---

THE PATIENT HISTORY

Indication for surgery	Allergies
Previous anesthetics	Drug abuse/addiction
Family health	Menstrual/obstetric history
Current drug use	Systems review

ficiency, which has the potential to result in prolonged paralysis after succinylcholine (Anectine) administration.

A family history of disease involving the cardiac and endocrine systems should be investigated. A family history of sudden cardiac death, myocardial infarction, and coronary artery disease should alert the anesthesiologist to the possibility of similar diseases, either overt or subclinical, in the patient. A family history of diabetes should also be investigated, as there is a high genetic predisposition to both insulin dependent–diabetes mellitus (IDDM) and non-insulin dependent–diabetes mellitus (NIDDM).

The anesthesiologist should ask the patient about current medication use, including the use of over-the-counter (OTC) medications. This is an important area to explore, for it is possible that these medications may interact with anesthetics, often by increasing or decreasing their potency and effectiveness. For example, drugs such as clonidine and verapamil decrease the required dose of volatile anesthetics. Magnesium, aminoglycoside antibiotics, quinidine, and lithium potentiate neuromuscular blocking agents. It is especially important to consider drugs used for heart disease, hypertension, immunosuppression, anticoagulation, and endocrine replacement.

In addition, knowledge of current medication usage can alert the anesthesiologist to order or evaluate laboratory tests. For example, if the patient is receiving warfarin (Coumadin) or aspirin therapy (anticoagulants), a coagulation profile should be obtained. If the patient is receiving diuretic therapy for control of hypertension, a serum potassium level should be obtained. If the patient is taking antidysrhythmia medications, a preoperative electrocardiogram (ECG) should be obtained.[27]

The anesthesiologist must also determine that the patient is using currently prescribed medications correctly. Is the patient taking the medication as ordered, or has the patient stopped taking the medication because of cost, side effects, or the feeling that ongoing therapy is not indicated? Has the patient increased the amount of medication with the belief that, if one is good, two must be better? Inquiry about medication use provides an ideal area for patient teaching and for referral of the patient back to the physician who prescribed the medication.

In addition to inquiring about medication use, the anesthesiologist should ask about medication intolerance and drug allergies. By being aware of medication intolerance and drug allergies, the anesthesiologist can avoid the use of these drugs and ideally maintain patient comfort, safety, and stability. The anesthesiologist should not only determine the drug or class of drug in question, but the patient's reaction to the drug. A true drug allergy produces an anaphylactic or anaphylactoid reaction, causing cardiopulmonary compromise, including hypotension, tachycardia, bronchospasm, and possible pulmonary edema. Medication intolerance usually results in side effects that are uncomfortable, but not life-threatening, to the patient, including nausea, constipation, diarrhea, or a rash.

If a medication intolerance or drug allergy is noted, the patient's chart should be so labeled, the patient should receive an allergy alert wrist bracelet, and the allergy should be noted on the anesthesia record. The PACU nurse should be told of the allergy in the postanesthetic report.

The anesthesiologist should also inquire about nondrug allergies, including allergies to foods, chemicals, and pollen. Patients with a history of allergic responsiveness have a greater potential of demonstrating hypersensitivity reactions to drugs administered during anesthesia.[11]

Although it may be difficult or embarrassing, the anesthesiologist should ask the patient about possible drug use, abuse, and addiction. Questions should be asked directly and matter-of-factly, and the patient should be encouraged to respond truthfully. Surprisingly, when patients are made aware of the anesthesiologist's need to know about drug use and abuse to maintain safety, most patients will respond honestly about their drug use.

The categories of drugs most likely to be used and abused include tobacco, alcohol, opioids, marijuana, and cocaine. Questions should be asked about all of these drugs.

Knowledge of a patient's smoking (tobacco) history is important. In people who smoke, 15% of the oxygen-binding sites on hemoglobin are occupied by carbon monoxide (CO), resulting in a decreased oxygen-carrying capacity of hemoglobin. As a further consequence, oxygen delivery and availability to tissues is reduced. In addition, smokers have a higher incidence of airway disease, including chronic obstructive pulmonary disease (COPD), emphysema, and bronchitis, which increases their risk of postoperative respiratory complications. Smoking can also paralyze cilia, compromising the ability of the patient to clear mucus after general anesthesia. Patients should be encouraged to stop smoking 6 weeks before admission and surgery to decrease perioperative morbidity.

When inquiring about alcohol use, the anesthesiologist should ask the patient to define approximate consumption in the typical day or week. Rather than making a judgment that intake is social, light, moderate, or excessive, the anesthesiologist should simply document the specifics, for example, glass of wine with dinner once or twice a week, 6-pack of beer nightly, fifth of bourbon daily.

Heavy alcohol consumption is often associated with alterations in other body systems, including increased nutritional deficits, dementia, cardiomyopathy, gastritis, cirrhosis, and hepatitis. Anesthetic requirements will be affected. Chronic alcohol use tends to increase the concentration of volatile anesthetic agents required; acute intoxication tends to decrease the concentration of volatile anesthetics required. Alcohol abusers also have a higher incidence of postoperative agitation.

Inquiry about patient use of marijuana, cocaine, and narcotics is also important. For the most part, marijuana and cocaine will not prove to be problematic unless the patient is under the influence of the substances at the time of surgery. Marijuana increases sympathetic nervous system activity, producing tachycardia and systolic hypertension. It is also associated with drowsiness, relaxation, and disinhibition. Cocaine prevents the uptake of norepinephrine back into postganglionic sympathetic nerve endings. Patients will have tachycardia, hypertension, and frequently an increased temperature secondary to vasoconstriction, increased skeletal muscle activity, and, perhaps, altered central regulation. Because of the relatively short half-life of the drug, these central effects are short-lived.[8]

The patient who uses narcotics should be evaluated carefully to determine the drug and dosage used. The intravenous narcotic user should also be evaluated for phlebitis, bacterial endocarditis, hepatitis, and acquired immunodeficiency syndrome (AIDS). In addition, there may be problems with nutritional status and basic health habits.

It is especially important to avoid the use of agonist-antagonists such as butorphanol or nalbuphine and narcotic antagonists such as naloxone.

In females, beginning with preteens, the anesthesiologist should inquire about menstrual and obstetric history. This includes obtaining the date of the patient's last menstrual period. The primary purpose for obtaining this information is to avoid possible maternal and fetal exposure to anesthetics during the first trimester of pregnancy. This type of question may be embarrassing for a preteenager or teenager to answer in the presence of care-givers. The anesthesiologist might elect to ask this question with care-givers out of the room.

Systems review

The last component of the patient history is the systems review. The anesthesiologist should ask specific questions designed to confirm the presence or absence of disease. It is especially important to target organ systems that affect the actions of anesthetics (pulmonary, hepatic, renal) and organ systems that can be affected by the anesthetics (central nervous, cardiovascular). Systems alterations may influence the choice of anesthetic agents, technique, intraoperative monitoring priorities, and the type of care administered in the PACU.

Cardiovascular system. The purpose of evaluating the patient's cardiovascular function is to determine the presence of preexisting disease, with the goal of decreasing perioperative morbidity. It is important to inquire about any history of cardiac problems, including hypertension, angina, dysrhythmias, and myocardial infarction. Patients may respond or understand questions better if asked about a history of high blood pressure, chest pain, palpitations, and heart attack. It is also important to inquire about any history of congestive heart failure and edema.

The anesthesiologist should also determine whether the patient has any history of having seen a cardiologist for a cardiac evaluation, of having been put on cardiac medications, or of having undergone cardiac surgery, including catheterization, pacemakers, angioplasty, or bypass surgery.[21]

It is important to ask these specific questions because the answers provide information about the degree of risk associated with surgery and anesthesia. Some preoperative variables are not alterable, including patient history, age, and overt disease. However, it may be possible to correct threatening conditions before the patient undergoes surgery, for example, hypokalemia-induced ventricular ectopy may be corrected with potassium supplementation, and congestive heart failure may be treated with diuretics, fluid restriction, and hemodynamic monitoring.

Knowledge of preexisting conditions can also alert the anesthesiologist and ultimately the PACU nurse when the report is given, to the potential risks of anesthesia and surgery. For example, patients who have had a myocardial infarction more than 6 months ago have a 6% risk of reinfarction. If the myocardial infarction occurred in the last 3 to 6 months, the reinfarction rate increases to 15%. However, if the myocardial infarction occurred in the last 3 months, the reinfarction rate is as high as 30%. The range has been reported as high as 86%. Unfortunately, reinfarction is also associated with a 50% risk of mortality. All of this is in comparision to the patient with no history of cardiac disease who runs a 0.1% to 0.7% chance of having a perioperative myocardial infarction.[23,33]

Patients with a history of hypertension are also at risk for postoperative problems secondary to the effect of hypertension on the kidney, carotid arteries, peripheral vessels, and myocardium.

The patient with a history of congenital heart disease can be placed on antibiotic prophylaxis before dental, respiratory, genitourinary, or gastrointestinal surgery to decrease the potential development of bacterial endocarditis.[16]

The anesthesiologist will plan the anesthetic to promote cardiovascular stability and safety. By communicating information about the patient's history to the PACU nurse, cardiovascular stability and safety can be promoted in the postanesthetic period as well.

Respiratory system. The purpose of evaluating the patient's respiratory status preoperatively is to determine the existence of preexisting disease, with the goal of decreasing perioperative morbidity. It is important to inquire about any history of dyspnea (at rest or exertional), coughing (productive or dry), hemoptysis, and asthma. If the patient has a history of asthma, it is important to determine the patient's history of bronchospasm (rare or frequent), medication use (as needed or continuous), and medication type (bronchodilator, steroids). The patient should also be asked about any history of smoking and recent and chronic respiratory infections.

In addition, the anesthesiologist should notice physical characteristics that are likely to influence or compromise respiratory function, both intraoperatively and postoperatively, including obesity, spinal or chest deformities, and overt airway deformities.

The anesthesiologist should also consider the patient's scheduled surgery, for it is well known that the type of surgery can contribute to postoperative pulmonary complications. The incidence of postoperative pulmonary complications increases with surgery involving the upper and lower abdomen and mediastinum. Abdominal surgery causes a decrease in diaphragmatic function. Mediastinal incisions compromise the mechanical function of the thoracic cage. Both contribute to the development of postoperative atelectasis and pneumonias. Care of the patient after thoracic and abdominal surgery is discussed in detail in Chapter 5.

The patient with a history of COPD is also at risk for postoperative pulmonary complications, including a decreased vital capacity and decreased diaphragmatic function. One study estimated that 60% of patients with COPD develop postoperative pulmonary complications when given no special postoperative respiratory care. In the same study, the incidence of postoperative complications dropped to 22% when antibiotics, bronchodilators, and chest physical therapy were included in the PACU routine.[12,30]

Ideally, patients with a history of asthma should be free from bronchospasm (wheezing) preoperatively. In addition, the anesthesiologist should have in mind a plan to treat bronchospasm if it develops. The PACU nurse will also be alert to the possibility of bronchospasm and should be prepared to institute appropriate therapy as ordered, including hydration, administration of bronchodilators, and chest physical therapy.[9,14]

The patient with normal pulmonary function runs a 6% to 10% risk of developing postoperative pulmonary complications. As the risk increases with preexisting pulmonary disease, and in consideration of the type of surgery performed, the PACU nurse can be aggressive in instituting postoperative pulmonary care, with the goal of decreasing postoperative morbidity and mortality.[30]

Central nervous system. Preoperative evaluation of the patient's neurologic functioning is done to assess the patient's ability to respond to questions, follow commands, and maintain ordered thought patterns. It is the appropriateness of the response and thought that must be evaluated. If a deficit is detected, careful assessment should be made to determine its extent. It should also be determined if the problem is one that can be corrected prior to surgery.

For example, if a deficit in communication is noticed, is it caused by a language barrier, necessitating a translator? If the problem is unresponsiveness secondary to electrolyte imbalance (hyponatremia, hyperglycemia, or hypoglycemia), the cause of the imbalance should be corrected. If the communication deficit is the result of a cerebrovascular accident (CVA, stroke), it may not be a correctable problem.

It should also be determined whether the patient has a history of neurologic compromise, including seizures, hydrocephalus, paralysis, or epilepsy. Awareness of the presence of neurologic compromise will influence the choice of anesthetic agents and techniques. For example, enflurane (Ethrane) increases seizure irritability by lowering the seizure threshold. Paralysis is a relative contraindication to regional (spinal, epidural, or caudal) anesthetics.

The PACU nurse should also be made aware of any preexisting neurologic deficits because neurologic assessments are a standard part of the PACU assessment. The PACU nurse should be told of patient deficits to allow for comparison postoperatively and to anticipate postoperative problems and patient needs.

For example, if the patient is a retarded or autistic child, a parent or care-giver might be invited into the PACU to assist the nursing staff in the care of the child. If the patient has a history of a seizure disorder, padded side rails should be readily available to increase patient safety. If the patient has a history of a cerebrovascular accident (CVA, stroke), the patient and/or family may be able to provide information specific to patient needs, such as suggestions for positioning, communication, or transferring.

Renal system. Because some 12 million people in the United States are affected by renal disease, it is important to include questions about preexisting renal disease during the preoperative assessment. Renal dysfunction is associated with a number of physiologic alterations, all of which have the potential to increase perioperative risk and affect postoperative care.

The patient with renal dysfunction is almost always chronically anemic, with an average hematocrit of 15% to 18% and hemoglobin of 5 to 8 g/dl. Anemia affects the oxygen-hemoglobin relationship in the body, causing a shift of the oxyhemoglobin dissociation curve to the right. Cardiac output increases to meet the oxygen supply needs of peripheral tissues. It will be important to avoid drugs that decrease cardiac output and to maintain oxygenation.[1,18]

Patients with renal dysfunction, especially those on dialysis, will have alterations in coagulation, including platelet dysfunction and systemic heparinization, which may compromise prothrombin and thromboplastin times. These alterations in coagulation may increase the potential for bleeding with surgical invasion and may influence an anesthesiologist's decision to use regional anesthesia in situations in which hypocoagulation exists as a contraindication.[22]

Patients in renal failure have alterations in hydration and electrolyte balance. Patients will present clinically with water retention, edema, hyperkalemia, hypocalcemia, and hypermagnesemia. The alterations in fluid and electrolyte status may compromise intraoperative stability of blood pressure, cardiac function, and vascular resistance.

Patients in renal failure are chronically acidotic because of retention of hydrogen ions. Acidosis further contributes to myocardial instability and increased oxygen demand and may require the administration of sodium bicarbonate if acidosis becomes severe.

Hypertension is a common finding in patients in renal failure. Hypertension may cause or contribute to cardiomegaly and congestive heart failure. Treatment may be via dialysis or with the use of systemic medications. In addition to hypertension, patients with chronic renal failure are prone to coronary artery disease and peripheral vascular disease. Control of blood pressure will be a priority intraoperatively and postoperatively.

Finally, secondary to the renal disease and to dialysis, patients are at an increased risk for infection. Sepsis is a leading cause of morbidity and mortality in patients with renal dysfunction. It is important for surgeons, anesthesiologists, and nurses to use meticulous sterile technique in all invasive procedures.

While the possibility of infection is a concern for every postsurgical patient, the presence of chronic hepatitis secondary to dialysis and repeated blood transfusions may increase risks to care-givers. Maintenance of universal body fluid precautions is essential.

Because of all of these acute physiologic alterations, postoperative priorities will include attention to ventilation (to maintain oxygenation and cardiac output), fluid management (to maintain cardiac output and electrolyte balance), and monitoring (to maintain hemodynamic status and to evaluate metabolism of renally excreted drugs).

Hepatic system. When one understands the physiologic role of hepatocytes, the functional cellular unit of the liver, it becomes clear why inquiry about hepatic and, ultimately, gastrointestinal function is so important. Hepatocytes contribute to or are responsible for glucose homeostasis, fat metabolism, protein synthesis, drug and hormone metabolism, and bilirubin formation and excretion. Hepatic dysfunction, therefore, will result in systemic effects.[32]

Impairments in glucose homeostasis may contribute to hypoglycemia. Alterations in fat metabolism may contribute to the development of metabolic acidosis. Alterations in protein syntheses may cause hypoalbuminemia, decreasing protein binding sites that may be necessary for drug binding. If drugs are unable to bind to protein, plasma concentrations of drugs will remain elevated, increasing the potential for drug reactions and adverse effects. Coagulation factors are produced in the liver, specifically prothrombin, fibrinogen, and factors V, VII, IX, and X. Hepatic disease may result in clotting abnormalities, increasing the risk of bleeding.[32]

Alteration in liver function will also prolong the effects of drugs that require hepatic metabolism for clearance, including diazepam (Valium), lidocaine (Xylocaine), meperidine (Demerol), morphine, and alfentanil (Alfenta).[32]

It is important to ask the patient about any history of hepatic (liver) disease or dysfunction, including any history of hepatitis, cirrhosis, and alcoholism.

Acute hepatitis is an inflammatory disease of hepatocytes, most often caused by a viral infection or ingestion (injection) of toxic drugs. Acute hepatitis may also be caused by sepsis, congestive heart failure, and, rarely, pregnancy.[32] The most significant problem of anesthetizing and operating on a patient with acute (active) hepatitis is the risk of disease transmission to health care providers. Because surgeons, anesthesiologists, and nurses in the operating room and PACU are in contact with body fluids (blood, saliva, vomitus), implementation of universal body fluid precautions is essential. It is also recommended that high-risk health care providers be immunized against hepatitis B.

Chronic hepatitis is the most serious form of hepatitis, often resulting in cirrhosis and hepatic failure. Liver function will be greatly compromised. Patients will require careful monitoring of fluid and electrolyte status and ongoing monitoring for bleeding, drug toxicity, and cardiovascular compromise.

Cirrhosis is a chronic liver disease whereby the hepatic parenchyema is destroyed and replaced with collagen. Normal physiologic functioning of the liver is compromised. Alcoholism is the most common cause of cirrhosis. Not only is physiologic functioning of the liver interrupted, but hepatic blood flow is also reduced, as blood meets increasing resistance in moving through the portal vein (portal hypertension). The patient will require monitoring for bleeding, drug toxicity, and cardiovascular compromise.

The PACU nurse should also be aware of the potential physiologic alterations that may occur secondary to liver disease. Caveats for caring for a patient with hepatic dysfunction will include monitoring, ongoing assessment, and judicious administration of all medications.[32]

While assessments of the cardiovascular, pulmonary, central nervous, renal, and hepatic systems are important, the patient should also be evaluated for alterations in musculoskeletal functioning and asked about any history of diabetes mellitus. Musculoskeletal alterations and diabetes mellitus have the potential to affect intraoperative and postoperative care.

Musculoskeletal alterations. It is important, particularly in the elderly patient, to inquire about the incidence of arthritis. Arthritis is a chronic inflammatory disease of joints; it is characterized by pain, swelling, and impaired mobility. If the patient is arthritic, all affected joints should be identified. Mobility restrictions may influence intraoperative and postoperative positioning, and, if the temporomandibular joint or cervical spine is affected, intubation and airway management may be difficult.

Any history of muscle disease should be explored. Muscular dystrophy is a hereditary disease characterized by painless degeneration and atrophy of skeletal muscles. Degeneration of cardiac and respiratory muscles will increase the risk of potential cardiopulmonary compromise intraoperatively and postoperatively. If general anesthesia is employed, the patient will probably be difficult to wean from the ventilator and will have difficulty coughing and deep breathing. Regional anesthesia may prove to be an ideal option to avoid respiratory compromise.

Myasthenia gravis is a chronic, autoimmune disease that compromises the neuromuscular junction. It is characterized by muscle weakness and fatigability and periods of exacerbation and remission. Multiple sclerosis is a chronic neuromuscular disease caused by demyelination of neurons. It is characterized by sensory and motor neurologic deficits and is episodic in its frequency and severity of exacerbation and remission. With both of these neuromuscular disorders, airway maintenance and ventilatory management will be the number one intraoperative and postoperative priority.

Diabetic patients. Diabetes mellitus causes the most significant alteration in endocrine functioning. A systemic disease characterized by a relative or absolute lack of insulin, diabetes mellitus is diagnosed clinically by its "classic" signs of polyuria, polydipsia, and fatigue, the manifestation of hyperglycemia, glycosuria, and cellular glucose deprivation.

Preoperative evaluation of the diabetic patient requires a determination of whether the patient is insulin-dependent and likely to develop intraoperative or postoperative ketosis. Additionally, in patients who have been in poor control or who have had diabetes mellitus for many years, the presence of long-term complications, including neuropathy, nephropathy, and retinopathy, should also be explored.

The anesthesiologist (or surgeon) will determine insulin use on the day of surgery. Some may prefer to hold all insulin, monitor frequent blood glucose readings (Accucheck), and to treat with insulin only as indicated by the blood glucose readings. Others may prefer to administer a portion of the usual insulin dosage, with ongoing, periodic blood glucose determinations. Regardless of the method chosen, the PACU nurse should be aware of the patient's diabetic status, and blood glucose monitoring should be continued postoperatively. The PACU nurse should be prepared to treat hyperglycemia with intravenous insulin and hypoglycemia with intravenous glucose.

Physical examination*

After completing the patient history, a physical examination of the patient should be performed. The physical examination will most likely not be a head-to-toe comprehensive assessment, but more likely an examination of anesthetic importance.

---

*For additional information about the relationship between anesthesia and coexisting disease, the reader is encouraged to obtain the reference: Stoelting R, Dierdorf S, and McCammon R: Anesthesia and co-existing disease, ed 2, New York, 1988, Churchill-Livingstone.

The anesthesiologist will assess the patient's airway for overt or covert abnormalities or restrictions in mobility. The function of the temporomandibular joints and the ability of the patient to hyperextend the neck will be observed to assess the risk of difficulties at intubation. The condition of the teeth will be noted, including the presence of dentures, loose teeth, or caps, particularly of the front teeth.

The anesthesiologist will assess cardiopulmonary function by inspection and auscultation; the assessment will include observation for overt signs of distress, poor color, and chest excursion and auscultation of heart and lung sounds. Any chest or spinal deviation will be noted, particularly if it is likely to have an impact on ventilation.

The anesthesiologist will probably assess the condition of veins or arteries that might be cannulated preoperatively. Peripheral pulses might be palpated.

If regional anesthesia is to be considered, the site of injection will be assessed to identify ease of landmark determination and the presence of any anatomic alterations that might interfere with the success of the injection.

If abnormalities were noted during the chart review or patient history, the physical assessment can be expanded as necessary.

Determination of physical status

After completion of the patient history and physical examination, the anesthesiologist will assign the patient a physical status rating. Defined by the American Society of Anesthesiologists, the assignment of a physical status rating is designed to be a predictor of perioperative risk and overall outcome. Information obtained from the patient history and physical examination will be used in the determination of a physical status rating. Table 2-1 defines the current physical status classifications. Theoretically, the higher the

Table 2-1. **American Society of Anesthesiology physical status classification**

Physical status	Definition	Example
I	Healthy patient with no systemic disease	Patient with no significant past or present medical history
II	Mild systemic disease without functional limitations	Patient with a history of asthma controlled with theophylline
III	Severe systemic disease associated with definite functional limitations	Patient with a history of chronic asthma controlled with theophylline, steroids, and inhalers as needed; not wheezing
IV	Severe systemic disease that is an ongoing threat to life	Patients with history of chronic asthma, poorly controlled with theophylline and steroids; Pao_2 50 mm Hg; wheezing; chest x-ray changes
V	Patient unlikely to survive for more than 24 hours with/without the surgery	Patient in status-asthmaticus, intubated, ventilated; isoproterenol (Isuprel) drip

physical status rating, the higher the risk of perioperative morbidity and mortality. However, the actual morbidity and mortality data remain somewhat controversial.[4,25,28,39]

In reviewing perioperative morbidity and mortality data, the majority of events are attributed to human error or mechanical or technical difficulties, not to patient variables. Furthermore, numerous factors in addition to anesthesia influence perioperative outcome. Despite the conflicting data, the assignment of physical status rating is well accepted. Because it does, to some degree, reflect perioperative outcome, it is a concept that should be understood by the PACU nurse.

Laboratory testing

Ideally, the ordering and obtaining of preoperative laboratory tests should be based on the individual patient history and physical examination, as opposed to arbitrarily being determined as "policy." Laboratory test results should serve as an adjunct to the history and physical examination data. The anesthesiologist should consider the potential of the laboratory data for altering perioperative outcome. If an abnormal result has the potential to increase perioperative morbidity or mortality, appropriate interventions should be instituted. Fig. 2-1 is an example of a preoperative patient checklist that may be used to suggest the ordering of laboratory tests.[25]

Conditions that have the potential to alter the surgical outcome or affect (compromise) surgical personnel and that may be diagnosed or evaluated by laboratory testing are identified in the box below.[24]

Factors in selecting type of anesthesia

Once the anesthesiologist has obtained preoperative patient data, there are a number of additional factors that must be considered when selecting the type of anesthesia. The first is age of the patient. For the adult patient going to surgery, depending on the type of surgery, there are a number of anesthetic options, including general anesthesia, re-

---

CONDITIONS DETECTABLE BY LABORATORY TESTING THAT MAY ALTER SURGICAL OUTCOME OR AFFECT SURGICAL PERSONNEL

Anemia	Ischemic heart disease
Diabetes mellitus	Cardiac dysrhythmias
Clotting disorders	Chronic obstructive pulmonary disease
Thrombocytopenia	Interstitial lung disease
Hepatitis	Congestive heart failure
Pregnancy	Nephrotic syndrome
Sexually transmitted diseases	Urinary tract infection

Modified from Robbins J and Mushlin A: Preoperative evaluation of the healthy patient, Med Clin North Am 63:1145, 1979.

M.D. Checklist for Ordering Preoperative Laboratory Tests

(Check indication if positive: Only one positive indication is needed per item.)

Patient's name: _____

Scheduled operation: _____

Test to be obtained	Indication for ordering test

Hb/Hct
- _____ Potentially bloody operation (blood to be cross-matched preoperatively)
- _____ Known anemia
- _____ Bleeding disorder
- _____ Hematologic malignancy
- _____ Radiation or chemotherapy
- _____ Chronic renal failure
- _____ Severe chronic disease
- _____ Other (specify): _____
- _____ _____

WBCs (differential will be automatic if abnormal WBC or Hb)
- _____ Infection
- _____ Disease of WBCs
- _____ Radiation or chemotherapy
- _____ Immunosuppressive therapy or steroid therapy
- _____ Hypersplenism
- _____ Aplastic anemia

_____ Check here if you wish differential in any case.
- _____ Collagen vascular disease
- _____ Other (specify): _____
- _____ _____
- _____ _____

PT/PTT
- _____ Known or suspected coagulation abnormality
- _____ Anticoagulant therapy or anticipated therapy
- _____ Hemorrhage or anemia
- _____ Thrombosis
- _____ Liver disease
- _____ Malabsorption or poor nutrition
- _____ Other (specify): _____
- _____ _____
- _____ _____

FIG. 2-1. Sample checklist for determining which preoperative tests should be obtained. Hb, hemoglobin; Hct, hematocrit; WBC, white blood cells; PT, prothrombin time; PTT, partial thromboplastin time; SMA 6 and SMA 12, simultaneous multichannel analysis of 6 and 12 blood

cont'd on p. 27.

PLATELETS	_____ Known platelet abnormality
	_____ Hemorrhage or purpura
	_____ Leukemia
	_____ Radiation or chemotherapy
	_____ Hypersplenism
	_____ Some anemias (aplastic, autoimmune, myelophthisic, pernicious)
	_____ Transplant rejection
	_____ Other

ELECTROLYTE PANEL	_____ Age 60 years or older
Sodium	_____ Use of diuretics
Potassium	_____ Renal disease
Chloride	_____ Other fluid or electrolyte abnormality (diarrhea,
Total CO_2	SIADH, diabetes insipidus, severe liver disease,
Creatinine	malabsorption, fever)
BUN	_____ Other (specify): _____
	_____ _____

CHEMISTRY PROFILE	_____ Age 60 years or older
Glucose	_____ Diabetes mellitus
Calcium	_____ Hypoglycemia
Phosphorus	_____ Pancreatic disease
Uric acid	_____ Pituitary disease
Total bilirubin	_____ Adrenal disease, steroid therapy
Total protein	_____ Liver disease or exposure to hepatitis
Albumin	_____ Radiation or chemotherapy
Cholesterol	_____ Parathyroid disease
SGOT	
LDH	
ALK. Phosphatase	
SGPT	

ECG (EKG)	_____ Age 40 years or older
	_____ Known or suspected cardiac abnormality
	_____ Other (specify): _____
	_____ _____

OTHER TESTS DESIRED	_____ Urinalysis
(specify indication):	_____ Rapid plasma reagin (syphilis screening test)
	_____ CPK isoenzymes

OTHERS	(Test name and indication):
_____ CXR	_____
_____	_____
_____	_____

FIG. 2-1, cont'd. components, respectively; SIADH, syndrome of inappropriate antidiuretic hormone; and CPK, creatinine phosphokinase. (From Roizen M: Routine preoperative evaluation. In Miller R: Anesthesia, ed 2, New York, 1986, Churchill Livingstone, Inc. With permission.)

gional anesthesia, intravenous sedation, or local anesthesia. The pediatric patient may well tolerate general anesthesia, but anatomic and cooperation factors may limit regional anesthesia and intravenous sedation as primary anesthetic tecnhiques.

The anesthesiologist should also consider the physical status of the patient. One variable to be assessed is the presence of preoperative disease. A number of anesthetics are metabolized and excreted via the kidney. If the patient has a history of renal dysfunction, the anesthesiologist may elect not to use these drugs, or, if the drugs are to be used, care must be taken to decrease the dosage and to monitor the effects of the drug more closely. The same holds true for drugs that are metabolized and eliminated hepatically when administered to a patient with hepatic dysfunction.

The anesthesiologist must consider not only renal and hepatic dysfunction, but findings of cardiopulmonary disease as well. Most anesthetics are associated with some degree of myocardial or pulmonary depression. In the presence of severe disease, the anesthesiologist must select the drugs and the technique most likely to promote cardiopulmonary stability. If the patient has severe impairment of vital signs, maintenance of stability becomes critical.

The anesthesiologist will consider the psychologic needs of the patient. If the patient is extremely agitated and uncooperative, regional anesthesia may prove difficult. If the patient is senile or demented, the anesthesiologist may want to avoid agents likely to further cloud sensorium.

Obesity must also be considered an important concern. The obese patient will be at risk for airway emergencies, particularly aspiration, intraoperatively and postoperatively. In addition, a number of anesthetic agents, including enflurane and gallamine, are extremely fat soluble. When administered to an obese patient, the drugs are readily taken up by fatty tissues. Fatty tissues have less perfusion than all other body tissues, therefore the drug is likely to remain in the body for a longer period of time.[5]

The anesthesiologist must consider the type of surgery to be performed. First, the anesthesiologist must determine where, anatomically, the surgery is to take place. Although anesthesiologists can safely anesthetize to higher anatomic levels with spinal and epidural anesthesia, coronary artery bypass surgery and craniotomies are not yet performed under regional anesthesia. The anatomic site of surgery will encourage or limit the choice of anesthetic technique and choice of anesthetic agents.

Also in consideration of the type of surgery, the anesthesiologist should determine whether the surgery will be performed on an inpatient or outpatient basis. Inpatients are candidates for most types of anesthetics and techniques. Outpatients traditionally have been limited to general anesthesia, intravenous sedation, and peripheral extremity nerve blocks. Rarely were spinal and epidural anesthetics administered to outpatients. Now outpatients are going home after spinal and epidural anesthesia. The use of these techniques in the ambulatory population will influence choice of agents and discharge criteria for these patients.

Other factors to be considered are the skill and requirements of the anesthesiologist. An anesthesiologist might have well-developed skills in managing airways that are difficult to access, using fiberoptic bronchoscopy, performing regional techniques, or practicing within a recognized specialty (for example, pediatric, neurologic, or cardiac anesthesia).

The skill and requirements of the surgeon must also be considered. In selecting the anesthetic, the anesthesiologist will consider such variables as speed and technical ability of the surgeon, the position the patient will be in for surgery, and the potential for postoperative sequelae.

Perhaps most important, the anesthesiologist should consider the patient's wishes concerning his or her anesthetic. Patients are getting better and better educated about their anesthetic options. Popular magazines and newspapers have published articles on patient-controlled analgesia and epidural infusions for total hip arthroplasty. Women undergoing childbirth preparation classes usually have one session devoted to anesthetic options in childbirth. The Illinois Society of Anesthesiologists has set up an exhibit in the Chicago Science and Industry Museum called Conquest of Pain, designed to explain concepts about anesthesia and the perioperative experience.

Some patients may specifically request a local or regional technique out of fear of losing personal control if given a general anesthetic. Others may flatly refuse a "needle in the back," fearing paralysis or having heard stories about headaches caused by spinal anesthetics. Patients have even requested specific anesthetic agents, or, for that matter, have requested that they not receive certain agents.

Ideally, the patient should be encouraged to take an active role in communicating with the anesthesiologist. It is recognized, however, that the anesthesiologist has many variables to consider when planning an anesthetic. The request of the patient is only one of these variables. If the request cannot be honored, the anesthesiologist should, ideally, explain the reason to the patient.

PREOPERATIVE VISIT BY THE PACU NURSE

In many hospitals, the PACU nurse will make a preoperative visit to see patients the evening before surgery. The purpose of this visit is to establish a nurse-patient relationship, to explain the purpose and routines of the PACU, and to identify any special patient needs that may have an impact on patient care in the PACU.

Ideally, the nurse who visits the patient preoperatively will be the nurse who directs or participates in the care of the patient postoperatively. Considering that most PACUs have staggered shifts to maximize unit coverage, this may not be possible. By meeting the patient and family before surgery, the PACU nurse can explain his or her role in providing postanesthetic care. The PACU nurse can identify the goals of the PACU: to provide acute postanesthetic, postoperative care to the surgical patient.

The PACU nurse can give the patient information about the average length of stay of patients in the PACU and the usual PACU routines. Not only does this help allay patient and family concerns, but it helps promote post anesthesia care nursing as a vital specialty in the continuation of the perioperative experience.

By reviewing the chart and meeting with the patient and family, the PACU nurse can determine if the patient has any unique needs that warrant a change in post anesthesia care. For example, if the patient speaks a language other than English or one that is not spoken by anyone in the PACU, the PACU nurse can arrange with a family member to translate. If the patient is dependent on hearing aids, the PACU nurse can arrange for the patient to go into surgery with the hearing aids in place or for the hearing aids to be brought to the PACU immediately after surgery for reinsertion.

The PACU nurse may or may not begin perioperative teaching, depending on the protocol of the hospital. In some hospitals, the nurse on the surgical unit does the teaching. However, in some hospitals, perhaps because of scheduling or staffing, it is the PACU nurse who will explain to the patient about awakening and encouraging movement, as allowed; deep breathing routines; the presence of drains (such as in surgical wounds) or breathing assistance devices (ventilators); the use of patient-controlled analgesia machines; and about other postanesthetic, postoperative routines.

It should be very clear within the hospital who is responsible for postoperative teaching. The goal is not to duplicate effort nor to overwhelm or confuse the patient. Hospitalization and impending surgery is enough of a stressor.

If the PACU nurse does make a preoperative visit, a note summarizing the visit should be made in the chart. If patient and family teaching was initiated, it is especially important that the content of the teaching be documented.

NPO STATUS

The anesthesiologist will usually request (order) that the patient have nothing to eat or drink, including water, after midnight on the day of surgery. This will be communicated to the nurses in the patient's chart in the preoperative orders or told to the patient directly the day before surgery when final confirmation of the surgery is made.

By having the patient on NPO (nothing by mouth) status, the risk of intraoperative vomiting and aspiration is minimized, as is the risk of postoperative nausea, vomiting, and aspiration. Aspiration greatly increases perioperative morbidity and mortality.

Intraoperatively, aspiration occurs because of the loss of protective airway reflexes secondary to the administration of central depressant medications (inhalation agents, narcotics, benzodiazepines). Postoperatively, aspiration occurs because protective airway reflexes are not yet fully restored to the preoperative level and the patient's altered sensorium does not recognize the warning signs of impending vomiting and the need to reposition oneself to protect the airway.

Aspiration appears clinically as bronchospasm, hypotension, and hypoxemia and may, if severe, develop into pulmonary edema and adult respiratory distress syndrome (ARDS). The severity of aspiration will increase with the volume of aspirate and the pH. A volume of 0.4 to 1.0 ml/kg is associated with an increase in perioperative morbidity and mortality, as is a pH of less than 2.5. Aspiration of gastric contents is essentially a chemical burn of the pulmonary system.[20]

The risk of aspiration can be decreased by keeping the patient on NPO status, by administration of H_2 histamine-receptor blocking agents (to increase gastric pH), and by administration of metoclopramide (Reglan) to increase gastric emptying. If the patient has eaten or drunk, despite instructions not to do so, the surgery will often be delayed or, if elective or nonemergent, cancelled and rescheduled. Lack of compliance in the maintenance of NPO status may be a sign of possible lack of compliance in other areas of instruction. Patient follow-up is important.

If the patient has eaten because surgery was unexpected (emergency), the anesthesiologist will use "rapid-sequence" induction (oxygenation, cricoid pressure, obtundation, rapid paralysis without fasciculations, and oral intubation).[20] This type of induction will help minimize the risk of aspiration. Once intubated, a nasogastric tube should be inserted to empty the stomach and to prevent aspiration on extubation.

The only exception to the NPO after midnight rule is usually made to allow the patient to take preoperative medications. These medications may be drugs routinely taken for a preexisting medical problem (dysrhythmias, hypertension, asthma) or single-dose preoperative medications ordered by the anesthesiologist. When taken with a small amount of water (30 to 60 ml), there is no evidence of any increased risk of perioperative morbidity. In fact, the morbidity may be increased in the patient who is denied routine medications. It is important for nurses working with patients in the preoperative period to clarify with the anesthesiologist which medications may be administered preoperatively (if any) and which medications will be held. The anesthesiologist will evaluate each patient individually to determine the advantages and potential disadvantages of the patient continuing with routine medications on the day of surgery.

USE OF PREOPERATIVE MEDICATIONS

The administration of preoperative medications ("on-call medications," "pre-ops") remains a controversial subject in the practice of anesthesia. There seems to be a consensus that premedications do serve a purpose. The argument, however, confronts the practice of routine administration of premedications. The trend is toward evaluation of each individual patient's needs prior to the ordering and administration of premedications. For example, the number one indication for premedication is reduction of anxiety. Hospitalization, surgery, fear of the unknown, fear of loss of control, and fear of pain are all frightening to patients. For some, the fear is overwhelming or incapacitating. If reduction of anxiety is the primary goal, the ideal premedication should be a benzodiazepine (midazolam, diazepam, lorazepam). These drugs induce sedation and are anxiolytic. Some anesthesiologists, however, prefer the use of barbiturates (secobarbitol).

Premedication may be given to increase gastric pH (H_2 receptor blocking agent) and/ or to promote gastric emptying. The overall goal of this indication for premedication is to decrease the risk of, and consequence of, aspiration. Medications that are indicated for this purpose include ranitidine (Zantac), cimetidine (Tagamet), famotidine (Pepsid) and metoclopramide (Reglan). Patients who would benefit from this type of premedication include those with a history of peptic ulcer disease or hiatal hernia.

Anticholinergics (atropine, scopolamine, glycopyrrolate) may be given preoperatively. Anticholinergics cause a drying of secretions, decreasing the risk of aspiration and airway irritability. These drugs are indicated in patients who have a preoperative problem with salivation (toddlers, small children) or for those patients whose oral mucous membranes are likely to be stimulated intraoperatively. Stimulation or irritation of oral mucosa can increase salivation tenfold, potentially placing the airway at risk. Anticholinergics may also be given to prevent bradycardia associated with anesthetic agents or with parasympathetic stimulation. Succinylcholine, usually given before intubation, may cause bradycardia. Intubation in infants greatly stimulates the parasympathetic nervous system, inducing bradycardia.

Other indications for premedication include the desire to decrease intraoperative anesthesia requirements and the desire to induce analgesia, especially when preoperative patient preparation may prove uncomfortable, as may be the case with placement of central or peripheral intravenous lines or the injection associated with regional blockade. An opioid (fentanyl, morphine, meperidine) is usually the medication indicated for this purpose.[36]

Premedications may be administered orally, intravenously, subcutaneously, or intramuscularly. There have been clinical trials with intranasal administration (midazolam, sufentanil) and transmucosal administration (oral transmucosal fentanyl citrate). Premedications may be administered by the patient (oral medications are usually self-administered, especially in the ambulatory patient population), by a general medical-surgical nurse before the patient is brought to the operating room or preoperative holding area, or by a PACU or operating room nurse or anesthesiologist once the patient has been brought to the operating room or preoperative holding area.

SUMMARY

Ideally, preparation and assessment of the patient for surgery should be a collaborative effort between representatives from the departments of anesthesia, surgery, and nursing. In addition, as the patient is the object of the health care team's attention, the patient should be told of the importance of sharing information and of compliance with preoperative instructions. The overall goal of the preoperative assessment is to provide for intraoperative and postoperative patient safety and to decrease perioperative morbidity and mortality.

REFERENCES

1. Bastron R: Anesthetic management of the patient with renal disease, ASA Annual Refresher Course Lectures 243:1-4, 1986.
2. Blery C et al: Evaluation of a protocol for selective ordering of preoperative tests, Lancet 1:139-141, 1986.
3. Boyle W and White P: Preoperative assessments and management of adults with pre-existing problems, Ambulatory Anesthesia Newsletter of the Society for Ambulatory Anesthesia 2:4, 1987.
4. Brown D (ed): Risk and outcome in anesthesia, Philadelphia, 1988, JB Lippincott Co.
5. Buckley F et al: Anaesthesia in the morbidly obese, Anaesthesia 38:840, 1983.
6. Carrieri V, Lindsey A, and West C: Pathophysiological phenomena in nursing: human responses to illnesses, Philadelphia, 1986, WB Saunders Co.
7. Clochesy J: Essentials of critical care nursing, Baltimore, 1988, Aspen Publishers, Inc.
8. Creger L and Mark H: Medical complications of cocaine abuse, N Engl J Med 315:1495, 1986.
9. Frownfelter D: Chest physical therapy and pulmonary rehabilitation, ed 2, Chicago, 1987, Year Book Medical Publishers Inc.
10. Hathaway D and Powell S: Innovations and excellence: preoperative assessment program, Perioper Nurs Q 3(2):56-64, 1987.
11. Hirshman C: Anaphylaxis and anesthesia, ASA Annual Refresher Course Lectures, 233:1-7, 1986.
12. Hotchkiss R: Perioperative management of patient with chronic obstructive pulmonary disease, Int Anesthesiol Clin 26:134-142, 1988.
13. Kaplan E et al: The usefulness of preoperative laboratory screening, JAMA 253:3576-3581, 1985.
14. Kersten L: Comprehensive respiratory nursing: a decision-making approach, Philadelphia, 1989, WB Saunders Co.
15. Knaus W, Wagner D, and Draper E: Relationship between acute physiologic derangement and risk of death, J Chronic Dis 38(4):295-300, 1985.
16. Mangano D: Perioperative cardiac risk evaluation, ASA Annual Refresher Course Lectures 115:1-7, 1986.
17. Marieb E: Anatomy and physiology, Menlo Park, 1988, Benjamin-Cummings Publishing Co.
18. Mazze R: Renal physiology and effects on anesthesia. In Miller R, editor: Anesthesia, ed 2, New York, 1986, Churchill-Livingstone, 1223-1248, 1986.
19. McConnell E: Clinical considerations in perioperative nursing: preventative aspects of care, Philadelphia, 1983, JB Lippincott Co.
20. Mecca R: Postanesthesia recovery. In Barash P, Cullen B, and Stoelting R: Clinical anesthesia, Philadelphia, 1989, JB Lippincott Co, pp 1397-1425.
21. O'Neill M and David D: Pacemakers in noncardiac surgery, Surg Clin North Am 63:1103, 1983.
22. Priebe H, editor: The kidney in anesthesia, New York, 1984, Little, Brown & Co, Inc.
23. Rao T, Jacobs K, and El Etr A: Reinfarction following anesthesia in patients with myocardial infarction, Anesthesiology 59:499-505, 1983.
24. Robbins J and Mushlin A: Preoperative evaluation of the healthy patient, Med Clin North Am 63:1145, 1979.
25. Roizen M: Routine preoperative evaluation. In Miller R: Anesthesia, ed 2, New York, 1986, Churchill-Livingstone, pp 225-254.
26. Roizen M: Preoperative patient evaluation: what's appropriate? ASA Annual Refresher Course Lectures 412:1-7, 1986.
27. Roizen M et al: Elimination of unnecessary laboratory tests by preoperative questionnaire, Anesthesiology 61:A545, 1984.

28. Savino J and Del-Guercio L: Preoperative assessment of high-risk surgical patients, Surg Clin North Am 65:713-791, 1985.
29. Squibb C: Outpatient surgical evaluations, Nursing Management 19(1):32L-32P, 1988.
30. Stein M and Cassara EL: Preoperative pulmonary evaluation and therapy for surgical patients, JAMA 211:787, 1970.
31. Stoelting R and Miller R: Basics of anesthesia, ed 2, New York, 1989, Churchill-Livingstone.
32. Stoelting R, Diendorf S, and McCammon R: Anesthesia and co-existing disease, ed 2, New York, 1988, Churchill-Livingstone.
33. Tarhan S et al: Myocardial infarction after general anesthesia, JAMA 220:1451, 1972.
34. Update: Universal precautions for prevention of transmission of HIV Hepatitis B Virus, and other bloodborne pathogens in health care settings, MMWR 37(24):377-382, 387-388, June 24, 1988.
35. Vacanti C, Van Houten R, and Hill R: A statistical analysis of the relationship of physical status to postoperative morbidity in 68,388 cases, Anesth Analg 49:564, 1970.
36. Vandam L and Desai S: Evaluation of the patient and preoperative preparation. In Barash P, Cullen B, and Stoeling R: Clinical anesthesia, Philadelphia, 1989, JB Lippincott Co, pp 407-438.
37. Vinsant M and Spence M: Commonsense approach to coronary care, ed 5, St Louis, 1989, The CV Mosby Co.
38. Wilson R and Crouch E: Risk assessment and comparison: an introduction Science 236:267, 1987.

Review Questions

1. *The purpose of the preanesthetic visit is to* ———————————.
    a. Obtain patient data to plan the anesthetic course
    b. Allow anticipation of perioperative problems
    c. Reduce perioperative morbidity and mortality
    d. All of the above
2. *The ideal patient interview* ———————————
    a. Will occur in the operating room just before induction
    b. Will occur when time and privacy can be ensured
    c. Can be eliminated if the patient chart is complete
    d. Will duplicate the surgeon's interview to assess patient reliability
3. *Reviewing previous patient anesthetic records* ———————————
    a. Will provide information about medications and techniques used and problems encountered
    b. Allows the anesthetic to be duplicated to avoid complications
    c. Is not useful and is often time consuming
    d. Is unnecessary
4. *Because each anesthetic is patient-specific, it is not necessary to inquire about family anesthetic experiences.*
    a. True
    b. False
5. *In the course of inquiry about use of medications, the patient should be asked about use of*
    ———————————
    a. Only prescription medications ordered by the surgeon performing surgery
    b. Only medications that can be given intravenously the day of surgery
    c. Prescription, over the counter, and illegal drugs
    d. Any drug prescribed since birth
6. *The most serious consequence of any anaphylactic drug reaction is* ———————————.
    a. Cardiopulmonary compromise
    b. Constipation
    c. Vomiting and diarrhea
    d. Pruritus
7. *Any report of a drug allergy by a patient* ———————————.
    a. Should be accepted and documented
    b. Should be discounted, because allergic reactions only occur once
    c. Should result in the patient being referred to an allergist immediately
    d. Should be explored to determine the type of reaction experienced
8. *Inquiries about a patient's use of illegal drugs* ———————————.
    a. Should never be made, because the drugs are not available in the hospital
    b. Makes the interviewer an accessory to illegal drug use
    c. Is against the law and a violation of patient privacy
    d. Should be made routinely and candidly

9. *A patient history of smoking (tobacco)* _____.
   a. Is inconsequential to an anesthesiologist
   b. Should alert care-givers to alterations in the oxygen-carrying capacity of hemoglobin
   c. Mandates the use of only regional anesthetic techniques
   d. Has no effect on perioperative morbidity and mortality

10. *To decrease the risk of complications caused by smoking, patients should stop smoking* _____.
    a. The night before surgery
    b. After the operation (to minimize psychologic stress preoperatively)
    c. 6 weeks before surgery
    d. Only if desired

11. *Cocaine* _____.
    a. Prevents the uptake of norepinephrine into postganglionic nerve endings
    b. Has a long half-life and prolonged central nervous system effects
    c. Produces bradycardia, hypotension, and hypothermia
    d. Decreases sympathetic nervous system responsiveness

12. *It is important to inquire about the possibility of a woman being pregnant before surgery* _____.
    a. To allow the father of the baby into the operating room
    b. Because, if the patient is pregnant, surgery must be cancelled
    c. To prevent maternal and fetal exposure to anesthetics
    d. Because, if the patient is pregnant, only regional anesthesia can be used

13. *A patient with a history of a recent myocardial infarction* _____.
    a. Is at no increased risk of reinfarction
    b. Is at an increased risk of reinfarction associated with high mortality
    c. Should only have regional anesthesia or intravenous sedation
    d. Is not a candidate for surgery

14. *Patients with a history of congenital heart disease may be placed on which prophylaxis to prevent endocarditis?*
    a. Antidysrhythmic
    b. Antiemetic
    c. Anticholinergic
    d. Antibiotic

15. *An expected laboratory finding in a patient with moderate to severe renal dysfunction would be a* _____.
    a. Hematocrit of 40%, a hemoglobin of 21 g/dl
    b. Hematocrit of 16%, a hemoglobin of 21 g/dl
    c. Hematocrit of 16%, a hemoglobin of 7 g/dl
    d. Hematocrit of 40%, a hemoglobin of 7 g/dl

16. *Other expected laboratory findings for a patient in renal failure include* _____.
    a. Hyperkalemia, hypocalcemia, hypermagnesemia
    b. Alkalosis, hyperoxygenation
    c. Hypokalemia, hypercalcemia, hypomagnesemia
    d. Hypercoagulation

17. *Hepatocyte function includes* ———————————————.
    a. Maintenance of glucose homeostasis
    b. Drug and hormone metabolism
    c. Fat metabolism and protein synthesis
    d. All of the above

18. *A patient with active, acute hepatitis* ———————————————.
    a. Should have only inhalation anesthesia and no intravenous medications
    b. Increases the risk of disease transmission to care-givers
    c. Will be hyperglycemic, hyperkalemic, and hypercalcemic
    d. Poses no risk to self or others

19. *The primary anticipated postoperative problem for a patient with muscular dystrophy is* ——————.
    a. Ambulation and proprioception
    b. Being able to discharge the patient to home
    c. Emergence delirium
    d. Respiratory compromise

20. *The "classic" signs of diabetes mellitus include* ———————————————.
    a. Alopecia, pruritis, and hypocalcemia
    b. Oliguria, hypotension, and bradycardia
    c. Hypoglycemia, hyperreflexia, and excitation
    d. Polyuria, polydipsia, and fatigue

21. *The following preoperative variable is unalterable and capable of influencing the anesthetic plan:*
    a. Age
    b. Hyperglycemia
    c. Hypokalemia
    d. Anemia

22. *Which of the following is a TRUE statement?*
    a. Patients should be encouraged to discuss their anesthetic with the anesthesiologist
    b. A patient's request for a particular anesthetic technique must always be honored to avoid legal ramifications
    c. Patients should be only recipients of information, not providers of information
    d. Patients do not need to consent to anesthesia and do not need to be seen by an anesthesiologist preoperatively

Answers

	5. c	10. c	15. c	20. d
	4. b	9. b	14. d	19. d
	3. a	8. d	13. b	18. b
22. a	2. b	7. d	12. c	17. d
21. a	1. d	6. a	11. a	16. a

CHAPTER 3

Knowledge of the anesthetic agents used intraoperatively, including their indications for use and physiologic sequelae, should be part of the working knowledge of every PACU nurse. The name PACU refers to post anesthesia, an explicit reminder of the importance of understanding anesthesia and its implications for nursing.

ANESTHETIC AGENTS

Chapter Objectives

After reading this chapter, the reader should be able to:

1. Discuss the concept of general anesthesia.
2. Understand basic concepts of pharmacokinetics and pharmacodynamics of anesthetic agents.
3. Describe differences among the inhalation agents in current use.
4. Identify nursing implications for the patient who has received an inhalation agent.
5. Identify the mechanism of action of the intravenous anesthetic agents or adjuncts.
6. Identify nursing implications for the patient who has received intravenous anesthesia.
7. Describe the different mechanisms of action of depolarizing and nondepolarizing muscle relaxants.
8. Discuss the role of antagonists in anesthesia.

OBJECTIVES OF GENERAL ANESTHESIA

Before any discussion of anesthetic agents, it is important to consider the goals of general anesthesia. The first goal is to provide amnesia or loss of consciousness and awareness. The second goal is to provide analgesia or pain control. For the patient about to undergo surgery, fear of pain is second only to fear of death. The third goal of general anesthesia is the elimination of somatic, autonomic, and endocrine reflexes, including coughing, gagging, vomiting, and sympathetic responsiveness. The fourth goal of general anesthesia is to achieve skeletal muscle relaxation. To achieve these objectives, the anesthesiologist will select the drug or drugs best suited to the individual patient, in consideration of the surgery to be performed.

MECHANISMS OF DRUG ACTION

Terms such as *pharmacokinetics* and *pharmacodynamics* are often considered foreign to nurses. However, it is important for nurses to understand the concepts behind drug action, distribution, and elimination so that they may better understand the clinical implications of anesthetic agents and thus enhance nursing care.

Pharmacokinetics is the study of what the body does to drugs, including absorption, distribution, metabolism, and excretion. Pharmacodynamics is the study of what the drug does to the body.

PHARMACOKINETICS OF INHALATION ANESTHETICS

The pharmacokinetics of inhalation anesthetics is the study of the absorption (uptake) of the anesthetic from alveoli into pulmonary capillary blood, the distribution of the agent in the body, and the eventual elimination by way of the lungs. Absorption, distribution, and elimination of the anesthetic agent from the alveoli into pulmonary capillary blood will be influenced by the blood-gas solubility coefficient, cardiac output, and the alveolar to venous partial pressure difference.[8,23]

Solubility of a drug reflects how readily or easily a drug is absorbed into solution (blood). Agents may be soluble (halothane, enflurane, isoflurane) or poorly soluble (nitrous oxide). It is important to understand that drugs in solution (dissolved in blood) exert no clinical effects. It is only when saturation occurs, that the drug begins to exert a partial pressure, causing clinical (physiologic) effects. When soluble agents are administered, a greater amount of the drug must be given to achieve and exceed saturation, slowing the onset of clinical effects. If the drug is poorly soluble, it rapidly begins to exert a partial pressure and rapidly produces clinical effects.

Cardiac output will also influence the uptake of anesthetic agents. A high cardiac output causes rapid delivery of blood to body tissues, where the drug moves out of blood, across tissue membranes. As the drug is pulled from blood, the saturation of blood is diminished, necessitating ongoing exposure to the drug to achieve saturation. Again, only when saturation is achieved and ultimately exceeded will the drug begin to exert a partial pressure and clinical effects. A low cardiac output will allow a more rapid attainment of saturation.

It is also important to understand that uptake of anesthetic agents also refers to uptake of the agents from blood by body tissues. Highly perfused tissues, also known as vessel-rich groups (VRGs), include the brain, heart, and kidneys. Although these organs make up only 10% of total body mass, they receive 75% of cardiac output. As a result, these organ tissues are rapidly affected by anesthetics. Poorly perfused tissues (skeletal muscles and fat) make up 70% of body mass but receive only 25% of cardiac output. These tissues have delayed uptakes of anesthetic agents.[21]

Just as vessel-rich groups rapidly absorb anesthetic gas from blood, elimination of the agent is also relatively rapid. Elimination of the drug from skeletal muscle and fat will be a much slower process.

PHARMACODYNAMICS OF INHALATION ANESTHETICS

Minimum alveolar concentration (MAC) is the term used to compare the pharmacodynamic effects of inhalation agents. MAC refers to the lowest concentration of inhalation anesthetic that will prevent skeletal muscle movement in response to surgical stimulation in 50% of patients. MAC reflects the partial pressure of the anesthetic agent at the site of action (the brain).

The objective of inhalation anesthesia is to achieve a constant and optimum brain partial pressure of the inhaled anesthetic. How inhalation agents work in the brain is a matter of some debate. Current theories suggest that inhalation agents alter neuronal activity in the central nervous system. Neuronal activities that may be involved include the release of neurotransmitters from the presynaptic neuron, the transport of neurotransmitters through the synapse, and the action of neurotransmitters on the postsynaptic receptor. It has been proposed that inhalation agents may interrupt neuronal transmission in the central nervous system, may depress excitatory transmission, or may prolong inhibitory transmission.[21,23]

INHALATION AGENTS

All of the modern inhalation agents have the ability to rapidly induce loss of consciousness and to allow a rapid recovery. Elimination is independent of hepatorenal function and occurs primarily via the lungs. As a result, elimination is also rapid. Each inhalation agent, however, has properties that distinguish it from the other agents, making some more appropriate for certain patients and surgical procedures than others.

Nitrous oxide

Nitrous oxide is the most widely used inhalation agent. Although it possesses analgesic properties, it is seldom used alone, as it can produce only light anesthesia when used independently. Nitrous oxide acts to potentiate most volatile anesthetics, allowing lesser concentrations to be used and therefore decreasing the negative effects of these agents. When administered, nitrous oxide is given with oxygen to prevent hypoxemia. Nitrous oxide does depress the myocardium, but less so than the volatile anesthetics. Right atrial pressure increases, but cardiac output, stroke volume, heart rate, and blood pressure remain constant.

Halothane

Halothane (Fluothane) is a bronchodilator, making the agent a useful one for patients with a preexisting pulmonary history, including asthma, smoking, or COPD. It is also useful for patients undergoing thoracic surgical procedures. On the negative side, halothane depresses the protective mucociliary function of the airway for up to 6 hours after surgery, placing patients at an increased risk for atelectasis and pneumonias. As a result, pulmonary care becomes more important in the PACU: special attention must be paid to coughing and deep breathing, elevating the head of the bed, and using sterile technique in suctioning. In addition, halothane depresses the pharyngeal reflex, increasing the risk of aspiration. Halothane is a myocardial depressant, decreasing heart rate, contractility, and cardiac output. In the PACU, the patient who has received halothane may have the "shakes," shivering unrelated to hypothermia. Halothane causes a slight neuromuscular irritation. The shaking is self-limited and usually resolves within a few minutes. Patients are usually treated with reassurance and distraction. Halothane was a very popular agent in the 1960s, but after it was blamed for the appearance of postoperative hepatic failure, its use diminished drastically. It is used frequently for pediatric anesthesia where hepatotoxicity does not appear.

Enflurane

Enflurane (Ethrane) is a vasodilator, dilating all major arterioles via direct smooth muscle relaxation. Cerebral blood flow increases, with a rise in intracranial pressure. In addition, enflurane lowers the seizure threshold, thereby increasing seizure irritability. As a result, enflurane is contraindicated in neurosurgical procedures. Vascular dilation lowers systemic vascular resistance; enflurane may be used to produce deliberate hypotension intraoperatively. Enflurane is extremely lipid soluble and may have a prolonged duration of action in the obese individual. Enflurane has been shown to cause less nausea and vomiting than the other halogenated agents and may be useful in patients at risk for postoperative nausea and vomiting (see Chapter 7).

Isoflurane

Isoflurane (Forane) is the most widely used volatile inhalation agent; its greatest strength lies in its stabilizing effects on the cardiovascular system. Because of its effects on the cardiovascular system, isoflurane is the agent of choice for patients who are unable to tolerate swings in myocardial function. Patients in this category include neonates and geriatric patients, critically ill patients, and patients likely to experience large blood or fluid losses intraoperatively.

Isoflurane increases heart rate without compromising cardiac output. Systemic vascular resistance is lowered because of direct smooth muscle relaxation. Because isoflurane is less soluble in blood than halothane or enflurane, recovery from isoflurane is more rapid.

Nursing implications

Regardless of the inhalation agent used intraoperatively, there are a number of implications for the PACU nurse. All of the inhalation agents are respiratory depressants. Because each is eliminated via respiration and ventilation, oxygen therapy is warranted in all postoperative patients having received inhalation anesthesia. Gases travel from high concentration to lower concentrations. The highest concentration of the inhalation agent is in the lungs of the PACU patient; therefore the movement is toward room air. The highest concentration of oxygen will be in the atmosphere; the movement of oxygen will then be into the lungs, via the nasal cannula or face mask. Stimulating the patient to awaken and breathe deeply will facilitate gas exchange.

As all of these agents affect the respiratory and cardiac systems, vital signs should be monitored routinely. The PACU nurse should also be aware that these agents do not have analgesic properties that continue in the PACU. Pain control is a priority for any patient receiving solely an inhalation anesthetic.

The organ system effects of the inhalation agents are summarized in Table 3-1.

Table 3-1. **Summary of organ system effects of inhaled anesthetics**

	Halothane	Enflurane	Isoflurane	Nitrous oxide
Cardiac effects				
Mean arterial pressure	↓	↓	↓	←→
Heart rate	↓	←→ ↑	↑	←→
Stroke volume	↓	←→ ↑	←→	←→
Cardiac output	↓ ↓	↓	←→	←→ ↓
Contractility	↓ ↓	↓ ↓	←→	↓
O_2 consumption	↓	↓	↓	↓
Right atrial pressure	↑ ↓	↑ ↓	↑ ↓	↑
Systemic vascular resistance	↓	↓ ↓	↓ ↓ ↓	↑
Pulmonary effects				
Airway resistance	↓	↓	↓	←→
Pulmonary vascular resistance	↓	↓	↓	↑
CNS effects				
Cerebral blood flow	↑ ↑	↑ ↑	↑ ↑	↑
Cerebral metabolic rate	↓	↓	↓	←→ ↑

Reprinted with permission from Julien RM: Understanding anesthesia, Stoneham, Mass, 1984, Butterworth Publishers.
*Significance: ←→, little or no change; ↑ or ↓, moderate increase; ↑ ↑ or ↓ ↓, marked increase or decrease; ↑ ↑ ↑ or ↓ ↓ ↓, profound increase or decrease.

PHARMACOKINETICS OF INTRAVENOUS ANESTHETICS

Pharmacokinetics of intravenous anesthetics describes the absorption, distribution, metabolism, and elimination of drugs in and from the body. As the drug is injected directly into the bloodstream, the process of absorption is bypassed. Unlike the inhalation agents that must be absorbed from the alveoli into pulmonary capillary blood, intravenous agents are directly introduced into the bloodstream. As a result, the onset of action of intravenous drugs is extremely rapid.

Distribution of the agents to organ tissues is dependent on organ blood flow. Highly perfused tissues (vessel-rich groups) are rapidly exposed to the intravenous drug. Less perfused tissues (skeletal muscle and fat) require a longer exposure to the agent to become affected. Movement of the drug from blood into organ tissues is termed the volume of distribution (V_D); it is dependent on a concentration gradient and the degree of lipid solubility of the drug.

Initially, the concentration of the drug is highest in blood and lowest in body tissues. Influenced by the variables of lipid solubility, ionization, and protein binding, the drug will move from blood across tissue membranes. Lipid-soluble drugs readily move across tissue membranes. Specific to ionization, all drugs are either weak acids or weak bases.

When injected into the bloodstream, a certain portion of the drug will dissociate into the bloodstream, into positively and negatively charged ions. The amount of charged and uncharged drug can be calculated using the Henderson-Hasselbalch equation. Without detailing the mathematics involved, the clinical significance is that only un-ionized (uncharged) drugs are capable of crossing cellular membranes and exerting a clinical effect.

Protein binding also influences the distribution of drugs in the body. When injected into the bloodstream, a certain amount of drug will bind to plasma proteins (including albumin). Only free drugs (unbound drugs) are capable of crossing cellular membranes and exerting clinical effects. Midazolam (Versed), for example, is 98% protein-bound, leaving only 2% of free drug available for action.

Volume of distribution (V_D) of a drug refers to the distribution of the drug throughout the body. Drugs that are water soluble (as opposed to lipid soluble), ionized (as opposed to un-ionized), and protein-bound (as opposed to free) have a difficult time crossing out of blood across the lipid membranes of cells. Therefore the drug remains in the bloodstream.

The average blood volume of a 75 kg adult man is 5500 ml. If 10 mg of a highly water-soluble drug is injected intravenously, the drug will be distributed throughout the circulating blood volume (5500 ml). As water-soluble drugs cannot cross lipid cellular membranes, the drug will remain in the bloodstream. Therefore the volume of distribution will be 5500 ml (10 mg/5500 ml).

However, if a lipid-soluble drug is injected, it will readily move from blood across cellular membranes and will be distributed to tissues throughout the body. Because less drug remains in the bloodstream, the volume of distribution is significantly greater. In the example from the last paragraph, every milliliter of blood exposed to the water-soluble drug contains 0.0018 mg of drug (10 mg/5500 ml). Because most of a lipid-soluble drug moves from the bloodstream into tissues, a milliliter of blood may contain as little as 0.000018 mg of the original 10 mg of lipid-soluble drug that was injected—giving the appearance of having been diluted in 550,000 ml of blood. In this case, the volume of distribution will be 550 L as compared with the 5.5 L distribution (1500 ml) of the water-soluble drug. The concept of volume of distribution will be of importance when drug elimination (clearance) is discussed.

In order for drugs to be metabolized, they must be in the blood. The drug may be pulled back into the blood as blood concentration levels fall lower than the concentration levels in organ tissues or, if the drug is water soluble, ionized, or protein-bound, it may remain in the bloodstream. The major organs of metabolism are the liver and, to a lesser degree, the kidney. The lungs and brain play a minor role. Obviously, patients with liver and/or renal disease will have prolonged metabolic times, which will lengthen the duration of drug action.

Elimination of drugs from the body is also referred to as drug clearance. The rate of drug clearance or elimination depends on the volume of distribution of the drug.

For example, the volume of distribution of thiopental (Pentothal) is 2.5 L/kg. The rate of clearance of pentothal is 3.4 ml/kg/min. For ease of calculation, assume the drug has been given to a 100 kg man. If the volume of distribution of thiopental is 2.5 L/kg and the man weighs 100 kg, the volume of distribution in this man is 2500 L or 2,500,000 ml. Because thiopental is cleared at a rate of 3.4 ml/kg/min, in this 100 kg man thiopental is cleared at a rate of 340 ml/min. Clearing the entire body (2,500,000 ml) of pentothal at a rate of 340 ml/min will require 7353 minutes, or 122 hours, or 5 days! As a general rule, five half-lives of a drug are required to clear 96% of the drug from the body.

PHARMACODYNAMICS OF INTRAVENOUS ANESTHETICS

Influencers of drug pharmacodynamics include patient variables such as age, weight, sex, and previous exposure to the drug selected for anesthesia and to other drugs. These variables are, to a large degree, beyond the control of the anesthesiologist administering the drugs; and it is virtually impossible to use formulas for drug administration. The anesthesiologist must observe and interpret clinical signs in patients to guide drug administration, titrating drug administration to the desired effect.

INTRAVENOUS ANESTHETICS

Intravenous anesthetics may be used to induce or provide anesthesia or may be used as adjuncts to inhalation anesthetic agents. In this chapter, induction agents, benzodiazepines, narcotics, and ketamine will be discussed, with a focus on clinical actions and implications for nursing.

Induction agents

Barbiturates. Although a number of drugs can be used for induction of anesthesia, it is the ultrashort-acting barbiturates thiopental (Sodium Pentothal) and methohexital (Brevital) that are used most commonly. Barbiturates are used as induction agents because they rapidly block wakefulness centers within the cerebral cortex and reticular activating system. Barbiturates will produce hypnosis (sedation) and amnesia, two main objectives of general anesthesia. Analgesia, the third main objective of general anesthesia, is not achieved.

Barbiturates are generally used to produce rapid, pleasant sleep induction prior to the administration of other slower, less pleasant anesthetic agents before the surgery or procedure. They may be used to supplement regional anesthesia or as the sole anesthetic for extremely short, minor procedures (for example, electroconvulsive therapy [ECT] or cardioversion).

Barbiturates can cause direct myocardial suppression, secondary to the action of the drugs in the central sympathetic apparatus in the medulla. Barbiturates cause respiratory depression as the medullary respiratory center decreases its sensitivity to increasing CO_2 levels, with resultant apnea. The depth of respiration is generally depressed more than the rate, causing progressive hypercarbia and hypoxemia. Dysrhythmias are a common side effect of hypercarbia. Laryngospasm is a potential problem with a barbiturate intubation, as laryngeal reflexes are not depressed until large amounts of barbiturates are given and deep levels of anesthesia have been achieved. For this reason, intubation is generally attempted only after the administration of both the barbiturate and a muscle relaxant, for example, succinylcholine.

Etomidate. Etomidate (Amidate) is an induction agent used as an alternative to thiopental. Unlike the barbiturates, etomidate produces little change in cardiovascular dynamics—and this is its greatest strength. Etomidate is useful for patients who need emergency surgery when there is not enough time for adequate volume replacement or there is a risk for extreme intraoperative blood loss. In addition, because etomidate decreases cerebral blood flow and cerebral oxygen consumption without decreasing arterial blood pressure, it may be the induction agent of choice in the neurosurgical patient with increased intracranial pressure.

Etomidate is associated with adverse effects, including pain on intravenous injection, myoclonia (transient skeletal muscle movements), hiccups, and adrenal (cortisol) suppression.

Recovery from etomidate is extremely rapid. As a result, the drug has little implication for PACU nurses.

Propofol. Propofol (Diprivan) is the newest induction agent. Classified as an intravenous hypnotic, propofol has a rapid onset of action (less than 30 seconds). Induction of anesthesia is smooth, and maintenance of anesthesia is controllable. Perhaps the most attractive benefit of propofol is that patients awaken rapidly, responsive and oriented, and without the "hangover" effect often associated with barbiturate administration. Table 3-2 highlights specific information for each of the induction agents.

Table 3-2. **Induction agents**

Drug	Induction dose	Important information
Thiopental (Pentothal)	3-5 mg/kg IV	Causes histamine release→vasodilation→ hypotension/flushing Patient may report "garlic taste" on IV administration Hepatic metabolism
Methohexital (Brevital)	1 mg/kg IV	Causes histamine release→vasodilation→ hypotension Lowers seizure threshold (epileptiform) Burns on IV administration Hepatic metabolism
Etomidate (Amidate)	0.3-0.5 mg/kg IV	Indicated when cardiovascular stability is essential Burns on IV administration May cause myoclonia/hiccups
Propofol (Diprivan)	2-2.5 mg/kg IV	Myocardial depressant—may decrease BP 20%-25% Avoid in patients with coronary stenosis, ischemia, hypovolemia Burns when given in small veins Hepatic metabolism

Table 3-3. **Benzodiazepines**

Drug	Primary use	Dosage	Elimination Half-Life (hours)	Important information
Diazepam (Valium)	Preoperative	2-15 mg IV 2.5-10 mg PO	20-40	Lipid-soluble; burns when given intravenously; IM absorption is unpredictable Renal excretion Little use intraoperatively or postoperatively because of long half-life
Midazolam (Versed)	Preoperative Intraoperative Postoperative	0.5-2.0 ml IV	1.5-3.5	Monitor for apnea when combined with narcotics Water-soluble; does not burn when given intravenously Decrease dosage when combined with narcotics Decrease dosage with elderly, debilitated, COPD, liver disease Hepatic metabolism
Lorazepam (Ativan)	Preoperative	2-4 mg IM/PO	10-20	Slow onset of action Pronounced sedation; long duration Renal metabolism Little use intraoperatively or postoperatively because of long half-life

Nursing implications. Because these drugs are extremely short acting and are generally given at the beginning of a surgical procedure, they generally have little implication for the PACU nurse. Recovery from induction agents is usually complete before the patient is admitted to the PACU. If induction agents are administered within the PACU (for example, for reintubation or ECT), the PACU nurse should be aware of the adverse effects of these medications, in particular, respiratory depression. Patients receiving anesthetic induction agents in the PACU are excellent candidates for pulse oximetry.

Benzodiazepines

Benzodiazepines are widely used for premedication before surgery, as agents for the induction and maintenance of anesthesia, as supplemental intravenous sedation during local and regional anesthesia, and for postoperative reduction of anxiety and/or agitation. Currently, three benzodiazepines are being used clinically: diazepam (Valium), midazolam (Versed), and lorazepam (Ativan). Each has very specific indications for use, cited in Table 3-3.

Nursing implications. Because benzodiazepines, particularly midazolam, are given postoperatively, as well as intraoperatively, it is important for the PACU nurse to be aware of drug-specific information. Of key importance is awareness that benzodiazepines potentiate narcotics. Apnea is more likely to occur after benzodiazepines are given to patients who have received narcotics.

Orthostatic changes have been observed in patients receiving benzodiazepines. It is important to exercise caution when repositioning a patient, for example, when moving an outpatient from a cart to a chair.

All benzodiazepines have amnestic properties. It is important for discharge teaching to include written instructions as an adjunct to verbal instructions. In addition, because these drugs cause sedation, patient safety should be maintained. Patients should be cautioned not to drive or operate machinery for 24 hours.

Narcotics

Narcotics are used preoperatively for sedation (morphine), intraoperatively for induction and maintenance of anesthesia (fentanyl [Sublimaze], sufentanil [Sufenta]), and postoperatively for pain management (morphine, fentanyl, demerol). The narcotics used primarily are the morphine derivatives, including morphine, fentanyl, sufentanil, and alfentanil (Alfenta). (Non-morphine narcotics are presented in Chapter 7 in the discussion on pain and pain management.) Specific information about these narcotics may be found in Table 3-4.

Nursing implications. Of primary importance with any narcotic is the need to ensure adequacy of ventilation, including a patent airway and equal, deep, bilateral breath sounds. Narcotics are central respiratory depressants, and when combined, as is commonly the case, with inhalation agents and benzodiazepines, the potential for respiratory depression increases tremendously. Secondary to respiratory depression is the risk of hypoxemia and hypercarbia. Narcotic respiratory depression is easily diagnosed by observing the respiratory rate. If the respiratory rate is less than 10 breaths per minute (in the adult patient), narcotic antagonists (naloxone [Narcan]) may be used. Ventilatory support may be warranted if naloxone is ineffective or contraindicated. If the respiratory rate is greater than 10 breaths per minute, narcotic antagonists will not be effective and could prove harmful, resulting in pain, tachycardia, and hypertension.

Naloxone (Narcan) should be available in the PACU, along with reintubation equipment, airways, and a ventilator.

Dissociative agents

Ketamine (Ketalar) is used for diagnostic and surgical procedures that do not require a muscle relaxant; it may be administered intravenously or intramuscularly. Ketamine may also be used for the induction of anesthesia prior to the administration of other agents or to supplement low potency agents such as nitrous oxide. Ketamine produces a state of unconsciousness described as dissociative anesthesia. The patient appears cataleptic, experiences profound analgesia that remains into the postoperative period, and is amnestic.

Table 3-4. **Narcotics**

Drug	Onset of action (minutes)	Peak (minutes)	Duration (hours)	Elimination Half-life (hours)	Important information
Morphine	1-2.5	10-20	3-7	2-4	High histamine release→ vasodilation→hypotension Nausea and vomiting common May be used IV or IM and via epidural bolus or infusion
Fentanyl (Sublimaze)	1-3	5-20	1-2	2-4	No histamine release Allows cardiovascular stability May be used IV or epidurally
Sufentanil (Sufenta)	0.5-2	5-15	1-2	2-3	5-10 times more potent than fentanyl No histamine release Direct myocardial suppression Causes decreases in BP and HR May be used IV, epidurally, or intranasally
Alfentanil (Alfenta)	0.5-1.5	5-15	0.25	1.6	¼ as potent as fentanyl Nausea and vomiting common Extremely short duration— ideal for short ambulatory surgical procedures

Ketamine produces cardiovascular stimulation via excitation of the central sympathetic apparatus. Elevation of blood pressure begins shortly after injection, reaching a maximum in minutes and returning to baseline 15 minutes after injection. The systolic and diastolic blood pressure peaks at 10% to 50% above preanesthesia levels. Ketamine is a respiratory stimulant, allowing normal airway reflexes to remain intact.

Nursing implications. The primary implication of ketamine for the PACU nurse is to monitor for and prevent emergent reactions. Pharmacologically, ketamine is a phencyclidine (PCP) derivative and may produce emergent reactions ranging from unpleasant dreams to hallucinations to emergence delirium. These emergent reactions are most commonly seen in patients between 16 and 65 years of age. As a result, ketamine will most commonly be used in pediatric and geriatric patients. It is important to minimize tactile and auditory stimulation of these patients, allowing them to awaken slowly on their own. If supplemental narcotics need to be given for pain, they should be titrated. The organ system effects of intravenous anesthetics are summarized in Table 3-5.

Table 3-5. **Summary of organ system effects of intravenous anesthetics**

	Induction agents			Benzodiazepines	Narcotics	Ketamine
	Propofol	Barbiturates	Etomidate			
Cardiovascular effects						
Myocardial contractility	↓ ↓	↓	O_1 ↓	O_1 ↓	O	↑
Cardiac output	↓ ↓	↓	O_1 ↓	O_1 ↓	O	↑
Mean arterial pressure	↓ ↓	↓	O_1 ↓	O_1 ↓	O	↑
Systemic vascular resistance	↓ ↓	↓	O_1 ↓	O_1 ↓	O	↑
Venous capacitance	↓ ↓	↑ ↑	?	O_1 ↑	O_1	↓
Pulmonary effects						
Minute ventilation	↓	↓ ↓	O_1 ↓	↓	↓ ↓	O_1 ↓
CO_2 sensitivity	↓ ↓	↓	O_1 ↓	O_1 ↓	↓ ↓	O_1 ↓
Respiratory rate	O_1 ↓	O_1 ↓	O_1 ↑	O_1 ↓	↓ ↓	O_1 ↑
Tidal volume	↓	↓ ↓	O_1 ↓	↓	↓	O_1 ↓
CNS effects						
Cerebral blood flow	↓	↓ ↓	↓	↓	O_1 ↓	↑ ↑
Cerebral metabolic rate	↓	↓ ↓	↓	↓	O_1 ↓	↑
Analgesia	O	O	O	O	↑ ↑	↑ ↑
Intracranial pressure	↓	↓ ↓	↓	O_1 ↓	O_1 ↓	↑ ↑

Modified from Julien R: Understanding anesthesia, Stoneham, Mass, 1984, Butterworth Publishers.
Significance: O = no change; O_1 ↑ or O_1 ↓ = little or no increase or decrease; ↑ or ↓ = moderate increase or decrease; ↑ ↑ or ↓ ↓ = marked increase or decrease.

NEUROMUSCULAR BLOCKING AGENTS

Neuromuscular blocking agents are used as an adjunct to general anesthetics to facilitate endotracheal intubation and to optimize surgical working conditions by providing relaxation of skeletal muscles. Neuromuscular blocking agents are considered adjuncts to general anesthetics as they provide no central nervous system depression nor analgesia.

Neuromuscular blocking agents work by interrupting the transmission of nerve impulses at the neuromuscular junction. Based on their mechanisms of action, neuromuscular blocking agents are classified as either depolarizing or nondepolarizing muscle relaxants.

Depolarizing muscle relaxants (such as succinylcholine) work by mimicking the action of acetylcholine. Depolarizing agents bind to cholinergic receptor sites on muscle cells, causing depolarization of the cellular membrane (Fig. 3-1). As long as the cell remains depolarized, it is incapable of responding to further stimulation of acetycholine, resulting in neuromuscular blockade.

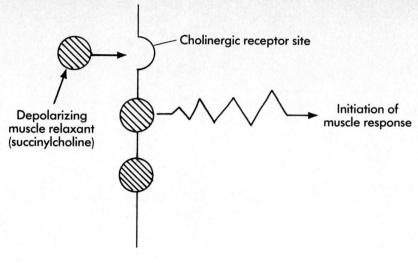

FIG. 3-1. Depolarization with succinylcholine.

Succinylcholine (Anectine) has a rapid onset (30 to 60 seconds) and a short duration of action (3 to 5 minutes), making it an ideal agent for intubation. Succinylcholine is metabolized by pseudocholinesterase (plasma cholinesterase), a plasma enzyme. Alterations in the efficacy or amount of pseudocholinesterase may result in an extended duration of neuromuscular blockade. The patient will be admitted to the PACU on a ventilator. The diagnosis of atypical pseudocholinesterase is made only after a healthy patient experiences prolonged neuromuscular blockade after a conventional dose of succinycholine. Although it is possible to obtain a serum assay of pseudocholinesterase, the problem is usually diagnosed clinically.

Although succinylcholine has the ideal characteristics of a rapid onset and short duration of action, adverse side effects include histamine release, bradycardia, hyperkalemia, increased intraocular and intracranial pressure, and myalgias (muscle aches).

Nondepolarizing agents compete with acetylcholine at the cholinergic receptor site. The high concentration of nondepolarizing muscle relaxant blocks the acetycholine from reaching the motor end plate of the muscle cell. Neuromuscular transmission is inhibited, resulting in neuromuscular blockade (Fig. 3-2).

As long as the cholinergic receptor site remains occupied by the nondepolarizing muscle relaxant, the cell is incapable of responding to stimulation by acetylcholine, and the neuromuscular blockade persists.

The onset of action of nondepolarizing agents ranges from 3 to 5 minutes. Their duration of action varies from intermediate duration (20 to 40 minutes) to long acting (50

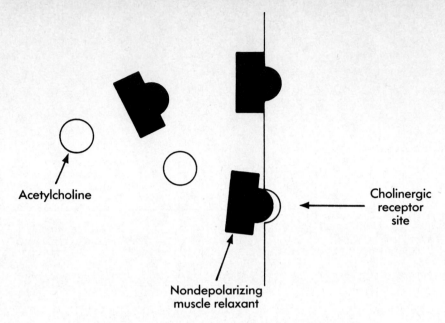

Acetylcholine

Cholinergic receptor site

Nondepolarizing muscle relaxant

FIG. 3-2. Mode of action of nondepolarizing muscle relaxants.

to 105 minutes). The decision as to which nondepolarizing agent will be used for a given patient will depend on the duration of the procedure to be performed, the route of elimination of the drug (in consideration of the patient's renal and hepatic function), and adverse effects of the drug and the patient's ability to tolerate them. Specific information on the currently used nondepolarizing neuromuscular blockers can be found in Table 3-6.

REVERSAL OF NEUROMUSCULAR BLOCKADE

Nondepolarizing muscle relaxants have the advantage of being pharmacologically reversible. Reversal agents or anticholinesterase drugs work to restore neuromuscular function via inhibition of acetylcholine, the neurotransmitter responsible for normal neuromuscular junction. As the concentration of acetylcholine increases, the odds in the competition for the motor end plate of the muscle cell change in favor of the acetylcholine. Acetylcholine ultimately displaces the nondepolarizing muscle relaxant, allowing for restoration of normal neuromuscular transmission. Anticholinesterase drugs used in anesthesia include neostigmine (Prostigmin), pyridostigmine (Regonol, Mestinon), and edrophonium (Tensilon).

Table 3-6.   **Nondepolarizing neuromuscular blockers**

Drug	Onset of action (minutes)	Duration of action (minutes)	Route of elimination	Adverse effects/ significant information
Atracurium (Tracrium)	3-5	20-40	Hoffmann* elimination	Slight histamine release Allows cardiovascular stability
Vecuronium (Norcuron)	3-5	20-40	Hepatic 80% Renal 20%	No histamine release Allows cardiovascular stability
d-tubocurarine (DTC)	3-5	60-150	Renal 40%-60% Hepatic 10%-40%	High histamine release → tachycardia→hypotension ↑ secretions→laryngospasm/ aspiration
Pancuronium (Pavulon)	3-5	60-150	Renal 60%-80% Hepatic 20%-40%	Vagolytic→tachycardia No histamine release
Metocurine (Metubine)	3-5	60-150	Renal 40%-60%	Slight histamine release Allows cardiovascular stability
Gallamine (Flaxedil)	3-5	60-150	Renal 90%	Highly vagolytic→tachycardia Cumulative effects with ↑ doses Fat soluble No histamine release

*Hoffmann elimination is a hepatorenal independent degradation of atracurium occurring spontaneously within plasma at a normal body temperature and pH.

Although these drugs are effective in reversing neuromuscular blockade, they are not without side effects. Anticholinesterase drugs stimulate muscarinic receptors, causing bradycardia, hypotension, bronchoconstriction, and excessive salivation. As a result, they are given concurrently with an anticholinergic agent, such as atropine or glycopyrrolate (Robinul). The anticholinergic agents prevent the muscarinic side effects of the anticholinesterase agents.

The anticholinesterase and anticholinergic drugs used in anesthesia are described in Tables 3-7 and 3-8. Ideally, when the drugs are selected, the onset and duration of action of the anticholinesterase will be matched with that of the anticholinergic.

Factors Influencing Reversal of Neuromuscular Blockade

Before administering anticholinesterase and anticholinergic agents, the anesthesia provider should consider factors that may interfere with reversal. First, is the patient ready to be reversed? An electronic nerve stimulator should be used to quantify the degree of recovery from neuromuscular blockade. Although nondepolarizing muscle relaxants do have a defined duration of action, patient variables may inhibit or prevent reversal. Antagonism of neuromuscular blockade may be difficult in the presence of impaired renal and hepatic function, hypothermia, respiratory acidosis ($Paco_2$ greater than 50 mm

Table 3-7. **Anticholinesterase drugs**

Drug	Onset of action (minutes)	Duration of action (minutes)	Usual dose	Important information
Neostigmine (Prostigmin)	6-8	60	0.5-2.5 mg IV	50% renal excretion May cause dysrhythmias—cardiac monitoring is essential Strong muscarinic effects
Pyridostigmine (Regonol, Mestinon)	12-15	90	10-20 mg IV	75% renal excretion Fewer muscarinic effects than neostigmine
Edrophonium (Tensilon)	2-4	60	10 mg IV	75% renal excretion Minimal muscarinic effects Must be given with atropine (glycopyrrolate causes bradycardia because of delayed onset of action)

Table 3-8. **Anticholinergic drugs**

Drug	Onset of action (minutes)	Duration of action (minutes)	Usual dose	Important information
Atropine	Rapid	40	2.0 mg IV	Tachydysrhythmias common May cause central anti-cholinergic syndrome as drug crosses blood-brain barrier
Glycopyrrolate (Robinul)	Slower	80	1.0 mg IV	Lower incidence of dysrhythmias Slow change in heart rate Does not cross blood-brain barrier

Hg), hypokalemia, metabolic alkalosis, and certain antibiotics (neomycin, gentamicin, clindamycin, streptomycin).[16] The electronic nerve stimulator quantifies the neuromuscular block to the individual patient.

Second, if the drugs used for reversal are likely to cause harmful side effects, they should not be used. Anticholinesterase agents cause muscarinic effects, which are offset by the concurrent administration of anticholinergic agents. Anticholinergic agents (atropine and glycopyrrolate) may cause tachydysrhythmias, thereby increasing oxygen demand. If the patient cannot tolerate these side effects without compromise, reversal should not be attempted.

Finally, reversal should not be attempted if the patient is to remain intubated and ventilated. Muscle relaxants allow for ease of ventilation, particularly in the patient requiring positive pressure ventilation for acute respiratory distress. If muscle relaxants are to be given to maintain paralysis in the postoperative period, the nurse should remember that neuromuscular blockers do not have central nervous system depressant effects. Patients who are paralyzed for ventilation should also be sedated to decrease awareness of immobility.

ANTAGONISTS
Physostigmine

Physostigmine (Antilirium) is used in anesthesia and post anesthesia care to antagonize the central anticholinergic syndrome caused by scopolamine and, to a lesser extent, atropine. As the anticholinergics block receptors in the central nervous system, patients may be restless, disoriented, and agitated. Physostigmine easily crosses the blood-brain barrier, antagonizing the anticholinergic agent at the central receptor site.

The administration of physostigmine necessitates monitoring of heart rate and blood pressure. Physostigmine can cause bradycardia and hypotension. Bradycardia may be treated with atropine. Nausea and vomiting are common side effects of physostigmine.

Physostigmine has also been shown to be effective in increasing the level of consciousness and awareness in patients sedated with volatile anesthetics and diazepam (Valium), although the mechanism of action is unclear.

Naloxone

Naloxone (Narcan) is a specific narcotic antagonist used in anesthesia and post anesthesia care to reverse narcotic-induced respiratory depression. Naloxone displaces opioid agonists (narcotics) from μ receptors. Because naloxone is lipid soluble, it rapidly crosses the blood-brain barrier, reaching a peak level in the brain almost immediately. Unfortunately, naloxone has a relatively short duration of action (30 to 45 minutes) compared with the longer acting narcotics, which are metabolized at a slower rate. It is possible that, as naloxone levels fall, narcotic-induced respiratory depression (renarcotization) may occur. Titration with supplemental doses of naloxone may be necessary.

Unfortunately, naloxone reverses respiratory depression and analgesia from narcotics. As a result, although the patient will demonstrate an improved ventilation pattern, complaints of surgical pain are common. Pain results in sympathetic stimulation and the release of catecholamines. As catecholamine levels increase, the patient will experience tachycardia, hypertension, increased peripheral vascular resistance, and ventricular dysrhythmias. Caution must be taken when administering naloxone to a patient with cardiac disease. Titration of naloxone until respiratory depression is reversed may decrease the severity of the sympathetic effects.

Flumazenil

Flumazenil is a specific benzodiazepine antagonist designed to reverse the relaxant, sedative, anticonvulsant, amnestic, anesthetic, and respiratory depressant effects of benzodiazepines. Designed to be administered intravenously or orally, reversal effects are seen within 1 to 2 minutes. Side effects are minimal, excepting slight, transient agitation. Of concern is the potential for the duration of action of the benzodiazepine to outlast the duration of action of flumazenil.

CONCLUSION

In this discussion of anesthetic agents, each agent or category of agents has been presented in isolation. It is to be remembered that often these drugs are given in combination with one another. It is not uncommon for a patient to receive a barbiturate (thiopental) and a depolarizing muscle relaxant (succinylcholine) for induction/intubation; an inhalation agent (isoflurane), a narcotic (fentanyl), a benzodiazepine (midazolam), and a nondepolarizing muscle relaxant (vecuronium) for the operative procedure; and an anticholinesterase agent (neostigmine) and an anticholinergic agent (atropine) for reversal at the end of a procedure. It is imperative that PACU nurses have an understanding of anesthetic agents, including their individual and cumulative effects.

REFERENCES

1. Barash P, Cullen B, and Stoelting R: Clinical anesthesia, Philadelphia, 1989, JB Lippincott Co.
2. Bevan D, Smith C, and Donati F: Postoperative neuromuscular blockade: a comparison between atracurium, vecuronium and pancuronium, Anesthesiology 69:272-276, 1988.
3. Biddle C and Gilliland C: The cardiovascular and pulmonary effects of inhalation anesthetic agents, Curr Rev Nurse Anesth 21(10):163-167, 1988.
4. Booij L: Neuromuscular blockade: an update, Curr Rev Nurse Anesth 1(10):3-7, 1987.
5. Brown B, Blitt C, and Vaughan R: Clinical anesthesiology, St. Louis, 1985, The CV Mosby Co.
6. Estafanous F: Opioids in anesthesia, Boston, 1984, Butterworth Publishers.
7. Glass P: Reversal of muscle relaxants, J Post Anesth Nurs 4(2):112-115, 1989.
8. Hug C: Pharmacokinetics of new synthetic narcotic analgesic. In Estafanous F: Opioids in anesthesia, Boston, 1984, Butterworth Publishers, pp 50-60.
9. Hull C: General principles of pharmacokinetics. In Prys-Roberts C and Hug C, editors: Pharmacokinetics of anaesthesia, London, 1984, Blackwell Scientific Publications, Ltd, pp 1-24.
10. Julien R: Understanding anesthesia, Menlo Park, Calif, 1984, Addison-Wesley Publishing Co, Inc.
11. Kitahata L and Collins J: Narcotic analgesics in anesthesiology, Baltimore, 1982, Williams & Wilkins.
12. Klanderia V and Pandit S: Drug review: use of midazolam hydrochloride in anesthesia, Clin Pharm 6:533-547, 1987.
13. Levy L and Pandit S: Is midazolam a dangerous drug? J Post Anesth Nurs 4(1):40-43, 1989.
14. Litwack K: Practical points in the use of midazolam, J Post Anesth Nurs 3(6):408-410, 1988.
15. Miller R: Anesthesia, ed 2, New York, 1986, Churchill-Livingstone.
16. Miller R et al: Anesthesiology 42:377-383, 1975.
17. Olsson G, Ledob C, and Wild L: Nursing management of patients receiving epidural narcotics, Heart Lung 18(2):130-138, 1989.
18. Pesci B: Neuromuscular blockade and reversal agents: a primer for postanesthesia nurses, J Post Anesth Nurs 1(1):42-47, 1986.
19. Prys-Roberts C and Hug C, editors: Pharmacokinetics of anaesthesia, London, 1984, Blackwell Scientific Publications, Ltd.
20. Reves J et al: Midazolam: pharmacology and uses, Anesthesiology 62:310-324, 1985.

21. Richter J: Mechanisms of general anesthesia. In Barash P, Cullen B, and Stoelting R: Clinical anesthesia, Philadelphia, 1989, JB Lippincott Co, pp 281-292.
22. Stoelting R and Miller R: Basics of anesthesia, ed 2, New York, 1989, Churchill-Livingstone.
23. Stoelting R: Pharmacology and physiology in anesthetic practice, Philadelphia, 1987, JB Lippincott Co.
24. White P: Propofol: pharmacokinetics and pharmacodynamics, Semin Anesth 7(suppl 1):4-20, 1988.

Review Questions

1. *Pharmacokinetics is the study of* _____.
   a. What the body does to drugs
   b. What the drugs do to the body
2. *An example of a poorly soluble inhalation agent is* _____.
   a. Halothane
   b. Enflurane
   c. Isoflurane
   d. Nitrous oxide
3. *To cause clinical effects, an inhalation agent must achieve and exceed saturation and exert a partial pressure. Which physiologic condition will cause this to occur most rapidly?*
   a. High cardiac output
   b. Low cardiac output
4. *Which of the following tissues is NOT a member of a vessel-rich group?*
   a. Skeletal muscle
   b. Brain
   c. Heart
   d. Kidneys
5. *Minimum alveolar concentration (MAC) is the term used to describe the concentration of inhalation agent required to prevent skeletal muscle movement in response to surgical stimulation in* _____ *of patients.*
   a. 25%
   b. 50%
   c. 75%
   d. 100%
6. *Halothane may be the agent of choice for a patient with COPD undergoing a lobectomy, because it is a* _____.
   a. Myocardial stimulant
   b. Bronchodilator
   c. Vasodilator
   d. Respiratory stimulant
7. *Enflurane is contraindicated in neurosurgical procedures because it is a(n)* _____ *and because it* _____.
   a. Vasoconstrictor, decreases cerebral blood flow
   b. Anticonvulsant, decreases cerebral blood flow
   c. Vasodilator, lowers seizure threshold
   d. Vasodilator, decreases intracranial pressure

8. *The greatest strength of isoflurane is* _____.
   a. That it does not cause respiratory depression
   b. Its high degree of solubility
   c. Its vasoconstrictive properties
   d. Maintenance of myocardial stability

9. *Barbiturates are used in anesthesia to provide* _____.
   a. Induction
   b. Analgesia
   c. Skeletal muscle stimulation
   d. Vasoconstriction

10. *Which of the following is NOT an induction agent?*
    a. Gallamine
    b. Etomidate
    c. Propofol
    d. Methohexital

11. *Common problems for patients receiving barbiturates include* _____.
    a. Hypotension and bradycardia
    b. Hypercarbia and hypoxemia
    c. Hypertension and tachycardia
    d. Dysrhythmias and hypertension

12. *The benzodiazepine with the shortest half-life is* _____.
    a. Fentanyl (Sublimaze)
    b. Diazepam (Valium)
    c. Midazolam (Versed)
    d. Lorazepam (Ativan)

13. *Naloxone must always be available when* _____ *is given to patients.*
    a. Ketamine
    b. Midazolam
    c. Scopalamine
    d. Fentanyl

14. *Alfentanil has a volume of distribution (V_D) of 0.86 L/kg and a rate of clearance of 6.4 ml/ kg/min. Calculate the time that will be required to clear the drug from the body of a 100 kg person.*
    a. 22.4 hours
    b. 1344 hours
    c. 0.93 hours
    d. 80.7 hours

15. *A major problem with pancuronium (Pavulon) is that it is* _____, *causing* _____.
    a. A vasodilator, hypotension
    b. Vagolytic, tachycardia
    c. Histaminic, hypertension
    d. Ultrashort acting, rapid recovery

16. *Agents used to reverse neuromuscular blockade are called* _____.
    a. Narcotic antagonists
    b. Antimuscarinic drugs
    c. Anticholinesterase drugs
    d. Anticholinergic drugs

17. *Which of the following blockades is reversible with antagonists?*
    a. Depolarizing blockade
    b. Nondepolarizing blockade

18. *An example of a depolarizing muscle relaxant is* _____.
    a. Succinylcholine
    b. *d*-Tubocurarine
    c. Pancuronium
    d. Vecuronium

19. *Succinylcholine is metabolized by* _____.
    a. The kidney
    b. The liver
    c. Hoffmann elimination
    d. Pseudocholinesterase

20. *Nondepolarizing blockade is best described as* _____.
    a. Prolonged depolarization
    b. Repolarization inhibition
    c. Sympathetic inhibition
    d. A competitive blockade

21. *Central anticholinergic syndrome caused by atropine or scopolamine may be reversed with*
    _____.
    a. Neostigmine
    b. Pyridostigmine
    c. Physostigmine
    d. Edrophonium

22. *Flumazenil is a specific* _____.
    a. Narcotic agonist
    b. Benzodiazepine antagonist
    c. Anticholinesterase agent
    d. Mixed agonist-antagonist

Answers

	20. d	15. b	10. a	5. b
	19. d	14. a	9. a	4. d
	18. a	13. d	8. d	3. b
22. b	17. b	12. c	7. c	2. d
21. c	16. c	11. b	6. b	1. a

CHAPTER 4

Local anesthetics are drugs that block the initiation and transmission of impulses in excitable tissues. Local anesthetics may be used topically, via infiltration, and for regional anesthesia; regional anesthesia includes peripheral nerve blocks, intravenous regional blocks, and spinal, epidural, and caudal anesthesia. It is the purpose of this chapter to highlight the pharmacology and physiology of local anesthetics and to discuss their use in anesthesia practice. Nursing implications of the various routes of administration shall be identified.

REGIONAL ANESTHETICS

Chapter Objectives

After reading this chapter, the reader should be able to:

1. Describe the mechanism of action of local anesthetics.
2. Discuss ways to classify local anesthetics.
3. Identify the signs and symptoms of local anesthetic toxicity.
4. Identify the uses of local anesthetics, including methods of administration.
5. Identify nursing implications for the patient who has received regional anesthesia.

PHYSIOLOGY AND PHARMACOLOGY OF LOCAL ANESTHETICS

Local anesthetics inhibit conduction of nerve impulses by preventing increases in cellular permeability to sodium ions. The decrease in sodium ion permeability slows the rate of cellular depolarization. A conduction blockade occurs because no action potential is generated.

With progressive increases in local anesthetic concentration, the transmission of autonomic, then somatic sensory, and finally somatic motor impulses are blocked. This produces autonomic nervous system blockade, anesthesia, and skeletal muscle paralysis in the area of the affected nerve.

Local anesthetics are classified pharmacologically as being either esters or amides, depending on a bond in the chemical construction of the local anesthetic molecule. The clinically significant differences between ester and amide local anesthetics involves their site of metabolism and potential for causing allergic reactions.

Ester local anesthetics include procaine, chloroprocaine, tetracaine, and benzocaine. Ester anesthetics are metabolized in plasma by the enzyme pseudocholinesterase. A by-product of metabolism is para-aminobenzoic acid (PABA). Some patients may react to PABA with a histamine-type allergic reaction, presenting with pruritus, erythema, and possibly bronchospasm and hypotension. Treatment includes maintenance of a patent airway, oxygenation, and the administration of diphenhydramine (Benadryl), broncho-dilators, and fluids.

Amide anesthetics include mepivacaine, lidocaine, prilocaine, bupivacaine, and etidocaine. Amide local anesthetics are metabolized in the liver by microsomal enzymes. Amide local anesthetics have only rarely been reported to have induced allergic reactions.

Local anesthetics are also classified according to their potency and duration of action. Low-potency, short-duration agents include procaine and chloroprocaine. Intermediate-potency, intermediate-duration agents include mepivacaine, prilocaine, and lidocaine. High-potency, long-duration agents include tetracaine, bupivacaine, and etidocaine. The pharmacologic properties of local anesthetics are summarized in Table 4-1.

It should be noted that the addition of a vasoconstrictor (for example, epinephrine) to the solution will slow systemic absorption of the local anesthetic. The duration of action of the drug is therefore prolonged, potentially by as much as 50%.

Side effects of local anesthetics

Systemic toxicity from local anesthetics is directly related to excess serum concentrations of the drug; it occurs most often because of an inadvertent intravascular injection of the drug. Presence of the anesthetic in blood means that the drug is carried to every cell and therefore may affect the function of many organs. The toxicity of local anesthetic agents is demonstrated primarily in the cardiovascular and central nervous systems. The uptake and distribution of local anesthetics with the potential for toxicity are represented schematically in Fig. 4-1.

Central nervous system effects. Because local anesthetics readily cross the blood-brain barrier, toxic levels may produce signs of central nervous system excitation, manifested by lightheadedness, dizziness, tinnitus, and inability to focus. Central nervous system depression follows, evidenced by muscular irritability and seizures. Apnea may result from seizure activity and central nervous system depression. Treatment includes

Table 4-1. Pharmacologic properties of local anesthetics

Agent	Chemical type	Potency	Duration (minutes)
Procaine (Novocain)	Ester	Low	60-90
Chloroprocaine (Nesacaine)	Ester	Low	30-60
Mepivacaine (Carbocaine)	Amide	Intermediate	120-240
Prilocaine (Citanest)	Amide	Intermediate	120-240
Lidocaine (Xylocaine)	Amide	Intermediate	90-200
Tetracaine (Pontocaine)	Ester	High	180-600
Bupivacaine (Marcaine)	Amide	High	180-600
Etidocaine (Duranest)	Amide	High	180-600

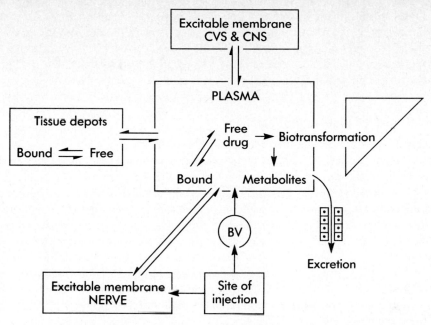

FIG. 4-1. Pharmacokinetic scheme of uptake, distribution, and elimination of local anesthetic drugs from the epidural space (site of injection). Uptake into nerve and blood vessels (BV) leads to redistribution into plasma, tissue depots, and potentially toxic sites in the cardiovascular system (CVS) and central nervous system (CNS). (From Bromage PR: Epidural analgesia, Philadelphia, 1978, WB Saunders Co.)

oxygenation and ventilation. Succinylcholine, barbiturates, and/or benzodiazepines may be used to stop seizure activity.

Cardiovascular effects. Local anesthetics may produce profound cardiovascular changes by direct cardiac and peripheral vascular action. All local anesthetics, with the exception of cocaine, cause peripheral vasodilation by direct relaxation of vascular smooth muscle. Local anesthetics cause a conduction blockade (their mechanism of action). This conduction blockade may cause conduction deficits in the myocardium, resulting in ventricular irritability, heart blocks, or asystole. Compromising myocardial contractility will negatively affect cardiac output. Treatment includes epinephrine, atropine, and possibly cardioversion. Bretylium is the drug of choice for ventricular ectopy. It should be noted that these signs and symptoms of local anesthetic toxicity progress along a continuum and are directly related to systemic anesthetic concentration. Treatment interventions, therefore, should be instituted on discovery of clinical manifestations to prevent the progression into life-threatening events. Table 4-2 summarizes the signs and symptoms of local anesthetic toxicity.

As the two most likely causes of systemic toxicity include an intravascular injection and administration of an excessive dose of local anesthetic, the best treatment for systemic toxicity is prevention.

As previously stated, local anesthetics may be administered topically, via infiltration, for peripheral and intravenous nerve blocks and for regional nerve blocks (spinal, epidural, and caudal blocks). Each technique shall be discussed.

Topical use of local anesthetics

Topical anesthesia results from the application of local anesthetics directly to a mucous membrane, serous membrane, or into an open wound. Local anesthetics may be applied to the eye, skin, tympanic membrane, rectum, oral mucosa, and tracheobronchial tree. Topical anesthetics are most often used for anesthesia of the tracheobronchial tree, to decrease laryngeal reflexes and coughing before laryngoscopy or bronchoscopy.

When applied to highly vascular mucous membranes, the onset of anesthesia is 5 to 10 minutes. When applied to skin, the onset is 30 to 60 minutes. Cocaine (4% to 10%), tetracaine (1% to 2%), and lidocaine (2% to 4%) are the agents most commonly used. Cocaine also has a unique advantage of producing vasoconstriction (unlike the other agents, which induce vasodilation). This vasoconstriction is useful in decreasing bleeding, as well as optimizing visualization of the surgical field.

Local infiltration

Local infiltration of local anesthetics is designed to achieve a sensory blockade without blocking a specific nerve. The agent is injected intracutaneously or subcutaneously

Table 4-2. **Signs and symptoms of local anesthetic toxicity**

	Cardiovascular effects	CNS effects
Mild	↑ PR interval	Lightheadedness
	↑ QRS duration	Dizziness
	↓ Cardiac output	Tinnitus
	↓ Blood pressure	Drowsiness
		Disorientation
Severe	↑ ↑ PR interval	Muscle twitching
	↑ ↑ QRS duration	Tremors of face and extremities
	Sinus bradycardia	Unconsciousness
	AV block	Generalized convulsions
	↓ ↓ Cardiac output	Respiratory arrest
	↓ ↓ Hypotension	
	Asystole	

Reprinted with permission, *Resident and Staff Physician* © June 1982, By Romaine Pierson Publishers, Inc.

and is designed to block nerve stimuli at its origin. Local infiltration is commonly used in anesthesia for intravenous and intraarterial catheter placement. Lidocaine is the agent most commonly used for local infiltration. The addition of epinephrine to the solution of local anesthetic will double the duration of action of the blockade.

Peripheral nerve block

Peripheral nerve blockade is achieved by the injection of a local anesthetic into or around a specific nerve or group of nerves, such as the brachial plexus. Nerve blocks may be used to provide intraoperative anesthesia and postoperative analgesia and for diagnosis and treatment of chronic pain. The box below identifies common nerve blocks and their indications for use.

COMMON PERIPHERAL NERVE BLOCKS

Head and neck

Trigeminal nerve: diagnosis and treatment of chronic pain
Cervical plexus: anesthesia for neck surgery (e.g., carotid endarterectomy or thyroidectomy)
Retrobulbar: anesthesia for opthalmic surgery

Upper extremity

Brachial plexus: anesthesia for forearm and hand surgery
Radial nerve: ⎫
Ulnar nerve: ⎬ simultaneous blocks providing anesthesia for hand surgery
Median nerve: ⎭

Trunk

Intercostal nerve: postoperative analgesia after thoraco-abdominal surgery
Paravertebral: segmental anesthesia, pain from herpes zoster or rib fracture
Stellate ganglion: diagnosis and treatment of reflex sympathetic dystrophy
Celiac plexus: analgesia from abdominal organ malignancy pain
Ilioinguinal: anesthesia for hernia repair
Penile: anesthesia for circumcision and urethral procedures
Lumbar sympathetic: treatment of sympathetic dystrophies or herpes zoster

Lower extremity (uncommon, usually accomplished via caudal, spinal, or epidural)

Psoas compartment: anesthesia for one leg
Sciatic nerve: anesthesia for sole of foot and lower leg
Lateral femoral cutaneous nerve: sensory anesthesia to obtain lateral high skin graft
Femoral nerve: anesthesia for knee surgery
Obturator nerve: anesthesia for knee surgery
Lumbar plexus: anesthesia for knee surgery
Ankle blockade: anesthesia for knee surgery

Intravenous regional block

Intravenous regional block (Bier block) is a technique used to provide anesthesia to the arm or leg via a distal intravenous injection of local anesthetic into an extremity whose circulation is occluded by a tourniquet. Surgery is then performed in a pain-free, bloodless field. The major concern in performing this type of block is the risk of systemic toxicity when the tourniquet is released, blood flow is restored, and absorption into central circulation occurs.

Epidural anesthesia

Epidural anesthesia involves the injection of a local anesthetic into the epidural space via either a thoracic or lumbar approach. Local anesthetics act by binding to nerve roots as they enter and exit the spinal cord. By using a low concentration of local anesthetic, sensory pathways are blocked, and motor fibers remain intact. Epidural anesthesia may be used as the sole anesthetic for a surgical procedure or for postoperative analgesia. Patients commonly receiving epidural catheters for postoperative pain relief include those undergoing major intraabdominal, gynecologic, obstetric, thoracic, and orthopedic procedures.

The local anesthetic may frequently be combined with narcotics (such as fentanyl [Sublimaze], sufentanil [Sufenta], and morphine [Duramorph]) for epidural anesthesia. Narcotics work by diffusing across the dura matter and into the outer surface of the spinal cord where they bind to opiate receptors in the substantia gelatinosa (Fig. 4-2).

Epidural anesthesia has the advantage of allowing segmental intraoperative anesthesia and continuous postoperative analgesia; and it often has positive benefits for the patient requesting an alternative to general anesthesia. The technique may also prove to be an ideal alternative for a patient unable to tolerate the respiratory and cardiovascular sequelae of general anesthetics.

There are side effects associated with the use of epidural anesthetics and narcotics. Of primary concern is the potential for respiratory depression secondary to the effect of epidural narcotics on the brainstem. Standing orders for naloxone will provide immediate intervention, as will reducing the dose of the infusion. Apnea monitoring may be a part of an institution's protocol for continuous infusions. Some institutions require intensive care monitoring of any patient with an epidural catheter in place.

Pruritus (itching) is also caused by a narcotic; more specifically, it results from histamine release. Treatment may include diphenhydramine (Benadryl), naloxone (Narcan), and reduction of the dose of infusion. Nausea and vomiting are also side effects of the narcotic, resulting from stimulation of the chemoreceptor trigger zone (vomiting center) in the medulla. Treatment includes an antiemetic, preferably one with minimal sedation as a side effect.

Urinary retention is an additional problem of epidural anesthesia. Local anesthetics block sympathetic and sensory pathways, both of which innervate the bladder. Catheterization is the treatment.

Side effects associated with epidural anesthesia are summarized in the box on the right.

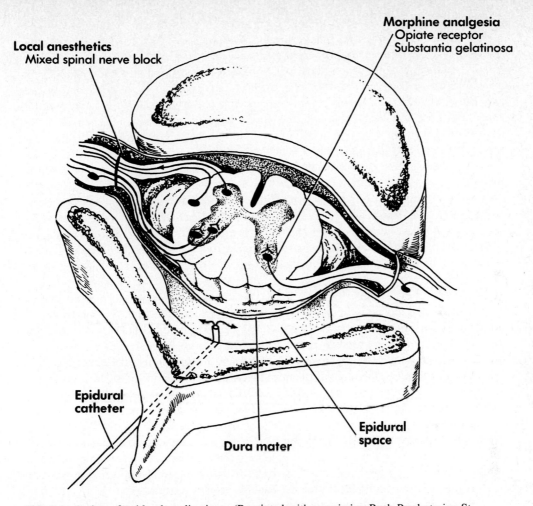

Morphine analgesia
Opiate receptor
Substantia gelatinosa

Local anesthetics
Mixed spinal nerve block

**Epidural
catheter**

Dura mater

**Epidural
space**

FIG. 4-2. Action of epidural medications. (Reprinted with permission Rush-Presbyterian-St. Lukes Medical Center Pain Center, Department of Anesthesia, Chicago, Il.)

SIDE EFFECTS ASSOCIATED WITH EPIDURAL ANESTHESIA

Respiratory depression	Nausea and vomiting
Pruritis	Urinary retention

There is an increasing role for epidural infusions for postoperative pain relief. PACU nurses may be responsible for establishing the infusion, bolusing the catheter, and monitoring for side effects and effectiveness of analgesia.

In establishing the infusion, the PACU nurse must first verify the anesthesiologist's order for the infusion and any additional medications. The use of a standardized physician order sheet will facilitate continuity in care. Fig. 4-3 is an example of such an order sheet. Once the infusate is obtained, the infusion system may be established. A volumetric infusion pump is used to deliver the solution under pressure and to allow the dosage to be regulated. Placing a buretrol in line between the infusate and the pump will provide a safeguard in case of pump failure. No more than a 2-hour supply of medication should be in the buretrol at one time. All connections between the infusate and the epidural catheter should be secured and taped, to prevent disconnections.

If the nurse is responsible for bolusing the epidural catheter, again, the order to do so and the medications to be used should be documented. Catheter placement should have already been verified by the anesthesiologist, with a test dose injection of local anesthetic plus epinephrine to rule out the potential for an intravascular injection or an intrathecal injection.

The epidural infusion is replacing the bolus in popularity because of the increase in patient safety and reduction in side effects. The side effects, particularly respiratory depression, are much more pronounced in patients receiving epidural boluses of narcotics. The infusion allows for continuous, small doses to be administered, rather than having higher doses administered at intervals. The continuous infusion also decreases the likelihood of peaks and valleys in pain control, seen commonly with bolus injections. Finally, the infusion minimizes demands on the medical and nursing staff.

Once the infusion is initiated or the bolus is given, the PACU nurse should monitor for side effects, instituting interventions as necessary. As the side effects of respiratory depression, pruritis, nausea and vomiting, and urinary retention have the potential to occur, the standardized order sheet can be used to specify interventions, allowing the nurse to rapidly reverse a potentially life-threatening complication (respiratory depression) or to increase patient comfort (treat pruritis, nausea, urinary retention).

The PACU nurse should also monitor the effectiveness of analgesia. If pain relief is not achieved, the patient may require an increase in the infusion, supplemental boluses, or intravenous administration of narcotics to provide optimum pain relief until the epidural level becomes therapeutic. If analgesic adequacy still remains inadequate, the catheter placement should be reevaluated. Some hospitals have established postoperative pain services managed by the department of anesthesia to provide follow-up of these patients.

Complications associated with epidural administration of anesthetic include accidental subarachnoid puncture and intravascular injection. During placement of the epidural needle, it is possible for the needle to be directed beyond the epidural space, into and through the dura. The subarachnoid puncture in and of itself is rarely problematic. However, because of the larger volume of injectate used in epidural anesthesia, the injection of this volume into cerebrospinal fluid will result in a high or total spinal anesthetic ef-

RUSH-PRESBYTERIAN-ST. LUKE'S MEDICAL CENTER
CHICAGO, ILLINOIS 60612
PHYSICIAN'S PRE-PRINTED ORDER SHEET
SIGNATURE AND TITLE REQUIRED WITH EACH ORDER

DATE & TIME		ANESTHESIA Post-op Epidural Analgesia	TRANSCRIBED BY	OB-TAINED BY	CHECK ✓ POSTED OR CANCELLED	
					P	C
		(PLEASE CIRCLE ORDERS TO BE IMPLEMENTED AND COMPLETE BLANKS WHERE APPROPRIATE)				
		1. Admit to PAR or SIT				
		2. Routine PAR or SIT VS				
		3. Discharge from PAR per anesthesia care team				
		4. On floor a) Apnea monitor _____ hours during bedrest, b) VS Q4°, respiratory rate Q 1°, c) IV per service or 1LD$_5$LR @ TKO #1, d) Tape 2 amps Narcan with syringe and needle @ bedside, e) Monitor for respiratory depression, f) If respiratory rate less than 8 per min., give .4 mg Narcan IV stat and call anesthesia.				
		5. Epidural solution - circle one. Buretrol to be used. a) MSO$_4$ 15 mg with Marcaine 150 mg in 150 cc NS, rate _____ cc/hr prn pain X 72 hr., b) Fentanyl 1500 microgram with Marcaine 150 mg in 150 cc NS, rate _____ cc/hr prn pain X 72 hr., c) Sufentanil 500 microgram with Marcaine 250 mg in 500 ccNS, rate 8 - 10 cc/hr/prn/pain.				
		6. Supplemental Medications a) MSO$_4$ 2 mg IV, IM, or SQ Q 2-4° prn pain, b) Emete-con 50 mg IM Q 4-6° prn nausea, c) Benadryl 25-50 mg po, IV, or IM Q 4-6° prn pruritus, d) If pruritus is unresponsive to 2 doses of Benadryl, give Narcan .080 mg IVP (dilute 1 amp Narcan with 4 cc NS in 5 cc syringe, give 1 cc of mixture. May repeat once Q 5 min.)				
		7. Nursing staff on floor call Pain Center (X26631) if any problems arise or catheter needs to be discontinued (8-4:30 p.m.). Call anesthesia on call after 4:30 p.m. and weekends (X26333).				
		8. All other pre-op orders, medications, and diet per service with the exception of narcotics.				

Signed _____ M.D.   Date _____

Nursing	Clerk	LLT

M/R FORM # 7869 8/87   1 of 1

FIG. 4-3. Postoperative epidural order sheet. (Courtesy Rush-Presbyterian-St Luke's Medical Center, Chicago, Il.)

fect. Profound hypotension should be expected. If total spinal anesthesia results, respiratory paralysis will develop.

Treatment will include fluid, Trendelenburg positioning, and intravenous doses of ephedrine (10 to 50 mg). If respiratory paralysis occurs, endotracheal intubation and mechanical ventilation will be necessary.

Because the epidural space is highly vascular, it is possible for the epidural needle to be placed intravascularly. Injection of the local anesthetic would then be systemic and potentially toxic. Central nervous system symptoms might include perioral numbness, shaking, or tremors. Treatment will include small doses of a central nervous system depressant, potentially a benzodiazepine or barbiturate. Cardiovascular symptoms usually present as hypotension. Treatment will include fluid administration and ephedrine intravenously.

To prevent the inadvertent subarachnoid or intravascular injection of local anesthetic, a test dose is used. The test dose consists of a local anesthetic (usually 2 to 3 ml of 2% lidocaine) and epinephrine (minimally 0.015 mg). The test dose is designed to rule out both subarachnoid and intravascular placement of the injectate. If the injection is subarachnoid, the lidocaine test dose will produce spinal anesthesia within 2 to 3 minutes. If the injection is intravascular, the epinephrine test dose will produce pronounced tachycardia within 1 minute.

Spinal anesthesia

Also known as intrathecal and subarachnoid anesthesia, spinal anesthesia involves the injection of a local anesthetic into the lumbar intrathecal space, usually below the level of L-2. Spinal anesthesia requires a smaller amount of local anesthetic than does epidural anesthesia, because the local anesthetic is coming into direct contact with the spinal cord and nerve roots. Sensory dermatome levels are usually used as targeted levels for spinal anesthesia. Dermatome levels are identified in Fig. 4-4.

Once injected, three types of blockade will be noted. A sympathetic block is the first block to occur, and it is caused by venous pooling (sympathetic nerves innervate blood vessels). Patients may react to the sympathetic blockade with hypotension. Hypotension may be minimized with preinjection hydration. Bolus injections of ephedrine (5 to 10 mg) or phenylephrine (Neo-Synephrine) (100 mg) may provide additional intervention.

The second block is the sensory block; it is assessed by dermatome level. A dermatome is an area of skin supplied by a single spinal nerve. Using a sharp object such as a needle, it is possible to verify the level of anesthesia. A sharp sensation reflects an area that is not blocked. A sensation of dullness or lack of sensation reflects an area under sensory blockade.

Motor block is the third block. Motor blockade is assessed by asking the patient to demonstrate return of function (for example, dorsiflexion, plantar flexion, bending knees, or lifting hips). Return of motor function is often identified as discharge criteria from the PACU.

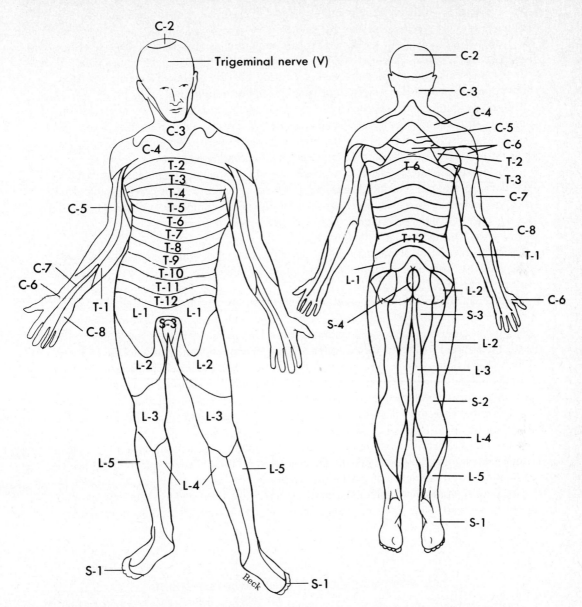

FIG. 4-4. Segmental dermatome distribution of spinal nerves. *C*, Cervical segments; *T*, thoracic segments; *L*, lumbar segments; *S*, sacral segments. (From Thibodeau G: Anatomy and physiology, St Louis, 1987, The CV Mosby Co.)

Spinal anesthesia may be advantageous for the patient who is unable to tolerate general anesthesia. Skeletal muscle relaxation is still achieved, and analgesia is pronounced, making spinal anesthesia an alternative to general anesthesia.

Spinal anesthesia is also associated with a number of complications. The side effects associated with spinal anesthesia are listed in the box below. Hypotension secondary to sympathetic blockade has already been discussed. The likelihood of hypotension is increased in patients with preinjection volume deficits or a high level of blockade.

Bradycardia may occur secondary to blockade of cardioaccelerator fibers and venous pooling. Atropine may be given if concomitant hypotension is a problem. Nausea and vomiting is also secondary to hypotension and is therefore treated with oxygen, hydration, and possibly ephedrine or atropine, not with an antiemetic.

Postdural puncture headache is considered to be a potential complication of spinal anesthesia. Postdural puncture headache is caused by a decrease in cerebrospinal fluid pressure secondary to a leak of cerebrospinal fluid via the dural puncture site. The headache is usually frontal or occipital, is worsened by erect posture, and may be accompanied by nausea, tinnitus, and photophobia.

The incidence of spinal headache appears greater in women, pregnant patients, young adults, and patients injected with a midline approach; the incidence is higher when a larger needle is used.

Treatment for postdural puncture headaches may be conservative or invasive. Conservative therapy includes analgesics, bedrest, and hydration. An abdominal binder is used to cause engorgement of the epidural veins. This increases cerebrospinal fluid pressure. Hydration is done to increase the volume of cerebrospinal fluid to the point at which production exceeds loss, thereby normalizing cerebrospinal fluid pressure.

An epidural blood patch may also be used, particularly if the patient is, or desires to be, ambulatory. Autologous blood (10 to 20 ml) is injected into the epidural space at the level of dural puncture. The blood patch "seals" the dural puncture. Relief is usually instantaneous with minimal complications.

A number of absolute and relative contraindications to spinal anesthesia have been identified. Absolute contraindications include patient refusal, patient uncooperativeness, and patients who are unable to give informed consent. Localized infection in the area to be injected is an absolute contraindication because of the risk of transmitting infection to the subarachnoid space. Increased intracranial pressure is another absolute contraindication because of the risk of herniation.

SIDE EFFECTS ASSOCIATED WITH SPINAL ANESTHESIA

Hypotension	Postdural puncture headache
Bradycardia	Urinary retention
Nausea and vomiting	

Relative contraindications include generalized sepsis, a history of bleeding disorders or use of anticoagulants, and a history of previous spinal neurologic disease (including multiple sclerosis, poliomyelitis, and paraplegia). If the patient reports a history of previous complications associated with epidural or spinal anesthesia, further evaluation is warranted.

Caudal anesthesia

Caudal anesthesia involves the injection of local anesthetics into the epidural space via the sacral hiatus (sacral canal). Caudal anesthesia is an unpopular technique in adults because of difficulty in palpating landmarks and the need for large volumes of injectate (averaging 3 ml/dermatome level). The popularity of caudal anesthesia is increasing in the pediatric population, as landmarks are more easily identified. Caudal anesthesia is useful for procedures of the lower extremity, perineum (circumcisions), and lower abdomen (herniorrhaphy).

NURSING IMPLICATIONS

Whatever technique is used, there are a number of nursing implications in caring for patients who have received local anesthetics. Initially, the nurse should be aware of the agent injected, as this will provide clues as to agent potency and duration of action. It is important to verify the addition of epinephrine to the solution, because epinephrine will prolong the duration of action of the local anesthetic. Local anesthetics that are commonly used to produce regional anesthesia are identified in Table 4-3.

Nurses should also be aware of the signs and symptoms of local anesthetic toxicity. It is unlikely that these signs and symptoms will occur for the first time in the PACU. They are most likely to occur at the point of the initial injection, usually in the operating room. Knowledge about the cause of toxicity is helpful in understanding its clinical presentation.

Table 4-3.   Uses of local anesthetics to produce regional anesthesia

Drug	Topical anesthesia	Local infiltration	Intravenous block	Peripheral nerve block	Epidural block	Subarachnoid Block
Procaine	No	Yes	No	Yes	No	Yes
Chloroprocaine	No	Yes	No	Yes	Yes	No
Tetracaine	Yes	No	No	No	No	Yes
Lidocaine	No	Yes	Yes	Yes	Yes	Yes
Mepivacaine	No	Yes	No	Yes	Yes	No
Bupivacaine	No	Yes	Yes	Yes	Yes	Yes
Etidocaine	No	Yes	No	Yes	Yes	No
Prilocaine	No	Yes	Yes	Yes	Yes	No

From Stoelting R and Miller R: Basics of anesthesia, ed 2, New York, 1989, Churchill Livingstone.

Finally, nurses should be prepared to treat any complications associated with a specific technique (for example, urinary retention, respiratory depression, and hypotension).

CONCLUSION

Regional anesthesia may be used for its anesthetic or analgesic properties. Successful understanding of the various techniques begins with an understanding of local anesthetics, including their pharmacology and physiology.

REFERENCES

1. Broadman L: Regional anesthesia and postoperative analgesia in pediatrics, ASA Refresher Course Lectures #165:1-7, 1986.
2. Bromage P: Epidural analgesia, Philadelphia, 1978, WB Saunders Co.
3. Brownridge P: The management of headache following dural puncture in obstetric patients, Anaesth Intensive Care 11:14-16, 1983.
4. Burden N and Iyer J: Local anesthesia: not always benign, J Post Anesth Nurs 2:1, 45-50, 1987.
5. Carpenter R and Mackey D: Local anesthetics. In Barash P, Cullen B, and Stoelting R: Clinical anesthesia, Philadelphia, 1989, JB Lippincott Co, pp 371-403.
6. Cohen M: Continuous epidural infusion for acute post-operative pain, Part I, Curr Rev Post Anesth Care Nurses 11(12):89-96, 1989.
7. Collier C: Epinephrine and epidural narcotics, Anesthesiology 60:168, 1984.
8. Cohen M: Continuous epidural infusion for acute post-operative pain, Part II, Curr Rev Post Anesth Care Nurses 11(13):96-104, 1989.
9. Cousins M and Bridenbaugh P: Neural blockade in clinical anesthesia and management of pain, Philadelphia, 1980, JB Lippincott Co.
10. Conklin K: Pharmacology of local anesthetics, J Am Assoc Nurse Anesth 55:1, 36, 1987.
11. Cousins M and Mather L: Intrathecal and epidural administration of opiates, Anesthesiology 61:276-310, 1984.
12. Covino B and Lambert D: Epidural and spinal anesthesia. In Barash P, Cullen B, and Stoelting R: Clinical anesthesia, Philadelphia, 1989, JB Lippincott Co, pp 755-786.
13. Drain C and Cristoph S: Assessment and management of postoperative pain. In The recovery room: a critical care approach to post anesthesia nursing, ed 2, Philadelphia, 1987, WB Saunders Co, pp 261-267.
14. Greene N: Physiology of spinal analgesia, ed 3, Baltimore, 1981, Williams & Wilkins.
15. Harrington T: An alternative treatment for spinal headache, J Fam Pract 15(1):172-177, 1982.
16. Holmes C: Intravenous regional neural blockade. In Cousins M and Bridenbaugh P, editors: Neural blockade in clinical anesthesia and management of pain, Philadelphia, 1988, JB Lippincott Co, pp 443-460.
17. Marx G: Cardiotoxicity of local anesthetics: the plot thickens, Anesthesiology 60:3-5, 1984.
18. Moore D: Regional anesthesia techniques, vol I, New York, 1979, Breon Laboratories.
19. Moore D: Regional block, ed 4, Springfield, Ill, 1981, Charles C Thomas, Publisher.
20. Mulroy M: Peripheral nerve blockade. In Barash P, Cullen B, and Stoelting R: Clinical anesthesia, Philadelphia, 1989, JB Lippincott Co, pp 787-818.
21. Perry S and Rogers W: Classical management of postop pain with narcotics, Infect Surg pp 115-123 February 1984.
22. Quaynor H and Corbey M: Extradural blood patch: why delay? Br J Anaesth 57:538-541, 1985.
23. Reiz S and Nath S: Cardiotoxicity of local anesthetic agents, Br J Anaesth 58:736-746, 1986.
24. Stoelting R: Pharmacology and physiology in anesthetic practice, Philadelphia, 1987, JB Lippincott Co, pp 148-168.
25. Stoelting R and Miller R: Basics of anesthesia, ed 2, New York, 1989, Churchill-Livingstone, pp 81-90, 173-200.
26. Strichantz G, editor: Local anesthetics, Berlin, 1987, Springer-Verlag.
27. Tucker G and Mather L: Clinical pharmacokinetics of local anaesthetics, Br J Anaesth 47:213-224, 1975.
28. Winnie A: Brachial plexus in anesthesia, Philadelphia, 1984, WB Saunders Co.
29. Wolfe M and Nicholas A: Selective epidural analgesia, Lancet 2:150, 1982.

Review Questions

1. *Local anesthetics generate a conduction blockade by* _____.
   a. Causing generation of an action potential
   b. Increasing sodium ion permeability and increasing cellular depolarization
   c. Decreasing sodium ion permeability and slowing cellular depolarization
   d. Destroying neural junctions

2. *Ester local anesthetics are metabolized by* _____.
   a. Pseudocholinesterase
   b. Catecholamines
   c. Hepatic microsomal enzymes
   d. Renal clearance

3. *Allergic reactions to local anesthetics are most commonly seen with* _____.
   a. Amide anesthetics
   b. Ester anesthetics

4. *The following agent is an example of a long-duration, high-potency local anesthetic.*
   a. Tetracaine (Pontacaine)
   b. Procaine (Novocain)
   c. Mepivacaine (Carbocaine)
   d. Lidocaine (Xylocaine)

5. *Cardiovascular symptoms of local anesthetic toxicity are caused by* _____.
   a. Inotropic and chronotropic effects of local anesthetics
   b. Central vasoconstriction and hypoxemia
   c. Enhanced conduction and peripheral vasoconstriction
   d. Peripheral vasodilation and conduction blockade in the myocardium

6. *Cocaine differs from other local anesthetics by causing* _____.
   a. No cardiac alterations
   b. No conduction blockade
   c. Bradycardia and hypotension
   d. Vasoconstriction

7. *Epidural narcotics produce analgesia primarily by* _____.
   a. Binding to spinal nerves
   b. Binding to receptors in the substantia gelatinosa
   c. Uptake in the epidural venous plexus
   d. Blocking sensory fibers

8. *Side effects seen with epidural narcotic administration are more severe and more commonly seen with* _____.
   a. Continuous epidural infusions
   b. Epidural bolus injections

9. *Nausea and vomiting seen in patients receiving epidural narcotics is caused by* _____.
   a. Stimulation to the chemoreceptor trigger zone
   b. An allergic reaction
   c. Hypotension
   d. A paralytic ileus

10. *Three types of blockade are seen in spinal anesthesia. The blocks occur in which order?*
    a. Sensory→motor→sympathetic
    b. Motor→sensory→sympathetic
    c. Sympathetic→motor→sensory
    d. Sympathetic→sensory→motor
11. *Hypotension as a consequence of spinal anesthesia is caused by* _____.
    a. Catecholamine release
    b. Histamine release
    c. Sympathetic blockade
    d. Blockade of cardioaccelerator fibers
12. *Postdural puncture headache is caused by* _____.
    a. Uncontrolled increases in intracranial pressure
    b. Hypoglycemia and hypotension
    c. A decrease in cerebrospinal fluid pressure
    d. Immobility after anesthesia and surgery

Answers

	10. d		5. d
	9. a		4. a
	8. b		3. b
12. c	7. b		2. a
11. c	6. d		1. c

CHAPTER 5

Patients admitted to the PACU are subject to physiologic alterations as a result of anesthesia and surgery. It is well accepted that the immediate postoperative period is critical to the recovery of the patient. Attention to detail and skills in postanesthetic, postoperative assessment and intervention are essential to prevent the potential morbidity and mortality associated with the surgical event. Anesthesia implies a transient alteration in perception and sensation; and post anesthesia recovery implies that patients will return to their preoperative status. The role of the PACU nurse is to assist the postsurgical patient in regaining and maintaining his or her highest possible level of functioning. To do so, the PACU nurse must be able to implement the PACU and postsurgical care plan, individualized for each patient. It is the purpose of this chapter to identify the components of the postanesthetic and postsurgical assessment. A systems approach will be used. The PACU and postsurgical care plan will be presented, and criteria for discharge will be identified.

POSTOPERATIVE AND POSTANESTHETIC ASSESSMENT

Chapter Objectives

After reading this chapter, the reader should be able to:

1. Identify the components of the initial PACU assessment.
2. Identify the purpose and components of the anesthesia report.
3. Discuss the benefits and limitations of currently used PACU assessment approaches:
   a. Head-to-toe
   b. Major body systems
   c. Scoring systems
4. Identify the components of the PACU care plan.
5. Discuss the purpose of the PACU care plan.
6. Discuss the relationship between the PACU care plan and the postsurgical care plan.
7. Using a systems approach, identify assessment criteria for postsurgical patients.
8. Identify the data used by the PACU nurse to determine whether a patient is ready for discharge.

ADMISSION TO THE PACU

The initial priority in admitting a patient to the PACU is assessment of airway and circulatory adequacy. The patient's airway is assessed for patency, respirations are counted, and high-humidity oxygen is applied. Pulse oximetry monitoring should be initiated. The patient is attached to the ECG monitor, and cardiac rate and rhythm is obtained. Finally blood pressure is measured. Only after the "A-B-Cs" of airway, breathing, and circulation have been attended to, can the PACU nurse and the anesthesiologist begin to communicate about patient specifics, including preoperative and intraoperative events.

ANESTHESIA REPORT

To ensure patient safety and continuity of care, the anesthesiologist must provide a verbal report to the PACU nurse, communicating specific patient information. The importance of this report is reflected in the American Society of Anesthesiologist's Standards for Postanesthesia Care:

Standard III: Upon arrival in the PACU, the patient shall be reevaluated and a verbal report shall be provided to the responsible PACU nurse by the member of the anesthesia care team who accompanies the patient. Information concerning the preoperative condition and the surgical/anesthetic course shall be transmitted to the PACU nurse.

Ideally, the report should include preoperative patient information, specific intraoperative anesthetic and surgical information, and anticipated postoperative problems. Table 5-1 identifies information that should be included in the admission report and the rationale for why it should be included.

The following is a sample report:

Mary Johnson is a 64-year-old female, status post cholecystectomy. Anesthesia included nitrous oxide, isoflurane, 2 cc of fentanyl, 1 milligram of midazolam. She was paralyzed with vecuronium, reversed with neostigmine and atropine. She was given 1.25 milligrams of droperidol at the end of the case, and one gram of Ancef at 8 a.m. Estimated blood loss was 100 cc. Fluid replacement included 1800 cc of crystalloids. No blood products were given. No urine output. No intraoperative problems. No significant history. She is allergic to aspirin. No postoperative problems are anticipated. The attending surgeon was Greene; the anesthesia team was George and Griffin.

The PACU nurse should document the anesthesia report onto the PACU record. Ideally the PACU record should allow for rapid, efficient documentation. Fig. 5-1 shows the documented anesthesia report from the clinical example just given.

Table 5-1. **Admission report**

Components	Rationale
Patient name	Provides means to identify patient
Patient age	Indicates recognition of physiologic differences associated with age
Procedure	Identifies the appropriate surgical care plan
Surgeon/anesthesiologist	Identifies responsible care-givers
Anesthetic agents	Identifies drug-specific priorities
Intraoperative medications	Allows for timing of next dose and identification of intraoperative problems
Estimated blood loss	Identifies potential need for transfusion and need to check laboratory values
Fluid/blood administration	Identifies potential for overload/volume deficit
Patient history	Identifies other potential problems
Patient allergies	Identifies medications that should not be administered
Expected problems	Identifies anticipated areas of difficulty

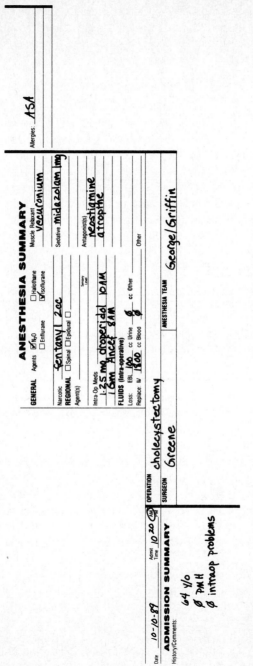

FIG. 5-1. Anesthesia summary. (Reprinted with permission of Rush-Presbyterian-St. Luke's Medical Center, Chicago, Il.)

The anesthesiologist should not leave the bedside until the PACU nurse accepts responsibility for the patient. Standard III-3 of the American Society of Anesthesiologists states: "The member of the anesthesia care team shall remain in the PACU until the PACU nurse accepts responsibility for the nursing care of the patient."

INITIAL PACU ASSESSMENT

On admission to the PACU, the patient's vital signs are obtained and communicated to the anesthesiologist. After a report is given, the PACU nurse will perform a more complete postanesthetic, postoperative assessment. The assessment should be performed rapidly and thoroughly, and it should be targeted to the needs of the postsurgical patient. The Standards of Care of the American Society of Post Anesthesia Nurses (ASPAN) includes a discussion of the need for and components of an admission assessment.

The head-to-toe assessment system is used in some PACUs. This approach provides a comprehensive approach to physical assessment. The organization of this approach is its major benefit. The PACU nurse begins with an evaluation of neurologic status and, moving downward, assesses respiratory, cardiovascular, gastrointestinal, and genitourinary functioning. This type of assessment system is easy to teach new practitioners in the PACU, because its organization provides a framework that encourages comprehensiveness (Fig. 5-2).

Unfortunately, the assessment system has also received much criticism for being cumbersome and excessive. The head-to-toe approach requires time. Practitioners may feel "locked in" to the order of the assessment and be unable to see the entire patient as a whole. In addition, documentation of the head-to-toe assessment is lengthy if all findings are recorded.

The major body systems approach has replaced the head-to-toe assessment system in many PACUs. This approach addresses the areas most affected by anesthesia and surgery. The PACU nurse assesses the admitting vital signs, and the "A-B-Cs" of airway, breathing, and circulation, beginning with the respiratory system. The respiratory assessment includes rate, rhythm, auscultation of breath sounds, and a pulse oximetry reading. The presence of airways is noted, along with the type of oxygen delivery system used.

Moving to the cardiovascular system, ECG rate and rhythm are noted. Some PACUs obtain an ECG admission rhythm strip to include in the chart. Blood pressure is obtained and compared with preoperative values. Body temperature and skin condition are noted.

The respiratory and cardiovascular admission assessments are by no means comprehensive. They are designed to verify adequacy. If the surgery involved the thoracic region or was vascular in nature, the assessment will be expanded during appraisal of the surgical system.

After respiratory and circulatory adequacy have been confirmed, the PACU nurse can then evaluate neurologic functioning. The patient's ability to respond to stimulation is assessed. Does the patient respond to verbal stimuli, to only tactile stimuli, or is the

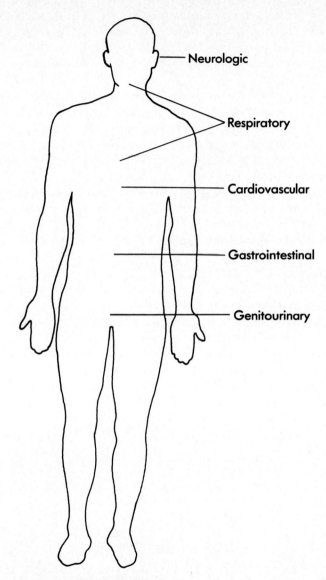

Neurologic

Respiratory

Cardiovascular

Gastrointestinal

Genitourinary

FIG. 5-2. Head-to-toe assessment.

patient unresponsive to both verbal and tactile stimulation? The quality of the patient's response to stimuli should also be evaluated. Are the patient's responses appropriate, or does he or she respond with bizarre, uncontrollable physical movement (delirium)? Is the patient able to follow commands appropriately? The patient should also be able to move all extremities purposefully and equally, unless he or she was unable to do so pre-operatively or as a result of surgery. The PACU nurse can assess this by asking patients to squeeze their hands against the nurse's hand and to dorsiflex and plantarflex their feet.

PACU patients will rarely be oriented to place and time. Patients should be capable of responding to their names and will probably know which hospital or surgical center they are in. It is unrealistic to expect the patient to be oriented to time. Anesthetic agents decrease awareness of time; patients have no idea how long the surgery actually took. Watches are removed preoperatively, and clocks in the PACU are often located out of sight of most patients.

Renal assessment will focus on intake and output. The anesthesiologist provides in-traoperative fluid totals in the verbal report. The PACU nurse will note and record all intravenous lines, irrigation solutions, and infusions going into the patient. The type of solution and rate of infusion will be recorded. All drains, catheters, and tubes for output will also be noted and recorded, as will the color and consistency of output. The major body systems assessment is summarized in Fig. 5-3.

All data obtained in the admission assessment should be documented. The PACU record should be organized in a way that facilitates documentation (Fig. 5-4). It should not take the PACU nurse longer to document the assessment than to perform it. The use of a checklist will minimize the need to write out the assessment data. A checklist may be used for normal, expected findings. The PACU nurse will then be required to document and describe only abnormal or unexpected findings.

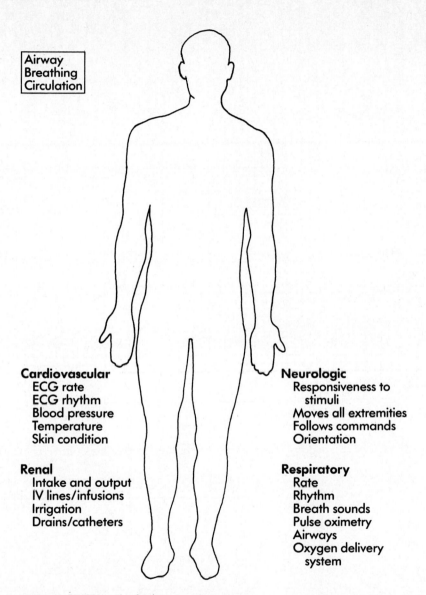

Airway
Breathing
Circulation

Cardiovascular
ECG rate
ECG rhythm
Blood pressure
Temperature
Skin condition

Renal
Intake and output
IV lines/infusions
Irrigation
Drains/catheters

Neurologic
Responsiveness to
  stimuli
Moves all extremities
Follows commands
Orientation

Respiratory
Rate
Rhythm
Breath sounds
Pulse oximetry
Airways
Oxygen delivery
  system

FIG. 5-3. PACU major body systems assessment.

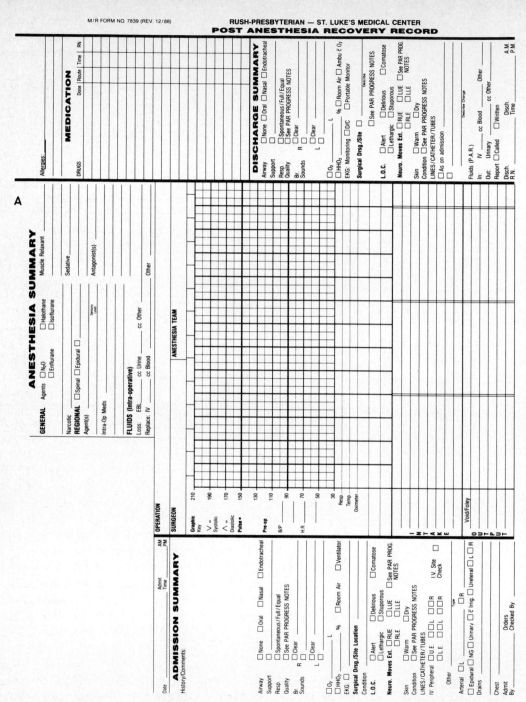

FIG. 5-4. A and B, Post anesthesia recovery record. (Reprinted with permission of Rush-Presbyterian-St. Luke's Medical Center, Chicago, Il.)

Time	Parameters O₂ or Vent.	ARTERIAL GASES							ELECTROLYTES					H6B/HCT		INITIAL	SIGNATURE & TITLE
		pH	pCO₂	pO₂	HCO₃	Total CO₂	BE	O₂ Sat %	NA	K⁺	CL₂	CA⁺⁺	Glucose	H6B	HCT		

TESTS/PROCEDURES

TEST	TIME DONE/SENT	COMMENTS OR RESULTS
EKG		
MODEL S		
SMA₆		

X-RAY EXAMINATION	TIME DONE
☐ CXR	
☐ PELVIS	

B

P.A.R. PROGRESS NOTES

_____
_____
_____
_____
_____
_____
_____
_____
_____
_____
_____
_____
_____
_____
_____
_____
_____
_____
_____
_____
_____

FIG. 5-4—cont'd.

Some PACUs have incorporated a postanesthetic scoring system as part of their admission assessment. The numeric scoring system with objectively defined criteria provides a consistent verification of patient status. The patient is usually scored (evaluated) on admission to the PACU and again at regular intervals until discharge.

The use of scoring systems to evaluate patient status began in 1953 with Apgar scoring to evaluate newborn infants.[5] In 1964, Carignan et al. proposed a postanesthetic scoring system that evaluated circulation, respiration, central nervous system, and gastrointestinal and renal function along a 6-point continuum (see the box on p. 89).[12] Unfortunately, the scale's complexity and the need to evaluate patients over an extended period of time prevented it from becoming a standard of care.

In 1970, Aldrete and Krovlik[3] proposed a postanesthetic scoring system that used physiologic assessment data already being obtained or observed by the PACU nurse. The Aldrete scoring system evaluated the patient's activity, respiration, circulation, consciousness, and color (Fig. 5-5).

Patients receive a numeric score of 0, 1, or 2 in each area, with 2 representing the highest level of functioning in each area. A score of 10 is the highest possible score. The Aldrete postanesthetic scoring system is the most widely accepted scoring system in PACUs today.

The Aldrete post anesthesia scoring system has been criticized for its use of color and blood pressure as criteria reflecting postanesthetic recovery. The inclusion of color is criticized on the grounds that it is a subjective finding. The inclusion of blood pressure has been criticized on the grounds that it is unrelated to recovery from general anesthesia. In addition, up to 40% or more of patients scheduled for surgery are outpatients, so only one preoperative (baseline) blood pressure may be obtained. This blood pressure may be unusually high in a patient anticipating surgery.

POSTANESTHETIC SCORING SYSTEM

	0	1	2	3	4	5
Circ.	BP stable Pulse always under 100	BP—change less than 30% Pulse 100-120	Vasopressors or digitalis	BP under 100 in spite of treatment	Decompensated	Severe shock
Resp.	Rate under 15 Breath-holding more than 25 sec.	Rate 15-20 Productive cough	Rate over 20, rales or temp. up to 100° F	Temp. over 100° F; partial atelectasis	Major atelectasis	Pneumonia
CNS	Amnesic, satisfied	Confused OR recalls induction	Dissatisfied with anesthesia for any reason	Extrapyramidal signs	Major neurologic complications	Coma
GI	Nothing	No more than 3 episodes of nausea	Nausea, vomited once only	Vomiting	Ileus	Evisceration or perforation
Renal	Voids over 800 ml	Over 800 ml per catheter	Voids 500-800 ml	500-800 ml per catheter	Under 500 ml	Anuria

From Carignan G: Postanesthetic scoring system, Anesthesiology 25(3):396-397, 1964.

POSTANESTHETIC RECOVERY SCORE

Study # _____
Name _____ Age _____ Sex _____ Hospital number _____
Date _____ Preanesthetic risk _____ Arrival time to RR _____
Type of surgery _____
Anesthetic agents _____
Muscle relaxants other than for intubation _____
Anesthesia time _____ Anesthesiologist _____

	At Arrival	1 Hour	2 Hours	3 Hours
ACTIVITY Able to move 4 extremities voluntarily or on command = 2 Able to move 2 extremities voluntarily or on command = 1 Able to move 0 extremities voluntarily or on command = 0				
RESPIRATION Able to deep breathe and cough freely = 2 Dyspnea or limited breathing = 1 Apneic = 0				
CIRCULATION BP ± 20% of preanesthetic level = 2 BP ± 20-50% of preanesthetic level = 1 BP ± 50% of preanesthetic level = 0				
CONSCIOUSNESS Fully awake = 2 Arousable on calling = 1 Not responding = 0				
COLOR Pink = 2 Pale, dusky, blotchy, jaundiced, other = 1 Cyanotic = 0				
TOTALS				

FIG. 5-5. Postanesthetic recovery score data sheet. (From Aldrete AJ: Anesthesia and analgesia 49(6):926, 1970.)

Steward[46] proposed a post anesthesia scoring system that evaluated only consciousness, airway, and movement. Robertson et al.[40] modified the Steward scale to emphasize the importance of a clear airway and the awake state as being essential for patient safety (see the box below). A score of 9 indicated complete recovery to the awake state.[40]

For any postanesthesia scoring system to be effective and useful, it must be simple to use. It should include routine assessment parameters so as not to add additional work for PACU practitioners. Criteria should be objective and applicable in all patient situations. It should complement and support patient care. Because of its objectivity, the post anesthesia scoring system may prove beneficial medicolegally.

POSTOPERATIVE ASSESSMENT

Consciousness	Score
Fully awake; eyes open; conversing	4
Lightly asleep; eyes open intermittently	3
Eyes open on command or in response to name	2
Responding to ear-pinching	1
Not responding	0
Airway	
Opening mouth or coughing, or both, on command	3
No voluntary cough, but airway clear without support	2
Airway obstructed on neck flexion but clear without support on extension	1
Airway obstructing without support	0
Activity	
Raising one arm on command	2
Nonpurposeful movement	1
Not moving	0

From Robertson G, MacGregor D, and Jones C: Br J Anesth 49(2):134, 1977.

PACU CARE PLAN

After the admission PACU assessment is completed, the PACU nurse will continue to apply the nursing process. The assessment data will be reviewed, analyzed, and evaluated. The conclusion about the meaning or importance of the assessment data provides the basis for nursing diagnosis.

The identification of an actual or potential alteration in functioning allows the PACU nurse to identify a conclusion, specifically to identify the problem and its most likely cause. The PACU nurse, using nursing diagnoses, will set goals for care and will direct nursing interventions toward resolution of the problem or elimination of the cause. The process of nursing diagnosis for the PACU nurse is presented in Fig. 5-6.

Nursing diagnoses that may be applied to the PACU patient include, but are not limited to:
- Ineffective breathing pattern
- Alterations in cardiac output
- Pain
- Altered thought processes
- Ineffective thermoregulation (hypothermia)

All of these nursing diagnoses have been approved by the North American Nursing Diagnosis Association. Examples of each diagnosis in the PACU care plan, along with their potential causes, are presented on the following pages.

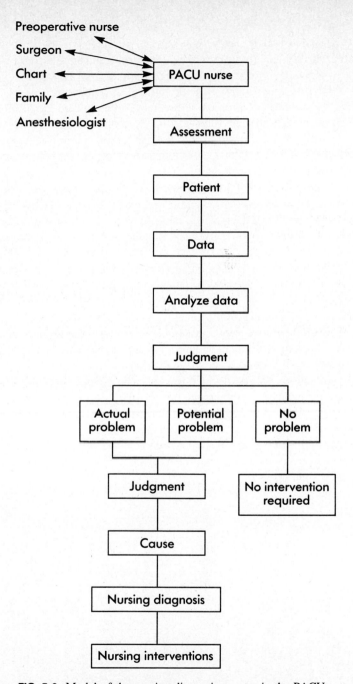

FIG. 5-6. Model of the nursing diagnosis process in the PACU.

Ineffective breathing pattern

If the PACU nurse makes a judgment that the patient is having difficulty in maintaining a patent airway, evidenced by obstruction, and in perfusing body tissues, evidenced by hypoxemia and/or hypoventilation, the diagnosis of ineffective breathing pattern can be made. The cause of the difficulty must also be determined.

Anesthetic agents can compromise adequate ventilation and perfusion. Inhalation agents and narcotics are respiratory depressants. Barbiturates decrease the sensitivity of the respiratory center to increasing carbon dioxide levels, thereby reducing respiratory drive. Muscle relaxants interfere with the functioning of the intercostal and diaphragmatic muscles required for inspiration.

The surgical procedure itself may compromise ventilation and perfusion. Thoracic surgery may have removed alveoli, the site of gas exchange, as occurs in a pneumonectomy. A chest tube may have been placed because of the development of a pneumothorax. A mediastinal incision to close the chest may be painful, causing the patient to hypoventilate.

Fluid overload may result in pulmonary edema, which interferes with alveolar gas exchange. Volume deficits may cause hypotension, which results in poor tissue perfusion.

Hypothermia and shivering may increase oxygen demand by 400% to 700% (see Chapter 7). The postoperative, postanesthetic respiratory emergencies of obstruction, hypoxemia, and hypoventilation, including signs and symptoms and management, are detailed in Chapter 8.

Nursing interventions will be directed toward maintenance of ventilation and perfusion and toward elimination of the cause. Actions may be independent nursing actions or may be interdependent, requiring collaboration with anesthesiologists or surgeons. Interventions are continued, and the patient's response to the interventions is evaluated and documented until nursing judgment confirms that the patient is, in fact, adequately ventilating and perfusing. The care plan for ineffective breathing pattern is summarized in the box on the right.

PACU STANDARDIZED CARE PLAN FOR INEFFECTIVE BREATHING PATTERN

POTENTIAL PATIENT PROBLEMS

Ineffective breathing pattern may result from:
- Anesthetic agents
- Medications (narcotics, sedatives, analgesics)
- Muscle relaxants
- Type of surgical procedure
- Fluid and blood loss and replacement
- Hypothermia/shivering
- Hypotension

DESIRED PATIENT OUTCOMES

Maintains ventilation and perfusion of lungs on discharge from PACU as evidenced by:
- Regular respiratory pattern
- Respiratory rate appropriate for age
- Clear bilateral breath sounds
- Absence of restlessness and confusion
- BP and pulse within baseline (preoperative range)
- Pulse oximetry >95% saturation or equal to baseline
- Arterial blood gases within normal parameters
- Ability to maintain patent airway

NURSING ORDERS

On admission to PACU and prn
1. *Identify cause or contributing factors*
   - Auscultate breath sounds bilaterally
   - Assess respiratory rate
   - Note breathing pattern
   - Assess level of consciousness
   - Monitor vital signs
   - Review laboratory data
2. *Provide interventions for causative factors*
   - Administer high humidity oxygen
   - Elevate head of bed unless contraindicated by surgery
   - Encourage patient to take deep breaths
   - Protect airway in the event of emesis
   - Use incentive spirometry to increase respiratory effort

Alterations in cardiac output

If the PACU nurse makes a judgment that the patient is having difficulty maintaining an adequate cardiac output, evidenced by hypotension, hypertension, or dysrhythmias, the diagnosis of alterations in cardiac output can be made. The cause of the difficulty must also be determined.

Anesthetic agents can compromise cardiac output. Drugs such as halothane, sufentanil, and succinylcholine are myocardial depressants.

Muscle relaxants such as pancuronium (Pavulon) and gallamine (Flaxedil)[1] are vagolytic and cause tachycardia. Preoperative medications, such as atropine, will cause tachycardia.

Hypoxemia and other ventilatory disorders will contribute initially to hypertension and ultimately to hypotension. Dysrhythmias, particularly ventricular, are commonly seen secondary to hypoxemia.

Orthostatic changes can result in hypotension and a reduction in cardiac output. Orthostatic changes may result from preoperative medications (diuretics and antihypertensive agents) or intraoperative medications (midazolam).

Fluid overload may cause hypertension and the development of congestive heart failure. Myocardial contractility will be diminished in failure states. Volume deficit, secondary to dehydration or hemorrhage, will result in a low cardiac output condition.

Peripheral pooling of blood occurs as the result of decreased peripheral vascular resistance, which may be caused by medications (enflurane, morphine sulfate, d-tubocurarine), spinal anesthesia, sepsis, or anaphylaxis.

Electrolyte imbalance, particularly disturbances of potassium, will affect myocardial contractility. Secondary to hypoxemia, hypokalemia is the most common cause of postoperative ventricular ectopy.

The surgical procedure itself may compromise cardiac output. A cardiac tamponade after a valve or bypass procedure will interfere with myocardial contractility. Baroreceptor stimulation after a carotid endarterectomy may cause hypertension.

Nursing interventions will be directed toward maintenance of adequate cardiac output and elimination of the cause. Actions may be independent nursing actions, or they may be interdependent, requiring collaboration with anesthesiologists or surgeons. Interventions will be continued, and the patient's response to the interventions evaluated and documented, until nursing judgment confirms that the patient is, in fact, maintaining an adequate cardiac output. The box on the right summarizes the care plan for alterations in cardiac output.

The postoperative, postanesthetic cardiac emergencies of hypotension, hypertension, and dysrythmias, including their signs and symptoms and management, are detailed in Chapter 8.

PACU STANDARDIZED CARE PLAN FOR ALTERATIONS IN CARDIAC OUTPUT

POTENTIAL PATIENT PROBLEMS

Decreased cardiac output may be caused by:
- Anesthetic agents
- Muscle relaxants
- Preoperative medications
- Poor lung ventilation
- Rapid position change
- Pain
- Fluid or blood loss or replacement
- Peripheral pooling of blood
- Electrolyte imbalance
- Surgical procedure

DESIRED PATIENT OUTCOMES

Maintains adequate cardiac output on discharge from PACU as evidenced by:
- BP within preoperative range
- Pulse strong and regular
- Skin warm and dry
- Oriented to person and place
- Hemoglobin >10
- Hematocrit >30
- Electrolytes within normal limits

NURSING ORDERS

On admission to PACU and prn
1. *Identify cause of contributing factors*
   - Monitor vital signs
   - Monitor EKG
   - Assess respiratory status
   - Monitor intake and output
   - Monitor CVP and/or Swan-Ganz catheter
   - Monitor drainage from surgical site
   - Monitor laboratory data
2. *Provide interventions for causative factors*
   - Administer fluid/blood products as indicated
   - Rewarm patient
   - Administer high humidity oxygen
   - Administer vasoactive agents as indicated
   - Use analgesics with caution
   - Position patient in Trendelenburg if symptomatic from hypotension
   - Maintain patency of intravenous lines

Pain

If the PACU nurse makes a judgment that the patient is experiencing physical or psychologic discomfort or pain, evidenced by complaints of pain or physiologic indication, the diagnosis of pain is made. The cause of the pain must also be determined.

Psychologic discomfort may be the result of disorientation, fear of the unknown, anxiety about the outcome of surgery, or alterations in body image that occur as a result of surgery. Separation from family members and significant others is frightening, particularly for children. Patients awaken in a room they have never seen before and in the presence of people they have never met before.

Physical discomfort or pain may be the result of surgical manipulation, positioning, shivering, or the presence of binders, tight dressings, or casts. Pain may also occur because of ineffective analgesia. The surgical procedure may have been performed without any analgesics included for postoperative pain control.

Nursing interventions will be directed toward increasing patient comfort and eliminating the cause. Interventions may be independent nursing actions, or they may be interdependent, requiring collaboration with anesthesiologist or surgeons. Interventions will be continued, and the patient's response to the interventions evaluated and documented until nursing judgment confirms that the patient is comfortable (or as comfortable as physiologic parameters allow). The care plan for pain management is summarized in the box on the right.

The postanesthetic and postoperative problem of pain, including its causes, signs, and symptoms and strategies for management, are described in Chapter 7.

PACU STANDARDIZED CARE PLAN FOR PAIN

POTENTIAL PATIENT PROBLEMS

Pain may result from:
- Psychologic response to surgery
- Separation from significant others
- Physical pain from surgery
- Immobility
- Position

DESIRED PATIENT OUTCOMES

Exhibits increased level of comfort on discharge from PACU as evidenced by:
- Verbalization of comfort or of decreased pain
- Vital signs within preoperative range
- Absence of restlessness

NURSING ORDERS

On admission to PACU and prn
1. *Identify cause or contributing factors*
   - Assess type and amount of anesthesia given
   - Assess physiologic response to pain, including:
     - Monitoring blood pressure
     - Monitoring pulse
     - Monitoring respiratory rate
   - Assess nonverbal response to pain
   - Positioning
   - Assess possible causes of pain
     - Patient report
     - Objective signs
2. *Provide interventions for causative factors*
   - Titrate pain medication
   - Provide comfort measures
   - Explain cause of pain to patient
   - Reposition patient if able
   - Involve family as PACU situation allows

Altered thought processes

If the PACU nurse makes a judgment that the patient is disoriented, delirious, or unresponsive, as evidenced by behavior, the diagnosis of alterations in thought processes is made. The cause of the alterations in thought processes must also be determined.

Anesthetic agents may contribute to central nervous system depression and unconsciousness. Ketamine may cause psychogenic reactions, including hallucinations and delirium. Benzodiazepines contribute to central nervous system depression.

Hypoxemia remains the "number one" cause of postoperative emergence delirium until proven otherwise. Postoperative agitation may also be the result of pain, discomfort, or extreme anxiety.

Patients with a history of substance abuse, including alcohol abuse, often awaken from anesthesia disoriented or delirious.

Viscous distention, including gastric and bladder distention, may contribute to postoperative agitation and uncooperativeness.

Nursing interventions will be directed toward restoration of appropriate neurologic functioning and elimination of the cause. Interventions may be independent nursing actions, or they may be interdependent, requiring collaboration with anesthesiologists or surgeons. Interventions will be continued, and the patient's response to the interventions will be evaluated and documented until nursing judgment confirms that the patient is reoriented and able to respond appropriately and to follow commands. The care plan for alterations in thought processes is summarized in the box on the right.

PACU STANDARDIZED CARE PLAN FOR ALTERED THOUGHT PROCESSES

POTENTIAL PATIENT PROBLEMS	DESIRED PATIENT OUTCOMES	NURSING ORDERS

Altered thought processes may be a reaction to:
• Anesthetic agents
• Hypoxemia
• Pain
• Viscous distention
• History of substance abuse
	Demonstrates appropriate neurologic functioning on discharge from PACU as evidenced by:
	• Orientation to self and place
	• Appropriate response to commands
	• Appropriate response to questions
	• Purposeful movement
	• Calm, comfortable appearance
		On admission to PACU and prn
		1. *Identify cause or contributing factors*
		  • Assess level of consciousness
		  • Evaluate type of anesthetic agents used
		  • Evaluate level of anxiety and/or pain
		  • Palpate abdomen/bladder for distention
		  • Evaluate patient's response to stimuli
		  • Evaluate patient's ability to follow commands
		  • Monitor pulse oximetry
		2. *Provide interventions for causative factors*
		  • Reorient patient to person and place
		  • Restrain patient (prn only)
		  • Use padded siderails (prn only)
		  • Administer high humidity oxygen
		  • Maintain patient safety
		  • Maintain staff safety
		  • If hypoxemia is ruled out, sedate patient

Ineffective thermoregulation (hypothermia)

If the PACU nurse determines that the patient is hypothermic, as evidenced by a body temperature of less than 96° F or 36.5° C, the diagnosis of ineffective thermoregulation is made. The cause of hypothermia should also be determined.

Anesthetic agents may contribute to hypothermia by altering hypothalamic thermoregulation. Muscle relaxants interfere with the body's ability to shiver as a heat-generating mechanism.

The length of time spent in the operating room will contribute to hypothermia. The average operating room temperature is 67°-68° F. Patients lose heat very quickly. The type of operating environment will influence heat loss. Laminar flow rooms and lithotripsy tanks contribute to rapid heat loss.

Pediatric and geriatric patients lose heat quickly. The type of surgical procedure will also influence heat loss. Anytime a body cavity is opened, the patient loses heat to the environment. Irrigation solutions that are stored at room temperature will cool patients. Rapid fluid and blood replacement will contribute to heat loss. Hypothermia is discussed in greater detail in Chapter 7.

Nursing interventions will be directed toward restoration of normothermia and elimination of the cause of hypothermia or continued heat loss. Nursing actions are usually independent, but may require collaboration with anesthesiologists or surgeons. Interventions will be continued and the patient's response to the interventions will be evaluated and documented until nursing judgment confirms that the patient is normothermic. The care plan for ineffective thermoregulation is summarized on the right.

Setting priorities

The PACU nurse must not only initiate the postanesthesia care plan, but he or she must also set appropriate priorities. With each patient admission, the PACU nurse must determine which problems require immediate attention. Obviously, actual problems will be given a higher priority than potential problems.

Airway will always be the first priority, both in assessment and in the implementation of the PACU care plan. If the PACU nurse determines that the patient is adequately ventilating and perfusing, then the patient will be evaluated for alterations in cardiac output. If cardiovascular stability is confirmed, then the PACU nurse will evaluate the patient for alterations in consciousness, comfort, and thermoregulation.

The challenge to nursing judgment occurs when priorities and patient needs seem to require equal attention. For example, on admission to the PACU, the patient is found to be intubated and unresponsive to verbal stimuli, with a heart rate of 120, blood pressure of 70/40, and a respiratory rate of 10. Temperature on admission is 94° F. The patient has alterations in airway, cardiac output, consciousness, and thermoregulation.

PACU STANDARDIZED CARE PLAN FOR INEFFECTIVE THERMOREGULATION

POTENTIAL PATIENT PROBLEMS	DESIRED PATIENT OUTCOMES	NURSING ORDERS
Ineffective thermoregulation may be associated with: • Anesthetic agents • Length of surgery • Age of patient • Type of surgery • Environment • Irrigation • Fluid replacement	*Maintains normal body temperature on discharge from PACU as evidenced by:* • Axillary temperature >96° F or >36.5° C • Oxygen saturation >95% or preoperative baseline • Vital signs within preoperative range • No shivering • Brisk capillary refill • Arterial blood gases within normal limits	*On admission to PACU and prn* 1. *Identify cause of contributing factors* • Measure body temperature • Review risk factors • Assess peripheral circulation • Obtain pulse oximetry reading • Observe for shivering • Monitor vital signs 2. *Provide interventions for causative factors* • Institute rewarming measures • Institute ongoing temperature monitoring

Airway and circulatory adequacy are essential for survival, so these needs will require immediate attention. The patient has a patent airway, maintained by an endotracheal tube. The patient is breathing with a rate of 10. With airway status confirmed, attention can then be directed toward the alterations in cardiac status. The cause of the decreased blood pressure should be determined, and treatment should be instituted. Alterations in cardiac output became the "number one" priority. Once circulatory adequacy is restored, interventions can be directed toward rewarming, patient stimulation, and extubation.

Interventions for all PACU problems will continue until nursing judgment determines that there are no longer alterations, actual or potential, in airway, cardiac status, consciousness, comfort, or thermoregulation. At that time, the PACU patient is considered ready for discharge. The patient will be discharged either to an inpatient bed or (if he or she is an ambulatory surgical patient) to phase II recovery and ultimately to home.

It is important to remember that the patient in the PACU is recovering not only from anesthesia but also from surgery. The patient requires postanesthetic and postsurgical assessment. The patient will be cared for under a postanesthetic and postsurgical care plan.

SURGICAL ASSESSMENT

In evaluating the patient in the PACU, attention must be directed toward the assessment of the body system affected by surgery. The combination of the postanesthetic assessment and the postsurgical assessment allows the PACU nurse to individualize care for each patient. The next section outlines surgical assessment criteria and nursing priorities for patients by surgical system.

Thoracic surgery patients

Patients scheduled for thoracic surgery may be undergoing diagnostic procedures (bronchoscopy, mediastinoscopy, node biopsy), treatment to correct pathologies (decortication, thoracoplasty, lobectomy, pneumonectomy), or procedures to repair mediastinal or vascular structures (thymectomy, tracheal resection, esophagogastrectomy). As all of the surgeries involve the airway or organs of ventilation, PACU assessment and care must be aggressively instituted.

PACU assessment of thoracic surgery patients. Inspection will be the first physical assessment skill used to evaluate the patient who has experienced thoracic surgery. Nursing observations begin the moment the patient is admitted to the PACU. The PACU nurse will observe the patient's level of consciousness. Is the patient awake, unresponsive, or agitated? The PACU nurse will observe the patient's breathing pattern. Is the patient breathing? Is the chest rising and falling? Is breathing spontaneous or assisted? The PACU nurse will note the presence or absence of artificial airways—endotracheal, nasal, or oral.

Observations will also be made about the respiratory rate. In the adult patient, a rate of 10 to 20 is considered normal. A rate greater than 20 is considered tachypnea. A rate less than 10 is considered bradypnea. If the patient is not breathing, the patient is apneic.

The PACU nurse will observe and make judgments about the respiratory pattern. The depth of respirations will be assessed as being shallow, regular, or deep. Chest movement will be assessed as being bilateral, equal, or restricted. The use of accessory muscles will be noted. Accessory muscle actions include nasal flaring, suprasternal retractions, intercostal retractions, and diaphragmatic breathing. The regularity of breathing will be assessed as being regular, irregular, or periodic.

Observations must also be made about overall chest wall anatomy. Does the patient have any chest wall deformities? Does the patient have any foreign bodies such as a chest tube, drains, or nasogastric tube?

If the patient has a chest tube, is it mediastinal or pleural? A mediastinal tube is designed for wound drainage, and it is usually put to continuous wall suction. A pleural tube is designed to reinflate the lung and/or drain a wound. A patient who is recovering from lobectomy (removal of one or more lobes of the lung) or segmentectomy (removal of bronchovascular segments of a lobe) will have chest tubes designed to promote lung reexpansion. A patient recovering from pneumonectomy (removal of an entire lung) will have the chest tube clamped and *not* put to suction.

The positioning of the patient is important. Usually the head of the bed is elevated 30 to 45 degrees. When turning a patient who is recovering from lobectomy or segmentectomy, the operative side should be in the uppermost position to promote lung expansion. If the patient has had a pneumonectomy, he or she should be positioned *operative side down* during turning, to promote maximum lung expansion of the remaining lung.

The PACU nurse will also use palpation to assess the thoracic surgery patient. Palpation will be used to identify any areas of tenderness or observed abnormalities. Swelling or bulges can be palpated to assess consistency or pain. The chest tube insertion site can be palpated for crepitus (also known as subcutaneous emphysema), which is caused by the presence of air trapped in subcutaneous tissue.

The PACU nurse may use percussion to determine if underlying thoracic tissues are air filled, fluid filled, or solid. Dullness will be heard when fluid or solid tissue replaces air-containing lung. Hyperresonance is heard over hyperinflated, emphysematous lung tissue.

Auscultation of breath sounds is part of the postanesthetic and postthoracic surgical assessment. Auscultation is used to estimate air flow through the tracheal-bronchial tree, to detect obstruction, and to assess the condition of surrounding lungs and the pleural space. Breath sounds should be auscultated bilaterally. Normal breath sounds are clear. Abnormal sounds may be superimposed over normal sounds.

Rales or crackles are heard when air moves through fluid-filled airways. Rales are noncontinuous, lessen with coughing, and are usually heard during inspiration. If the PACU nurse is unfamiliar with the sound of rales, rubbing hair between one's fingers next to the ear will produce the sound.

Rhonchi are low-pitched, continuous snoring sounds usually heard on expiration as air moves through narrow airways. Rhonchi may be heard in patients with bronchitis, emphysema, and congestive heart failure.

Wheezing is a high-pitched, continuous sound that may be heard throughout the respiratory cycle. Wheezing occurs as air moves through narrow airways. Wheezing may be heard in patients with asthma, bronchitis, and chronic obstructive pulmonary disease (COPD).

A friction rub may be heard as the visceral and parietal pleura rub together. Patients will usually complain of pain on inspiration. It is most clearly heard around the diaphragm. A friction rub may be heard in patients with pleurisy, tuberculosis, and pneumonia.

Nursing priorities for thoracic surgery patients. Three nursing priorities can be identified for the patient who is recovering from thoracic surgery. The first goal of the PACU nurse is to optimize respiratory function. The second goal is to assist the patient in liquefying and mobilizing secretions. The third goal of the PACU nurse is to promote ventilation of available lung tissue and to reexpand the lungs. Nursing interventions that may be used to assist the patient to an optimal level of functioning are identified in Table 5-2.

Table 5-2.   Nursing interventions for the thoracic surgery patient

Nursing action	Purpose
Deep breathing	Maintain patent airway
	Maximize ventilation
	Decrease pulmonary complications
Coughing	Maintain patent airway
	Mobilize secretions
	Prevent atelectasis
Turning	Maintain patent airway
	Maximize ventilation
	Decrease pooling of secretions
	Increase excursion
Suctioning	Remove secretions
	Increase oxygenation and ventilation
	Decrease pulmonary infection
Postural drainage	Maintain patent airway
	Increase drainage from lungs
Chest physical therapy	Loosen secretions
	Promote oxygenation
Intermittent positive pressure breathing (IPPB)	Maintain slow, deep inspiration
	Decrease work of breathing
	Increase lung expansion
	Mobilize secretions
Spirometry	Maintain slow, deep inspiration
	Prevent atelectasis
	Visual feedback of effort
Mechanical ventilation	Promote oxygenation/ventilation
	Decrease work of breathing
	Increase lung expansion

Cardiac surgical patients

Patients may be candidates for cardiac surgery for the correction of congenital anomalies (atrial or ventricular septal defect, transposition), for treatment of coronary artery disease (coronary artery bypass graft), to repair damage in a patient after myocardial infarction (pacemaker implant), or for treatment of valvular disease (valve replacement). Although each surgery has unique intraoperative concerns, postoperatively care priorities are similar, focusing on ventilation, perfusion, and the prevention of complications.

PACU assessment of cardiac surgical patients. Admission of the patient after cardiac surgery requires cooperation between nursing, anesthesia, and surgical personnel because several tasks of admission must be accomplished simultaneously. Airway and oxygenation needs require that the patient be placed on a ventilator. The patient will be anesthetized and paralyzed and will require ventilatory support for a number of hours after surgery, perhaps even overnight. Breath sounds should be auscultated bilaterally to ensure that the endotracheal tube has not become dislodged or has not slipped into the right mainstem bronchus during transport.

The patient should be attached to the ECG monitor, and an admission rate and rhythm should be obtained. It is important to obtain a baseline rhythm strip to include in the chart for comparison if dysrhythmias develop later in the postoperative period. The patient should also have arterial line monitoring connected and calibrated. A cuff pressure should be obtained for comparison. It may be difficult to obtain a cuff pressure if the patient is hypothermic or vasoconstricted. If the patient has a Swan-Ganz catheter in place, it too should be connected and calibrated, and baseline readings should be obtained.

The chest tube(s) (usually mediastinal, occasionally pleural) should be connected to suction immediately in case bleeding should start. The sternal dressing (and leg dressings if after bypass) should be inspected for bleeding.

After these initial tasks and observations have been completed, the PACU nurse should complete the admission assessment by palpating peripheral pulses to assess the patency of the vessels and the adequacy of cardiac output. Skin temperature should also be assessed by thermometer and palpation. Rewarming should be initiated if the patient is hypothermic ($<96°$ F or $36.5°$ C).

Urine output should also be assessed and monitored. It is not unusual to detect blood in the urine, because of lysis of red blood cells by the cardiopulmonary bypass pump. A large urine output, secondary to the administration of intraoperative diuretics, may alert the PACU nurse to the possible need for potassium supplementation.

Finally, the PACU nurse should obtain laboratory specimens for measurement of arterial blood gases, CBC, platelets, coagulation studies (PT/PTT), electrolytes, and cardiac enzymes. The PACU nurse should also arrange for the patient to have a 12-lead ECG and chest x-ray examination.

Nursing priorities for cardiac surgical patients. The overriding goal of the PACU nurse in providing care to the patient after cardiac surgery is maintaining adequate oxygen transport. Maintenance of adequate oxygen transport is dependent on pulmonary function, hemoglobin level, and cardiac output.

The PACU nurse should assess and maintain ventilation (pulmonary function). A number of variables may compromise pulmonary function, including a preoperative history of pulmonary dysfunction, and the intraoperative use of high-dose narcotics and muscle relaxants. Patients will often be ventilated overnight and will be extubated only after demonstration of adequate pulmonary function and neurologic awareness.

The PACU nurse should also assess and monitor the patient's hemoglobin level. Hemoglobin is required for oxygen transport. A fall in hemoglobin may occur because of hemorrhage, hemodilution, or lysis of red blood cells secondary to cardiopulmonary bypass. An evaluation of coagulation studies is mandatory. With significant postoperative bleeding, the cause may be loss of surgical integrity or alterations in coagulation. Chest tube output of greater than 50 to 75 ml after the first hour is cause for further evaluation.

Maintenance of oxygen transport is dependent on an adequate cardiac output. Maintenance of cardiac output is dependent on stroke volume and heart rate. Stroke volume is dependent on *preload, afterload,* and *contractility.* These three terms are defined in the box on the right.[36]

Heart rate changes include tachycardia and bradycardia, both of which can decrease cardiac output. Bradycardia may occur secondary to disruptions in the conduction system; it may be seen in patients recovering from valve surgery or in patients who have had an intraoperative myocardial infarction. Beta-blockers may also produce bradycardia. Tachycardia is caused by sympathetic stimulation, which may be caused by pain, anxiety, hypovolemia, and hyperthermia.

Maintenance of stroke volume is dependent on preload. Right ventricular preload is measured by central venous pressure (CVP). Left ventricular preload is measured by pulmonary capillary wedge pressure (PCWP). Preload may be decreased as a result of fluid shifts, PEEP, or tamponade. Clinically, the patient will have hypotension, tachycardia, oliguria, and decreased CVP and PCWP readings. Treatment is aimed at increasing the circulating volume.

The exception to this is cardiac tamponade. Clinical signs of hypotension, tachycardia, and oliguria will occur, but the CVP and PCWP will rise and will ultimately equal each other. Cardiac tamponade is caused by an accumulation of blood in the pericardium. As blood accumulates, the effectiveness of the myocardial pump declines. Treatment usually consists of a return to the operating room and reexploration for the cause of bleeding.

Increased preload may occur in cases of fluid overload. The patient will have elevated CVP and PCWP readings and, often, hypertension. Treatment involves fluid restriction to less than 100 ml per hour, diuretics, and electrolyte monitoring.

Afterload is measured by systemic vascular resistance (SVR), which is calculated as

$$\frac{\text{Mean Arterial Pressure} - \text{Central Venous Pressure}}{\text{Cardiac Output}} \times 80$$

In cases of increased SVR, the myocardium must empty against increased resistance, thereby increasing myocardial work. Hypertension is the most common cause of increased SVR; it may result from increased sympathetic tone, hypothermia, and baroreceptor response. Treatment will include rewarming and the use of vasodilators, including morphine, nitroglycerin, and sodium nitroprusside (Nipride).

Finally, treatment will be directed toward the development of any dysrhythmias. Dysrhythmias are usually transient; they may be caused by underlying disease, electrolyte imbalance, cardiac manipulation, hypoxemia, hypothermia, or acid-base disturbances. Treatment is directed toward the cause. If the dysrhythmia is life-threatening, cardiopulmonary resuscitation and advanced life support should be instituted. Treatment of life-threatening dysrhythmias is reviewed in Chapter 8.

Neurosurgical patients

Patients may require neurosurgical intervention to decrease intracranial pressure (ventroperitoneal shunt), to repair damage from trauma (evacuation of hematoma, burr hole), to remove intracranial growths (craniotomy), or to reconstruct congenital malfor-

___ **FACTORS AFFECTING STROKE VOLUME** ___

Preload:	The force that stretches the ventricle during diastole. The degree of stretch depends on the volume of blood filling the ventricle. The greater the ventricular volume, the greater the force of contraction required to empty the ventricle (Starling's law).
Afterload:	The degree of pressure opposing cardiac ejection; this pressure is imposed by vascular resistance, blood pressure, and blood viscosity.
Contractility:	The rate and force of cardiac ejection

mations (cranioplasty). Neurosurgical procedures may also involve the spinal cord (discectomy, removal of spinal cord tumor).

PACU assessment of neurosurgical patients. Although a neurologic assessment is part of the PACU admission assessment, the neurosurgical patient will require a more in-depth assessment of neurologic functioning. Ideally, a complete assessment will have been made preoperatively and documented in the patient's chart. The PACU nurse will then be able to compare postoperative findings with the preoperative baseline.

The neurologic assessment begins with an evaluation of the patient's level of consciousness. The anesthesia team will usually try to bring the patient to the PACU as awake as possible to allow for a more complete and accurate evaluation. The PACU nurse should first assess the patient's response to verbal stimuli, for example, by asking the patient to follow a command. The appropriateness of the response should be evaluated. If the patient does not respond to verbal stimuli, tactile stimulation should be tried. A sternal rub or pressure on the patient's fingernail-bed may cause the patient to respond. Again, is the response appropriate and purposeful? If not, is any change or posturing noted? Decorticate (flexion of arms across the chest) and decerebrate (extension of arms) posturing is a sign of neurologic deterioration.

Before determining true unresponsiveness, fluid and electrolyte balance should be checked, hypothermia corrected, anesthetics metabolized or reversed, and oxygenation adequacy confirmed (oximetry or blood gas).

A change in level of consciousness may raise suspicions of bleeding, hypoxia, and edema (increased intracranial pressure).

Vital signs should be obtained. Changes may be seen in pulse, blood pressure, and respirations because of neurologic influence. A slow, bounding pulse may be indicative of increased intracranial pressure. A rapid, thready pulse may be a late sign of decompensation. A widening pulse pressure may indicate increased intracranial pressure. Abnormally deep and slow patterns of respirations interspersed with periods of apnea (Cheyne-Stokes) usually indicate cerebral damage. Apneic or ataxic (irregular) breathing is seen with damage to the pons and medullary respiratory center.

The PACU nurse should also evaluate the patient's pupils for size, equality, and reaction to light. Pupil size may range from pinpoint to dilated. Use of a visual scale will aid in assessment (Fig. 5-7). Reactivity is rated as sluggish to brisk.

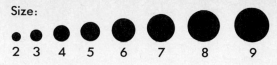

Size:

2 3 4 5 6 7 8 9

FIG. 5-7. Pupil sizes.

Sensorimotor functioning should also be assessed. The patient will be asked to smile, frown, and to stick out his or her tongue. Hand grasp and strength should be assessed, as should the patient's ability to dorsiflex and plantarflex the feet. Equality of the right and left sides should be evaluated.

Formal assessment of cranial nerve functioning may be part of the PACU assessment. Table 5-3 identifies the 12 cranial nerves and the tests for their assessment. Most PACU nurses do not perform a formal cranial nerve assessment, but instead incorporate many of the cranial nerve assessment tests into the routine PACU neurologic examination.

The PACU nurse should also evaluate and monitor the patient for signs of increased intracranial pressure, including restlessness, increasing systolic blood pressure, widening pulse pressure, bradycardia, and apneic or irregular breathing. The patient may also have an intracranial pressure monitor in place to detect early increases in pressure. The neurosurgeon should be notified immediately of any of these signs.

If seizure activity is noted, the PACU nurse should carefully observe the type of seizure. Focal seizures are localized areas of motor activity. Tonic-clonic or grand mal seizures are generalized convulsions. Respiratory adequacy should be assessed during and after the seizure. The patient should be protected from injury during seizure activity. Anticonvulsants (phenytoin [Dilantin]) may be ordered.

Nursing priorities for neurosurgical patients. The goal of the neurologic assessment is to provide an objective account of patient functioning. Each assessment is compared with the preoperative (baseline) assessment and the assessment immediately preceding the current one. Documentation should be kept up to the minute. Any acute changes should be immediately reported to the neurosurgeon.

Pain management is also a priority. The PACU nurse must be careful not to administer agents that cause sedation or that may cloud neurologic parameters. Narcotics such as morphine cause pupillary constriction, making assessment difficult. Codeine is the agent of choice because it is associated with minimal sedation, does not cause respiratory depression, and does not mask pupil signs.

Renal and urologic surgical patients.

Patients may be candidates for urologic or renal surgery to repair a congenital finding (hypospadius, epispadius, circumsion), to correct problems with voiding (cystoscopy, dilation, urethrotomy, prostactectomy), to correct problems that cause swelling in the urogenital area (hydrocelectomy, spermatocelectomy, torsion), or to correct problems that cause changes in urine concentration or output (transplant, cystostomy). Sur-

Table 5-3. **Cranial nerve assessment**

Cranial nerve	Function	Test for assessment
I Olfactory	Sensory	Ask patient to identify smell (e.g., alcohol on swab).
II Optic	Sensory	Hold up fingers, ask patient to count. Assess vision in each eye.
III Oculomotor	Motor	Check pupil constriction to light.
IV Trochlear	Motor	Assess patient's ability to look downward and inward.
V Trigeminal	Sensory	Assess facial response to touch.
	Motor	Assess patient's ability to clench jaw.
VI Abducens	Motor	Assess lateral deviation of eye.
VII Facial	Sensory	Check taste on anterior two thirds of tongue.
	Motor	Assess patient's ability to smile, frown, and elevate eyebrows.
VIII Acoustic	Sensory	Whisper sentence into patient's ear. Ask patient to repeat sentence. Assess both ears.
IX Glossopharyngeal	Sensory	Check taste on posterior tongue.
	Motor	Ask patient to swallow. Check gag reflex.
X Vagus	Sensory	Ask patient to speak.
	Motor	Ask patient to swallow.
XI Spinal accessory	Motor	Ask patient to shrug his shoulders against resistance.
XII Hypoglossal	Motor	Ask patient to stick out his tongue.

gery may also be indicated in cases of urologic trauma, which are caused by either injury or the presence of a foreign body.

PACU assessment of genitourinary patients. Inspection will be the first physical assessment skill used to evaluate the patient who has experienced renal and urologic surgery. On admission, the surgical site (or dressing) will be inspected, with notation of the type and location of dressings, presence of drains, and presence and type of drainage.

The dressing may be abdominal, suprapubic, or lateral. If the surgery was transurethral, as with a cystoscopy or prostatectomy, no dressing will be present. The meatus should be inspected for bleeding. A suprapubic, ureteral, or urethral (bladder) catheter may be placed. Catheters are designed to collect urine and wound drainage and to allow for monitoring of output. They may also be placed to provide traction at the surgical site, to decrease bleeding, and to promote healing. The color and amount of drainage should be noted. If the drain is part of an irrigation system, as it is for prostatectomy patients, the PACU nurse should verify the solution and rate of infusion and maintain accurate output records, separating urine from irrigation output. The output catheters should be assessed for patency.

Palpation may be used to assess bladder distention. The catheter may be palpated to dislodge clots and to maintain catheter patency.

Percussion and auscultation are not used in the surgical assessment of the renal and urologic patient.

Nursing priorities for renal and urologic surgical patients. The PACU nurse should make patency of the output system the first postoperative priority. Catheters should be assessed for patency. Output (drainage) should be assessed for color and consistency. If an irrigation system is part of the drainage system, flow should be monitored and maintained. Internal irrigation may contribute to hypothermia. Temperature monitoring and rewarming, as necessary, is important. Irrigation may also contribute to hyponatremia. Postoperative electrolyte levels should be obtained. Maintenance of intake and output is essential. If the patient has no catheter, any attempts to void should be noted. Most ambulatory surgical patients will be required to void prior to discharge.

Ice packs may be ordered to decrease swelling. Likewise, after procedures like hydrocelectomy, varicocelectomy, or spermatocelectomy, a scrotal support may be ordered to prevent edema and to decrease discomfort.

Nurses should recognize that patients may experience embarrassment from the procedure and the continued assessment required postoperatively. Care should be provided professionally and directly. If the patient asks specific questions, answers should be provided.

Peripheral vascular surgical patients

Patients may be scheduled for peripheral vascular surgery to increase perfusion to an extremity or organ (endarterectomy) or to circumvent abnormalities in a blood vessel (aneurysm repair, bypass, vein stripping). PACU assessments and care must be directed toward the maintenance of vascular patency and perfusion.

PACU assessment of vascular surgical patients. The overall goal of the PACU nurse in caring for the peripheral vascular surgical patient is maintenance and ongoing assessment of circulatory integrity and perfusion. Assessments must be made at regular intervals and documented. The assessment must be compared with the baseline (preoperative) assessment and with previous postoperative assessments.

The vascular assessment begins with observation of the surgical dressing, any drains, and any drainage. Any sign of bleeding should be evaluated and documented. Skin color is also visually assessed. Skin color may be described as pink or ruddy (a sign of venous congestion) or as mottled, dusky, or pale (signs of inadequate perfusion).

Palpation is perhaps the most useful skill in the assessment of the peripheral vascular surgical patient. Skin should be palpated to assess temperature. Cool or cold extremities or digits (fingers and toes) are a sign of circulatory compromise. Warm extremities are a sign of good perfusion.

Capillary refill of the affected extremity should be assessed and compared with that of the unaffected extremity. Capillary refill should be brisk and equal to that of the unaffected extremity.

Pulses should also be palpated for their presence and quality. The location of the peripheral pulses is shown in Fig. 5-8. To aid in future assessments, the location of the pulse may be marked with a magic marker. Pulses distal to the operative site should be assessed, and their presence or absence should be noted. If a pulse is absent, the vascular surgeon should be notified immediately. The quality of the pulses should also be described. Words such as *weak, normal quality,* and *bounding* may be used.

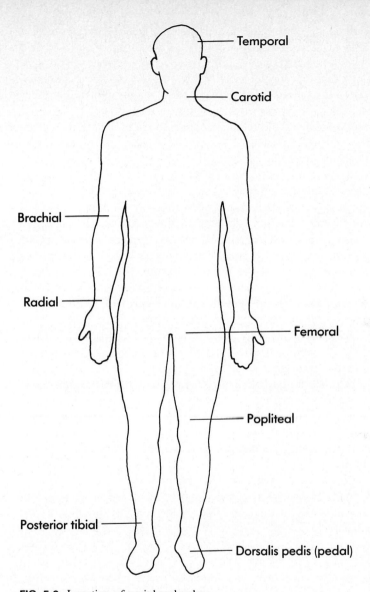

FIG. 5-8. Location of peripheral pulses.

If the peripheral pulses distal to the operative site cannot be palpated, a Doppler monitor should be used to auscultate pulse flow. Once again, if located, the site should be marked with a magic marker to facilitate ongoing evaluation. If distal pulses are not found with palpation or Doppler monitor, the surgeon should be notified immediately.

The PACU nurse should also ask the patient about pain in the affected extremity. Pain is an indicator of possible circulatory impairment.

If the surgery involved the cerebral circulation (as in a carotid endarterectomy), it is important for the PACU nurse to also assess neurologic function (see the discussion titled *Neurosurgical Patients*).

Vital signs should be monitored in all vascular surgical patients. Hypertension in the carotid endarterectomy patient may cause hemorrhage, hematoma formation, or edema and may compromise the surgical suture line integrity. Pharmacologic intervention (hydralazine, sodium nitroprusside, labetalol) may be ordered. Hypotension may be problematic in the peripheral vascular surgical patient. Hypotension compromises blood flow through the graft and bypassed artery, making it difficult to palpate pulses. Perfusion will also be compromised. The treatment will usually be intravenous fluids, and it may include use of colloids, such as hetastarch, to increase intravascular volume.

Nursing priorities for peripheral vascular surgical patients. The goal of the PACU nurse caring for the peripheral vascular surgical patient is to promote circulatory integrity and perfusion. Circulatory assessments must be made at regular intervals, and the surgeon must be notified immediately of any changes in pulses, skin color, skin temperature, or vital signs.

Postoperative bleeding should be evaluated carefully. Hematoma formation may compromise vascular integrity, or, as with the carotid endarterectomy patient, it may compromise airway patency. Excessive bleeding may indicate loss of vascular integrity along a suture line, requiring return to the operating room, or it may indicate alterations in coagulation, secondary to intraoperative anticoagulation with heparin. The PACU nurse should obtain a coagulation profile (prothrombin time and partial thromboplastin time). Alterations may be treated with protamine sulfate.

If the patient is recovering from carotid endarterectomy, neurologic functioning should also be evaluated and documented. Acute changes should be reported to the surgeon immediately.

Orthopedic surgical patients

Patients may be candidates for orthopedic surgery for the correction of trauma or injury (fixation), for diagnosis of injury (arthroscopy), for removal or replacement of bone destroyed by disease or trauma (arthroplasty), or for repair of structural defects (laminectomy). Surgery may also be indicated to realign structures (osteotomy, spinal fusion, rod placement) or to remove dysfunctional or diseased structures that cause pain or restrict mobility (amputation, disarticulation).

PACU assessment of orthopedic surgical patients. Inspection is the first skill used in the assessment of the orthopedic surgical patient. The site of surgery should be assessed for the type of dressing, presence of drains and/or drainage, and extremity status.

Whether the extremity is casted or ace-wrapped, the digits (fingers or toes) should be assessed for color, capillary refill, sensation, and mobility. Pale skin color may reflect arterial insufficiency. The operative side should be compared with the unaffected side. Capillary refill is assessed by the nurse depressing the patient's fingernail or toenail until blanching occurs. The nail is then released, and the speed of color refill is observed. Refill should occur in less than 3 seconds. The operative extremity should be compared with the unaffected extremity. If capillary refill is sluggish, peripheral pulses, if accessible, should be palpated. Skin temperature should also be assessed, and the temperature of the operative side should be compared with that of the unaffected side. An abnormally cool extremity should be reported to the surgeon. Pain may also be a sign of circulatory inadequacy. The surgeon should be notified immediately if circulatory inadequacy is suspected.

Deficits in sensation or mobility should raise concern about the possibility of nerve damage. Nerve function tests commonly used to assess the postoperative orthopedic patient are described in the box below. If the patient is unable to respond to sensory testing or to perform the motor function tests, the PACU nurse should notify the surgeon immediately.

Nursing priorities for orthopedic surgical patients. Of primary importance is the need to maintain surgical and anatomic alignment. Casts may be used to immobilize an extremity and promote healing. Traction may be used to maintain positioning and promote healing.

Depending on the procedure, some position changes should be avoided. For example, adduction, external rotation, and acute hip flexion are contraindicated in the patient recovering from hip arthroplasty. Adduction and external rotation are contraindicated in

---

TESTS OF NERVE FUNCTION

Radial

Sensory: Pinch web space between thumb and index finger.
Motor: Hyperextend thumb or wrist.

Median

Sensory: Pinch distal surface of index finger.
Motor: Oppose thumb and little finger; flex wrist.

Ulnar

Sensory: Pinch distal end of little finger.
Motor: Abduct all fingers.

Perineal

Sensory: Pinch lateral surface of great toe and medial surface of second toe.
Motor: Dorsiflex ankles; extend toes.

Tibial

Sensory: Pinch medial and lateral surfaces of sole of foot.
Motor: Plantarflex ankles; flex toes.

the patient after total knee arthroplasty. The PACU nurse should also maintain positioning. The surgeon may order a postoperative x-ray examination to confirm alignment or prosthetic placement.

The surgeon may order elevation of the extremity to minimize or prevent swelling. If the extremity is casted, pillows or blankets should be used to avoid placing hard surfaces against a wet cast. The extremity should be elevated above the level of the heart. If the arm is casted, the placement of a sling will facilitate elevation of the extremity. The sling can be attached to an IV pole and secured. Ice packs may also be ordered to decrease swelling and pain.

Ongoing monitoring of extremity color, capillary refill, sensation, and mobility should continue throughout the patient's PACU stay. A final assessment should be made before discharge from the unit. All assessments should be documented; any deviations should be reported immediately to the surgeon.

The dressings should be assessed for drainage. "Bleed-throughs" on casts should be circled and timed. Drainage in Hemovacs or other wound drainage systems should be noted and recorded. If an autotransfusion device has been placed (Solcotrans), the patient should be autotransfused when drainage exceeds specified parameters (usually 400 ml in 4 hours or less).

Although compartment syndrome is an uncommon problem in postoperative patients, it is important that PACU nurses be aware of the potential for patients to develop it. Compartment syndrome develops when pressure in a fascial compartment increases and venous return is occluded. Subsequently, although pulses may be present, perfusion is interrupted. Muscle and nerve ischemia ensues, and, if untreated, progesses to necrosis.

Compartment syndrome can occur in any of the fascial compartments of the limbs. In the upper extremity, it occurs most commonly in the anterior (flexor) compartment of the forearm. In the lower extremity, it is most common in the anterior and deep posterior compartments.

The patient may have extreme pain during stretch of the involved compartment or pain that is not responsive to analgesics. Classically, the diagnosis is based on five "Ps": pain, paresthesias, pallor, paralysis, and pulselessness. The PACU nurse should remember, however, that pulselessness is an extremely poor prognostic sign and is indicative of severe compromise.

Treatment of compartment syndrome involves prompt recognition of symptoms. Nonsurgical intervention may include cast removal or splitting of the cast. Surgical intervention will be decompression via a fasciotomy.

Gastrointestinal surgical patients

Patients scheduled for gastrointestinal surgery may be undergoing diagnostic procedures (biopsy, endoscopy) or procedures to correct pathophysiologic conditions, including obstruction, ulceration, herniation, perforation, and inflammation. Surgery may also be necessary to correct congenital malformations (tracheal-esophageal fistula, imperforate anus, pyloric stenosis). Surgery may involve the esophagus, stomach, biliary, or hepatic system, the small and large intestines, and the rectum or anus.

PACU assessment of gastrointestinal surgical patients. Inspection will be the first physical assessment skill used to evaluate the patient who has undergone gastrointestinal surgery. The surgical site dressing will be evaluated for location, type, presence of drains, drainage, and bleeding. Drains may be placed to self-suction (Hemovac drains, Jackson-Pratt drains), to wall-suction (nasogastric drain, Davol drain), or to a dressing (Penrose drain). Occasionally an abdominal drain may include an irrigation port for fluid irrigations.

Palpation may be used to assess abdominal distention. It is also used to maintain drain patency. Percussion is used to assess abdominal or gastric distention. Auscultation may be used to confirm placement of the nasogastric tube.

Nursing priorities for gastrointestinal surgical patients. Most patients who have undergone gastrointestinal surgical procedures will have a nasogastric (NG) tube in place. The NG tube is designed to provide gastric decompression. The PACU nurse should place the NG tube to low intermittent suction. Proper functioning of the tube will prevent reflux, nausea and vomiting, and abdominal distention. The PACU nurse should check with the surgeon prior to irrigating or repositioning the NG tube. The NG tube may be placed in close proximity to an anastomosis. Repositioning of the tube could cause perforation or disruption of surgical integrity.

It is also important to maintain NPO status. Good mouth care should be given. The PACU nurse should check with the surgeon before giving the patient ice chips.

The PACU nurse should evaluate respiratory adequacy. Large abdominal incisions are painful. In addition, the incision may be in close proximity to the diaphragm. The patient may hypoventilate secondary to pain. Hypoventilation can predispose the patient to atelectasis and pneumonia. Pain management is important. Intravenous narcotics may be used, or paravertebral nerve blocks (such as the intercostal nerve block) may be used to decrease splinting and promote ventilation. Local anesthetics may be injected along incision lines.

To prevent thrombus formation and the development of pulmonary embolism, antiembolism stockings (TED hose) or sequential compression devices may be ordered. Encouraging the patient to perform active range of motion exercises will promote venous return. Subcutaneous heparin will further decrease the risk of venous stasis.

Fluid status should be evaluated. Loss of intravascular volume ("third-spacing") is not usually seen until the second or third postoperative day. Accurate intake and output records are important.

Obstetric surgical patients

The pregnant woman who requires surgery may fall into one of three categories: nonobstetric surgery during pregnancy, surgery for delivery, or surgery for the termination of pregnancy. Even though pregnancy and the physiologic changes that accompany it are common factors, each type of patient has different postsurgical needs.

Operative concerns for the parturient. The management of the obstetric patient includes assuring maternal safety, preventing preterm labor, preventing fetal asphyxia, and avoidance of the administration of harmful drugs.[35,41] Knowledge of the physiologic changes that occur in pregnancy is vital to the medical team administering care to the patient.

The many physiologic changes that occur in pregnancy are identified in the box on the right. The major organ systems affected are respiratory, cardiovascular, and gastrointestinal. Knowledge of the changes in these systems has implications for the anesthetic management of these patients.

The pregnant woman has a marked increase in her metabolic demand. Alveolar ventilation is increased to meet this demand for oxygen by increases in both tidal volume and respiratory rate. The enlarging uterus elevates the diaphragm, thus decreasing the functional residual capacity. The results of these respiratory changes are that induction and emergence from anesthesia is rapid and that the pregnant patient will become hypoxic sooner than the nonpregnant patient.

Blood volume and cardiac output are also increased to meet increased metabolic demands. Maintenance of cardiac output is essential for maternal stability and for preventing fetal distress. The parturient may become hypotensive if she is placed in a supine position, where the uterus and pregnancy obstructs the vena cava and aorta (supine hypotensive syndrome). The patient should be positioned in a left lateral tilt to displace the uterus and prevent vena caval occlusion.

The pregnant patient is considered at risk for aspiration because of increased gastric acidity, increased esophageal reflux, and delayed gastric emptying. The airway must be protected for surgical procedures.

Intrauterine fetal distress is avoided by the maintenance of maternal oxygenation and cardiac output. Fetal oxygenation is dependent on maternal oxygenation. Continuous fetal heart rate monitoring will provide an indication of compromised fetal oxygenation.

Prevention of preterm labor is also important. The cause of preterm labor may be associated with surgical manipulation or with anesthetic agents. Intraabdominal procedures requiring uterine manipulation or retraction have been cited as a cause of preterm labor. Although no study has found any particular anesthetic agent or technique to increase the incidence of preterm labor, agents such as ketamine and anticholinesterase agents such as neostigmine and edrophonium do increase uterine tone, which may induce preterm labor. Uterine activity should be monitored intraoperatively with an external tocodynamometer to detect the onset of uterine activity.

Avoidance of harmful drugs in pregnancy is also a priority. To produce a defect, a teratogenic drug must be given in an appropriate dosage, during a particular developmental stage of the embryo, in a species of individual with a particular genetic susceptibility.[35] Almost all anesthetics are harmful (teratogenic) in some animal species. The generalizability of these studies to the human embryo has not been determined.

PACU assessment of obstetric patients. The obstetric patient may be admitted to the PACU after delivery (caesarean section), after nonobstetric surgery, and after termination of pregnancy (abortion). Because of the surgical outcome and the differences in

___ **PHYSIOLOGIC ALTERATIONS IN PREGNANCY** ___

Respiratory system

40% increase in tidal volume
15% increase in respiratory rate
20% increase in oxygen consumption
30% decrease in compliance
35% decrease in resistance

Cardiovascular system

35% increase in blood volume
40% increase in cardiac output
30% increase in stroke volume
15% increase in heart rate
15% decrease in peripheral vascular resistance

Central nervous system

40% decrease in anesthetic requirement (MAC)
40% reduction in local anesthetic requirement for spinal anesthesia
Increased neurosensitivity to local anesthetics

Gastrointestinal system

Incompetence of gastroesophageal reflex
Delayed gastric emptying
Decreased gastric pH

Renal system

Progressive increase in glomerular filtration rate (up to 50%)
Increased renal blood flow

the degree of fetal dependency (total to none), assessment parameters will differ for each type of admission.

Assessment of patients after caesarean section. During the first 2 hours after delivery, the mother will begin the return (physiologically) to the nonpregnant state. Aggressive nursing care and attention to detail can help to prevent postdelivery complications. Assessment begins immediately on arrival to the PACU. Baseline vital signs should be obtained.

Assessment of bleeding is also a priority. The PACU nurse should palpate the fundus of the uterus to note consistency and position. Immediately after delivery, the fundus is located approximately 2 cm below the umbilicus. The uterus should be firm to palpation. Bleeding secondary to uterine atony will require uterine massage, and, if unsuccessful, administration of oxytocin to stimulate uterine contraction.

Almost all patients recovering from a caesarean section will have an indwelling urinary catheter. The drainage color should be monitored. If the urine turns bloody, a bladder perforation should be suspected, and the obstetrician should be notified.

Hemorrhage after delivery is characterized by a blood loss of 500 ml or more. It is a serious complication after delivery, and it is associated with an increase in maternal morbidity. If uterine atony is discovered, the obstetrician should be notified immediately, and uterine massage should be instituted.

The PACU nurse should also note the presence of lochia. Lochia is the vaginal discharge, consisting of blood, tissue, and mucous, that appears after childbirth. Immediately after delivery, lochia rubra (distinctly bloody vaginal flow) is noted. Flow should be moderate. Lochia rubra will last an average of 3 days after delivery. A flow rate of greater than 100 ml (evidenced by a saturated perineal pad) is considered excessive and should be monitored at frequent intervals. The PACU nurse should also check under the woman's buttocks for bleeding, as vaginal bleeding may pool in a distended vagina and flow downward.

Incision pain and the incisional dressing should also be assessed. Uterine contractions may also contribute to postoperative pain. Analgesic therapy may be indicated.

Ongoing monitoring of vital signs and assessment for bleeding will continue for an average of 2 hours. If the woman remains stable, she is then returned to her postdelivery room.

Assessment of the pregnant patient who has undergone nonobstetric surgery. Obviously, assessment of the patient who has nonobstetric surgery will depend on the type of surgery performed. However, because the woman is still pregnant, postoperative assessment criteria will be directed toward the mother and the fetus.

To continue with intraoperative priorities, the PACU nurse will work to maintain maternal stability and to prevent fetal distress and preterm labor. Maternal monitoring of ECG, blood pressure, and pulse oximetry is imperative. Oxygen therapy will be instituted to prevent maternal hypoxemia.

Maintenance of cardiac output is important. To prevent supine hypotension, the patient should be positioned in the left lateral tilt position. Fetal heart tones should be monitored continuously if possible. The normal fetal heart rate is 120 to 160 beats per minute. Fetal bradycardia should cause the PACU nurse to immediately assess maternal oxygenation and to notify the obstetrician.

Uterine contraction monitoring should also be continued in the PACU using a tocodynometer. Any evidence of uterine contraction should be reported to the obstetrician.

It is important to protect the mother and fetus from x-rays in the PACU. Lead aprons may be used to shield the patient from the x-ray, or the patient may be moved to a more distant part of the PACU for x-ray shooting.

Assessment of the patient recovering from abortion. Normally, surgery designed to terminate a pregnancy occurs within the first trimester. The women admitted to the PACU will demonstrate many of the physiologic changes associated with pregnancy, but without the intensity or severity of those that occur in the second and third trimesters.

Vital signs should be obtained. The PACU nurse should also monitor for bleeding. Uterine tone and vaginal discharge should be assessed. A perineal pad should be placed. To encourage uterine contraction and to decrease bleeding, intravenous oxytocin (Pitocin) may be administered.

The PACU nurse should also check the chart for maternal blood type. If the mother is Rh-negative and the father is Rh-positive, RhoGAM must be administered. RhoGAM is designed to prevent Rh isoimmunization by preventing the formation of maternal antibodies to the Rh-positive factor.

Nursing priorities for the obstetric patient. Nursing priorities for the obstetric patient mimic the anesthetic priorities: maintenance of maternal stability, prevention of fetal distress, and prevention of preterm labor. Ongoing maternal assessment is mandatory. If the woman is still pregnant in the PACU (after nonobstetric surgery), fetal monitoring is also mandatory.

In addition to physiologic monitoring, the PACU nurse will probably need to attend to psychosocial needs. After delivery, the mother may wish to be with her baby and the baby's father. Ideally this should be facilitated, unless it is precluded by maternal instability. Patients who have undergone nonobstetric surgery may have high anxiety levels because of concern for their babies. A patient who has undergone a termination of pregnancy may have emotions ranging from relief, to guilt, to concern about the future. The PACU nurse should remain supportive, empathic, and nonjudgmental.

Gynecologic surgical patients

Patients scheduled for gynecologic surgery may undergo diagnostic procedures (laparoscopy, laparotomy, biopsy), procedures to remove growths or organs (oophorectomy, salpingectomy, hysterectomy, vulvectomy), or procedures to correct anatomic deviations (hymenectomy, Marshall-Marchetti operation, tuboplasty). Surgery may also be scheduled to terminate or prevent pregnancy (tubal ligation, dilation and curettage).

PACU assessment of gynecologic surgical patients. Inspection will be the first skill used to assess the patient who is recovering from gynecologic surgery. The surgical site should be inspected, and the condition of dressings should be noted. A diagnostic laparoscopy patient may have only two lower abdominal Bandaids. An abdominal hysterectomy patient may have a large suprapubic dressing. The presence of drains (Hemovac drains or Jackson-Pratt drains) should be noted; and an assessment of the type and quantity of output should be made. Drains are used to facilitate wound drainage and to decrease swelling. A urinary catheter may be placed to promote bladder emptying. The color of output should be noted. Occasionally the Foley catheter may contain blue dye (methylene blue). Methylene blue dye is injected into the bladder intraoperatively to observe for any movement of the dye into the uterus. If dye is found in the uterus, a perforation should be suspected.

Nursing priorities for gynecologic surgical patients. Wound care and assessment of drainage will be a priority for the patient who is recovering from gynecologic surgery. The PACU nurse should evaluate and document evidence of bleeding.

If the incision is abdominal, pain may interfere with respiratory adequacy. Hypoventilation may occur secondary to splinting. Pain management is important. Elevation of the head of the patient's bed will promote respiratory excursion. High-humidity oxygen will promote gas exchange.

Antiembolism stockings (TED hose) or sequential compression devices (SCD) may be ordered to decrease venous stasis and to reduce the incidence of pulmonary embolism, which may occur secondary to immobility. Subcutaneous heparin may also be ordered to decrease venous stasis and to promote anticoagulation.

Plastic surgery patients

Patients may have plastic surgery to reconstruct a congenital or acquired abnormality or for cosmetic reasons to enhance appearance. Surgery may be to skin (grafts, flaps, dermabrasion, z-plasty), to the face (blepharoplasty, rhytidectomy, rhinoplasty, mentoplasty, cleft lip, cleft palate), to the thorax (reduction or augmentation mammoplasty), or to the abdomen (abdominoplasty, liposuction). Despite the anatomic variations, PACU care has some clear similarities for any patient recovering from plastic surgery.

PACU assessment of plastic surgical patients. If the surgery involves or has the potential to involve or threaten the airway (as with a rhinoplasty, cleft lip or palate repair), the PACU nurse must first assess the patient for airway patency and adequacy. Breath sounds should be auscultated bilaterally. High-humidity oxygen should be applied, especially in patients who are mouth-breathers. Suction equipment should be available at the bedside.

The surgical site should be assessed for the presence of drains, drainage, or edema. The dressing should be intact, and any drainage should be noted. Drains should be patent and should be placed to self-suction or to wall-suction. Admission findings should be documented. If changes occur later in the postoperative period, baseline data can be used for comparison.

Nursing priorities for plastic surgical patients. Maintenance of a patent airway and oxygenation will be a priority in any patient undergoing surgery in or around the airway. The PACU nurse should continually monitor respiratory effort and adequacy. Airway protection equipment (airways, suction, Ambu-bag) should be immediately available.

A major nursing priority should mirror the surgeon's priority: promotion of wound healing without infection or inflammation. Ice or iced saline pads may be placed to decrease swelling and to keep suture lines free of coagulated blood and serum. Positioning the head of the patient's bed upward promotes drainage of secretions and decreases swelling after facial procedures. If a graft was performed on an extremity, the extremity is usually elevated to decrease swelling.

To prevent wound infection, the PACU nurse should use good handwashing techniques before touching dressings, suture lines, and saline pads. Infection can compromise healing and cause disfigurement.

Ophthalmic surgical patients

Patients scheduled for ophthalmic surgery may be undergoing procedures to correct congenital abnormalities (strabismus repair, ptosis repair, lacrimal duct probing), to repair damage (scleral buckle, retinal detachment), to correct pathophysiologic conditions (enucleation, iridectomy, keratoplasty), or for cosmetic reconstruction (blepharoplasty). Surgeries may be scheduled for the pediatric, adult, or geriatric patient.

PACU assessment of ophthalmic surgical patients. Assessment of the patient who has undergone ophthalmic surgery is rooted in skills of inspection. On admission to the PACU, the patient will usually wear an eye patch, covered with a metal or rigid plastic shield. The PACU nurse should confirm that the dressing is secure. Care should be taken not to dislodge the dressing when applying the oxygen mask or when repositioning the patient.

Nursing priorities for ophthalmic surgical patients. The goals of nursing care for ophthalmic surgical patients include ongoing evaluation and prevention of the postoperative problems of coughing, nausea, and vomiting.

It is important for the patient to avoid coughing and/or bucking against the endotracheal tube. Ideally, the patient will be extubated in the operating room. During surgery, many patients will be given intravenous sedation, rather than general anesthesia, which necessitates intubation. Coughing may increase intraocular pressure and may disrupt the integrity of the suture line.

Vomiting may also increase intraocular pressure and threaten surgical integrity. If the patient complains of nausea, the PACU nurse should obtain an order for and should promptly administer an antiemetic.

Dressing care has already been addressed. However, the effects of decreased vision secondary to the surgery and the eye patch must be considered. Visual impairment may contribute to disorientation and postoperative agitation. The patient may have an increased level of anxiety or fear of injury, potential or actual. Gentle reorientation will assist the patient in regaining awareness and maintaining a personal sense of well-being.

There will be times when it becomes important for the PACU nurse to maintain patient positioning. Patients who have undergone cataract surgery may assume a position of comfort and choice. Patients who have undergone a scleral buckle, vitrectomy, or retinal surgery will have their position specified by the surgeon. For this type of surgery, the surgeon will often inject air or an expandable gas behind the retina. The patient will be positioned so that the air, when it rises, will hold the retina against the choroid (blood supply). Patients may even arrive in the PACU face down.

Moderate to mild discomfort is expected and may be treated with analgesics. Severe eye pain may be indicative of increased intraocular pressure and/or hemorrhage. The ophthalmologist should be notified immediately.

Ear, nose, and throat surgical patients

Indications for ear, nose, and throat (ENT) surgery include the need to remove diseased or damaged tissue (radical neck dissection, tonsillectomy), the need to promote healing by decreasing or removing infection (myringotomy, nasal antral window), reconstruction (submucous resection, tympanoplasty), and the need to maximize the airway (tracheal dilation, tracheostomy). Despite the fact that surgery may involve three anatomically distinct areas, all surgeries are performed in or through the patient's airway. As a result, nursing interventions and assessment parameters will be similar.

PACU assessment of ear, nose, and throat patients. Immediately on admission to the PACU, the patient's airway should be assessed. The presence of a patent airway should be confirmed by the presence or absence of an artificial airway, auscultation of bilateral breath sounds, evaluation of respiratory rate and effort, and oxygen saturation (pulse oximetry). Vital signs should be obtained, and oxygen therapy should be instituted.

The secondary priority should be assessment of the operative site. The presence or absence of a dressing should be noted. If a suture line is visible, it should be intact. The surgical site should be assessed for drainage and the presence of drains and packing. Any swelling or discoloration should also be noted. Careful, accurate documentation of the admission assessment is important, because baseline data may be needed for comparison if problems develop later in the postoperative period.

Nursing priorities for ear, nose, and throat patients. The first priority in caring for the patient who is recovering from ENT surgery is maintenance of the airway. The airway may be threatened as a result of edema, laryngospasm, or bleeding. Ideally, maintenance of the airway stems from a preventative approach rather than a treatment approach.

If the patient has no artificial airway in place (as will most likely be the case with ear and nasal surgery), maintenance of the airway is achieved through positioning and ongoing assessment of respiratory adequacy. Usually the patient will be maintained in a semi-Fowler's position (head of the bed elevated). This position minimizes eustachian tube edema (especially after mastoid procedures), decreases nasal swelling, and promotes sinus drainage. In addition, the semi-Fowler's position promotes respiratory excursion.

Assessment of respiratory adequacy requires ongoing observation for signs and symptoms of airway obstruction. Signs and symptoms of obstruction include snoring, increased respiratory effort, absent breath sounds, and decreasing oxygen saturation. If the PACU nurse suspects obstruction, interventions include repositioning the patient, stimulating the patient to take deep breaths, and opening the patient's airway by a jaw thrust on the mandible, chin lift, or placement of an artificial airway.

If the patient has an artificial airway in place (including endotracheal tubes, tracheostomy tubes, or nasal airways), placement of the airway should be confirmed by repeated ausculation of breath sounds. A chest x-ray examination may be performed to confirm positioning of the endotracheal tube.

It is important for the PACU nurse to also evaluate the need for additional airway safety equipment at the bedside. If the patient has a new tracheostomy, a spare tracheal airway is usually kept at the bedside. If the patient's jaws are wired shut, as may be the case in a fracture repair, a wire cutter should be at the bedside. Reintubation equipment and a tracheostomy set should be readily available.

Oxygen therapy is also a priority. Because tracheal or mouth breathing replaces nasal breathing after ENT surgery, the oxygen should be humidified. Monitoring of oxygen saturation (pulse oximetry) is recommended.

Management of bleeding and secretions is also a priority. Tissue in the airway is extremely vascular, and as a result, bleeding may become a problem postoperatively. If wound drainage devices are in place (Hemovac or Jackson-Pratt drains), their patency should be evaluated and the adequacy of suction maintained. If the wound has packing in place, as is common after nasal surgery, some bleeding is to be expected because the packing acts as a wick to remove blood from the operative site. The cover dressings may need to be changed or reinforced. The packing should be left in place.

If the patient is bleeding into the mouth or oropharynx, suctioning may be required. Suctioning should be done gently with a soft, flexible catheter. If the tracheostomy or endotracheal tube needs to be suctioned, sterile technique must be maintained to prevent infection.

Secretions may also be problematic after surgery. Normally, 20 to 50 ml of saliva per hour is produced. However, irritation of the oral mucosa may cause an increase to 200 ml per hour. Again, if the patient is unable to clear the secretions independently, gentle suctioning may be required.

Postoperative edema may occur as a result of surgical manipulation and bleeding. Edema may threaten the patient's airway. To prevent edema formation, ice packs will be ordered for up to 48 hours postoperatively. Steroids may be ordered to decrease inflammation. Steroids are commonly ordered for patients recovering from tonsillectomy, radical neck dissection, or maxillary fracture repair (Le Fort procedures). Voice rest may be ordered to decrease vocal cord irritation.

The surgeon should be notified in the event of airway compromise, excessive bleeding, secretion, or edema.

An additional postoperative priority is prevention and treatment of nausea and vomiting. Nausea and vomiting may occur because of changes in equilibrium (common after middle ear surgery) or because of swallowed blood, intolerance of anesthetic agents, pain, or hypoxia. Prevention of nausea and vomiting increases patient comfort and promotes patient safety by decreasing the risk of aspiration. Nothing should be administered by mouth until the gag and swallow reflex are confirmed and an order is given to provide fluids. Many patients will be kept NPO for a specified period of time postoperatively.

Finally, the PACU nurse should also attend to patient needs for communication. If on voice rest or if a tracheostomy tube or endotracheal tube is in place, the patient should be provided with a means to communicate. A pencil and paper will facilitate communication. A picture board with words and pictures for common patient needs — such as pain, bathroom, family, need to turn — may also be used. Intubated patients and any patient who is unable to communicate may be extremely anxious. By providing explanations and a means to communicate and by frequent questioning about needs, the nurse will do much to promote psychologic comfort for the ENT patient.

ASSESSMENT FOR DISCHARGE

Before discharging the patient from the PACU, the PACU nurse should complete a discharge assessment. If the PACU care plan is used as an organizing framework, recovery from anesthesia can be assessed and documented.

Respiratory ventilation and perfusion is evaluated by the presence of a patent, unassisted airway, clear bilateral breath sounds, an appropriate respiratory rate for age, and the achievement of the PACU's pulse oximetry saturation criteria (usually greater than 95%).

Cardiac stability should be present as evidenced by a stable cardiac rate and rhythm and a stable blood pressure. Comparison with preoperative ECGs and blood pressures may be useful in determining acceptable discharge parameters.

The patient should have a body temperature of at least 96° F or 36.5° C before discharge. All active rewarming should be discontinued.

The patient's neurologic status should be assessed. Although the patient may not be alert, he or she should respond to name, be appropriate in response, and be able to follow commands. Movement of extremities should be assessed and documented. If the patient is going to be discharged with a spinal blockade in place, the sensory level should be assessed and documented.

The degree of postoperative pain should also be assessed. Ideally, the patient will be as pain-free as physiologic stability allows. If the patient is to be discharged with an epidural infusion or with patient-controlled analgesia, the systems should be implemented.

The PACU nurse should also assess surgical stability. The patient should have immediate postoperative needs taken care of (x-ray, traction, blood transfusion, laboratory tests) before discharge. The patient should be free of complications expected for the type of surgery performed. The surgical discharge assessment should be documented.

The PACU nurse should review the postanesthetic and postoperative orders prior to discharge. Evaluation of documentation also includes the presence of a signature from the anesthesiologist indicating clearance for discharge. The PACU nurse should then provide a PACU report to the receiving nurse (or family member) and make appropriate arrangements for transport.

If the patient does not meet surgical and anesthesia discharge criteria, consideration must be given to discharging the patient to an intensive care unit for continued care, to retaining the patient in the PACU, or, if the patient's baseline status has been achieved, to documenting that and returning the patient to a surgical floor.

REFERENCES

1. Abels L: Critical care nursing: a physiologic approach, St Louis, 1986, The CV Mosby Co.
2. Aldrete J: Assessment of recovery from anesthesia, Curr Rev Recov Room Nurses 1(21):163-167, 1980.
3. Aldrete AJ and Krovlik D: The postanesthetic recovery score, Anesth Analg 49(6):924-933, 1970.
4. American Society of Post Anesthesia Nurses: The post anesthesia nursing review for certification, Richmond, Va, 1986, ASPAN.
5. Apgar V: A proposal for a new method of evaluation of the newborn infant, Anesth Analg 32:260-267, 1953.
6. Baden J and Brodsky J: The pregnant surgical patient, Mt Kisco, NY, 1985, Futura Publishing Co, Inc.
7. Beard K, Jick H, and Walker A: Adverse respiratory events occurring in the recovery room after general anesthesia, Anesthesiology 64:269, 1986.
8. Berger J: Transurethral resection of the prostate, Curr Rev Post Anesth Care Nurses 10(17):130-135, 1988.

9. Biddle C: The cardiovascular system during pathophysiologic states, Curr Rev Post Anesth Care Nurses 11(10):73-80, 1989.
10. Brenner B and Rector F (editors): The kidney, ed 2, Philadelphia, 1981, WB Saunders Co.
11. Bushong M: Principles of postanesthetic recovery room management: criteria for patient discharge, Curr Rev Recov Room Nurses 1(10):75-78, 1979.
12. Carignan G, Kerri-Szanto M, and Lavelle J: Post-anesthetic scoring system, Anesthesiology 25(3):396-397, 1964.
13. Carpenito L: Handbook of nursing diagnosis, ed 2, Philadelphia, 1987, JB Lippincott Co.
14. Carrieri V, Lindsey A, and West C: Pathophysiological phenomena in nursing, Philadelphia, 1986, WB Saunders Co.
15. Cullen D: Recovery room management of the surgical patient, Curr Rev Recov Room Nurses 3(19):147-151, 1981.
16. Cullen D and Cullen B: Post anesthetic complications, Surg Clin North Am 55:987, 1975.
17. DeWeese D and Saunders W: Textbook of otolaryngology, ed 6, St Louis, 1982, The CV Mosby Co.
18. Doenges M and Moorhouse M: Nurse's pocket guide: nursing diagnoses with interventions, Philadelphia, 1985, FA Davis Co.
19. Donlon J: Anesthesia for ophthalmic surgery, Curr Rev Post Anesth Care Nurses 11(5):33-40, 1989.
20. Epstein B: Recovery from anesthesia, Anesthesiology 43:285, 1975.
21. Farman J: The work of the recovery room, Br J Hosp Med 19:606, 1978.
22. Farrell J: Illustrated guide to orthopaedic nursing, Philadelphia, 1986, JB Lippincott Co.
23. Feeley T: Postoperative care of the adult patient, Curr Rev Recov Room Nurses 9(3):19-26, 1987.
24. Fonseca R and Davis W: Recontructive preprosthetic oral and maxillofacial surgery, Philadelphia, 1986, WB Saunders Co.
25. Frost E and Andrews I (editors): Recovery room care: International Anesthesiology Clinics, Boston, 1983, Little, Brown & Co, Inc.
26. Gadalla F: Postanesthesia care after obstetric surgery, Curr Rev Post Anesth Care Nurses 10(16):123-127, 1988.
27. Gordon M: Manual of nursing diagnosis, 1986-87, New York, 1987, McGraw-Hill, Inc.
28. Greundemann B and Meeker M: Alexander's care of the patient in surgery, St Louis, 1983, The CV Mosby Co.
29. Hathaway R: Nursing care of the critically ill surgical patient, Rockville, Md, 1988, Aspen Publishers, Inc.
30. Humphrey L and Rogers M: Cardiac physiology: an update, Curr Rev Post Anesth Care Nurses 11(3):19-23, 1989.
31. Israel J and Dekornfeld T (editors): Recovery room care, Chicago, 1987, Year Book Medical Publishers, Inc.
32. Jaffe N: Cataract surgery and its complications, ed 3, Philadelphia, JB Lippincott Co.
33. Kim M, McFarland G, and McLane A (editors): Pocket guide to nursing diagnoses, St Louis, 1984, The CV Mosby Co.
34. Kleinbeck S: Simplifying postoperative assessments, AORN J 38:344, 1983.
35. Levinson G and Shnider S: Anesthesia for surgery during pregnancy. In Shnider S and Levinson G (editors): Anesthesia for obstetrics, ed 2, Baltimore, 1987, Williams & Wilkins, pp 188-205.
36. Litwack K, Hicks F, and Brooks D: Practical points in the care of the patient post cardiac surgery, J Post Anesth Nurs 5(2):106-111, 1990.
37. Luczun M: The surgical patient with coronary artery disease, Curr Rev Post Anesth Care Nurses 10(15):115-199, 1988.
38. Luczun M: Handbook of postanesthesia nursing, Rockville, Md, 1987, Aspen Publishers, Inc.

39. Mitchell P: Concepts basic to nursing, ed 2, New York, 1977, McGraw-Hill, Inc.
40. Robertson G, MacGregor D, and Jones C: Evaluation of doxapram for arousal from general anesthesia in outpatients, Br J Anaesth 49(2):133-139, 1977.
41. Shnider S and Levinson G (editors): Anesthesia for obstetrics, ed 2, Baltimore, 1987, Williams & Wilkins.
42. Schoen D: The nursing process in orthopaedics, Norwalk, Conn, 1986, Appleton-Century-Crofts.
43. Smith J and Watkins J: Care of the postoperative surgical patient, Boston, 1985, Butterworth Publishers.
44. Smith J: Complications of surgery in general, Philadelphia, 1984, Baillière Tindall.
45. Stevens S and Becker K: How to perform a picture perfect respiratory assessment, Nursing' 88 18(1):57-63, 1988.
46. Steward D: A simplified scoring system for the post-operative recovery room, Can Anaesth Soc J 22(1):111, 1975.
47. Tarhan S (editor): Anesthesia and coronary artery surgery, Chicago, 1986, Year Book Medical Publishers, Inc.
48. Thomas S (editor): Manual of cardiac anesthesia, New York, 1984, Churchill Livingstone, Inc.
49. Traver G (editor): Respiratory nursing: the science and the art, New York, 1982, John Wiley & Sons, Inc.
50. Walker S and Love C: Nursing role in management: postoperative client. In Lewis S and Collier I (editors): Medical-surgical nursing: assessment and management of clinical problems, ed 2, New York, 1983, McGraw-Hill, Inc, pp 291-309.
51. Wetchler B: Postanesthesia scoring system: discharging ambulatory surgery patients, AORN J 41(2):382-384, 1985.
52. Yao F and Artusio J: Problem-oriented patient management, Anesthesiology, Philadelphia, 1983, JB Lippincott Co.

Review Questions

1. *Post anesthetic scoring systems* ⸻.
   a. Provide absolute criteria for admission to the PACU
   b. Provide objective criteria for patient assessment
   c. Provide clearance for discharge from the PACU
   d. Are outdated and no longer used in the PACU

2. *The use of a PACU care plan* ⸻.
   a. Allows the PACU nurse to set priorities
   b. Facilitates organization of nursing care
   c. Allows the PACU nurse to recognize competing patient demands
   d. All of the above

3. *In the patient who is recovering from a pneumonectomy, the chest tube is* ⸻.
   a. Designed to reinflate the lung
   b. Placed to low continuous wall suction
   c. Clamped and not put to suction
   d. Not necessary because the lung has been removed

4. *When a patient who is recovering from pneumonectomy is turned, he or she should be positioned* _____.
   a. Operative side up
   b. Operative side down
5. *Subcutaneous emphysema is caused by* _____.
   a. Air trapped in subcutaneous tissues
   b. Smoking
   c. Chronic bronchitis
   d. Allergic rhinitis
6. *Rales heard during auscultation* _____.
   a. Are an example of normal bronchovesicular breath sounds
   b. Are caused by air moving through narrow airways
   c. Are caused by air moving through fluid-filled airways
   d. Are the result of the visceral and parietal pleura rubbing together
7. *Preload is defined as* _____.
   a. The rate and force of cardiac ejection
   b. The force that stretches the ventricle during diastole
   c. Opposition to cardiac ejection
   d. Blood pressure, vascular resistance, and blood viscosity
8. *Systemic vascular resistance is calculated as* _____.
   a. Stroke volume × Heart rate
   b. $\dfrac{\text{Central venous pressure (CVP)} - \text{Wedge (PCWP)}}{\text{Heart rate}}$
   c. $\dfrac{\text{Mean arterial pressure (MAP)} - \text{Central venous pressure (CVP)}}{\text{Cardiac output (CO)}} \times 80$
   d. $\dfrac{\text{Blood pressure} \times \text{Heart rate}}{\text{Central venous pressure (CVP)}}$
9. *Checking pupil constriction is an assessment of the* _____.
   a. Optic nerve
   b. Abducens nerve
   c. Glossopharyngeal nerve
   d. Oculomotor nerve
10. *Codeine is the agent of choice for pain management in the neurosurgical patient because*
    _____.
    a. It does not mask pupil signs
    b. It decreases agitation
    c. It controls seizure activity
    d. It may be taken by mouth
11. *Internal irrigation in the genitourinary patient may contribute to* _____.
    a. Hypothermia
    b. Hyponatremia
    c. Fluid overload
    d. All of the above

12. *Ruddy skin color in the peripheral vascular surgical patient is a sign of* _____.
    a. Inadequate perfusion
    b. Pulselessness
    c. Hematoma formation
    d. Venous congestion

13. *Hypertension in the peripheral vascular surgical patient* _____
    a. May compromise surgical integrity
    b. Decreases perfusion to the grafted area
    c. Makes it difficult to palpate pulses
    d. Causes venous stasis

14. *An orthopedic patient is asked to dorsiflex his or her ankles so that* _____ *may be assessed.*
    a. Perineal nerve functioning
    b. Tibial nerve functioning
    c. Median nerve functioning
    d. Radial nerve functioning

15. *Supine hypotensive syndrome in the pregnant patient is caused by* _____.
    a. Postpartum hemorrhage
    b. Uterine obstruction of the vena cava and aorta
    c. Hypoxemia
    d. Fetal distress

16. *Postpartum hemorrhage is usually the result of* _____.
    a. Multiple births
    b. Uterine atony
    c. Heavy lochia
    d. Bladder perforation

17. *The normal fetal heart rate is* _____
    a. 160 to 200 beats per minute
    b. 60 to 100 beats per minute
    c. 120 to 160 beats per minute
    d. Unaffected by maternal oxygenation

18. *RhoGAM is administered* _____.
    a. To increase uterine contraction
    b. To prevent preeclampsia
    c. To prevent Rh isoimmunization
    d. To decrease pain associated with labor

19. *The patient recovering from retinal surgery* _____.
    a. May assume any position of comfort
    b. Should never receive pain medication
    c. Should cough frequently to increase intraocular pressure
    d. Should be positioned according to the surgeon's instructions

20. *Ear, nose, and throat (ENT) procedures are always associated with an element of risk because* _____.
    a. Surgeries are performed in or through the airway
    b. The surgical fields are highly vascular
    c. Of the risk of infection
    d. Most procedures are done in pediatric patients
21. *Increased salivation after ear, nose, and throat (ENT) surgery* _____.
    a. Is an early sign of infection
    b. Is caused by irritation of the oral mucosa
    c. Is never a normal finding
    d. Is not a problem and may be ignored
22. *Ice packs may be ordered after surgery* _____.
    a. To decrease swelling
    b. To decrease pain
    c. To decrease disfigurement
    d. All of the above
23. *Prior to discharge from the PACU, the patient* _____.
    a. Should be alert and oriented to person, place, and time
    b. Should not require ongoing pain management
    c. Should be breathing, warm, and comfortable and have a heartbeat
    d. Must have an oxygen saturation of 100%.

Answers

	20. a	15. b	10. a	5. a
	19. d	14. a	9. d	4. b
23. c	18. c	13. a	8. c	3. c
22. d	17. c	12. d	7. b	2. d
21. b	16. b	11. d	6. c	1. b

CHAPTER 6

The image of the patient who requires hemodynamic monitoring is often one of a "sick" patient with a "bad" disease. Although physiologic instability may be an indication for instituting hemodynamic monitoring, there are proactive, as opposed to reactive, reasons for instituting hemodynamic monitoring. These reasons include providing a means for early detection of clinical changes, providing for continuous patient monitoring, and as a mechanism to improve or promote patient safety.

HEMODYNAMIC MONITORING

Chapter Objectives

After reading this chapter, the reader will be able to:

1. Identify the indications for arterial blood pressure monitoring.
2. Identify nursing considerations for the patient with arterial pressure monitoring.
3. Identify the indications for placement of a central venous pressure line.
4. Identify nursing considerations for the patient with a central venous pressure line.
5. Identify the indications for placement of a pulmonary artery (Swan-Ganz) catheter.
6. Discuss the parameters that may be obtained and derived from pulmonary artery pressure monitoring.
7. Identify nursing considerations for the patient with a pulmonary artery catheter.

ARTERIAL BLOOD PRESSURE

Arterial blood pressure monitoring is used to provide continuous, direct arterial systolic, diastolic, and mean pressure monitoring. An arterial catheter is placed in a peripheral artery (radial, brachial, or femoral) and is connected by a fluid-filled pressure line to a transducer that converts the pressures into readable values and wave forms on an oscilloscope monitor.

The arterial line allows for continuous blood pressure monitoring, which is useful in monitoring unstable patients, in regulating vasoactive drug therapy, and in measuring blood pressures in patients in whom indirect monitoring via cuff is difficult or impossible (such as burn, trauma, or obese patients).

The arterial line also provides ready access for blood sampling, negating the need for frequent venipunctures. This is useful when frequent blood gas sampling is necessary to guide therapy or in times of metabolic derangement, for example in the patient who requires glucose analysis, electrolyte monitoring, osmolarity monitoring, or acid-base regulation. Frequent blood sampling may also be required to monitor the adequacy of anticoagulation (heparin) therapy and protamine antagonism.

The normal systolic reading in the adult is 90 to 140 mm Hg. The normal diastolic pressure is 60 to 90 mm Hg. The normal mean pressure is 70 to 110 mm Hg. A mean pressure of greater than or equal to 60 mm Hg is required for adequate perfusion of vital organs. It should be noted, that whenever normal values are quoted, each individual patient may have his or her own normal values that may fall above or below population averages.

Placement of an arterial line is associated with a number of complications, including exsanguination (if the catheter becomes disconnected from the pressure tubing or if it is dislodged), thrombus formation, infection (particularly if sterile technique is not used in placement and for blood sampling), and air embolism (if air is flushed into the catheter).

Postoperative implications

When the patient arrives in the PACU, the PACU nurse should attach the arterial line to the monitoring transducer. The line should be calibrated, and the waveform tracing should be confirmed. A poor (dampened) waveform may indicate a loose connection, failure to calibrate, or a lack of pressure in the pressure bag or transducer tubing.

The PACU nurse should verify all connections. The insertion site should be covered and secured with a sterile dressing. The affected extremity should remain visible at all times so that bleeding will be observed. Restraints may be used as necessary to prevent the patient from accidentally or purposefully pulling out the line. Sterile technique—including protecting the access port cap—should be used whenever blood is drawn. The insertion site should be observed for swelling, pain, redness, or tenderness. The extremity distal to the site of catheter placement should be observed for circulatory adequacy, including the presence of capillary refill, sensation, mobility, and temperature.

CENTRAL VENOUS PRESSURE

Central venous pressure (CVP) is a measure of preload; it is used to reflect the venous return to the heart. It is often referred to as a measure of right heart function, although it may be used as an adjunct to infer total myocardial function. The CVP actually measures the pressure in the great veins (superior vena cava, subclavian, jugular) as blood returns to the heart. The normal CVP using a manometer is 6 to 12 cm H_2O. Low values may indicate hypovolemia or venous dilation. Higher than normal values may indicate volume overload, cardiac dysfunction, or pulmonary hypertension.

The CVP catheter is used to monitor fluid replacement and the adequacy of central venous return. When CVP data is considered along with heart rate, blood pressure, and urine output, decisions can be made about fluid therapy (including restriction and replacement). The CVP catheter is particularly helpful during surgery to monitor active bleeding and volume replacement; postoperatively it is used primarily to assess dehydration, to monitor fluid and blood replacement, and to detect changes in cardiac function. Because of its large size and direct access into central circulation, the CVP line may be used for the administration of cardiac medications.

CVP monitoring is also used to provide venous access for intravenous therapy when peripheral veins are thrombosed or collapsed. This may be useful for patients who have a history of long-term intravenous therapy, vascular disease, or intravenous drug abuse or for patients who are vasoconstricted secondary to medications, hypothermia, or acute volume loss.

CVP access also allows for medication administration for drugs or solutions known to be irritating or harmful when given peripherally, including antibiotics, potassium, vasoactive solutions, chemotherapy, or hyperalimentation. CVP access may also be used for hemodialysis.

Finally, the CVP access route may also be used to provide an access route for placement of a pulmonary artery catheter (Swan-Ganz) or intravenous pacemaker.

The CVP line is usually placed preoperatively to allow for baseline preoperative readings to be obtained and to minimize the costs of increased operating room time. The catheter may be placed via the basilic, subclavian, external jugular, or internal jugular vein. The internal jugular route has the highest success rate in placement, however, it is also associated with the highest rate of carotid artery puncture. Other complications vary with the route of placement but include pneumothorax, hematoma, infection, tissue trauma, air embolism, and thrombophlebitis.

Postoperative implications

When the patient is admitted, the PACU nurse should obtain from the anesthesiologist the indication for CVP placement and the range of preoperative and intraoperative readings. It is also important to inquire about possible complications that may have occurred during catheter placement. For example, to rule out or to assess the extent of a pneumothorax, a chest x-ray should be taken to confirm catheter placement. If a carotid puncture occurred, the site of insertion should be monitored for swelling and signs of respiratory or neurologic compromise.

After the patient is admitted, a CVP reading should be obtained as part of the admission vital signs. The CVP reading should be compared with preoperative and intraoperative values. The one-time reading is not as useful as "trending" the data over time in consideration of the surgery, fluid and blood replacement, drug therapy, and other physiologic influences. The reading should also be interpreted in consideration of heart rate, blood pressure, and urine output.

Care should be taken to obtain the reading with the manometer at the level of the right atrium; therefore the head of the patient's bed should be flat for readings. The head may be raised again after the reading is obtained. To prevent a possible air embolism, the PACU nurse should ensure that air does not enter the manometer or CVP tubing.

PULMONARY ARTERY CATHETER

A pulmonary artery catheter (Swan-Ganz, Edwards Laboratories) is a multilumen catheter that is placed through the right side of the heart into the pulmonary artery. It is used to assess the cardiac and hemodynamic status of the patient by providing information about right and left heart function, the effectiveness of the heart as a pump, preload, and afterload (Fig. 6-1).

The placement of a pulmonary artery catheter is indicated in patients with known or suspected cardiac dysfunction, including those with a history of myocardial infarction, coronary artery or valve disease, or cardiac surgery. It is also indicated in patients with compromised oxygenation, including those in acute respiratory failure and those with pulmonary edema or a pulmonary embolism. It is indicated in patients in whom fluid status monitoring is essential for physiologic stability, including patients who are recovering from trauma, patients who are in shock, and patients with sepsis. The pulmonary artery catheter also is indicated for any high-risk surgical patient.

Highly sophisticated pulmonary artery catheters may also be used. Pulmonary artery catheters are available with pacing capabilities and with oxygenation monitoring capabilities (co-oximetric catheters).

The pulmonary artery catheter may be placed via the internal jugular, subclavian, brachial, or femoral vein. Each is associated with complications: internal jugular placement is associated with carotid puncture; subclavian placement is associated with pneumothorax; and brachial and femoral placement are associated with plexus injury.

The pulmonary artery catheter allows for continuous monitoring of right atrial and pulmonary artery pressures. The right atrial pressures reflect preload or venous return to the heart during systole. This is also referred to as central venous pressure (CVP). CVP readings are obtained by opening the proximal lumen of the catheter to the transducer and the monitor. The normal right atrial (CVP) pressures are 0 to 8 mm Hg. The CVP may be increased in right ventricular failure, volume overload, aortic and tricuspid valve dysfunction, pulmonary hypertension, constrictive pericarditis, and tamponade. The CVP may be decreased in states of hypovolemia or during venous dilation.

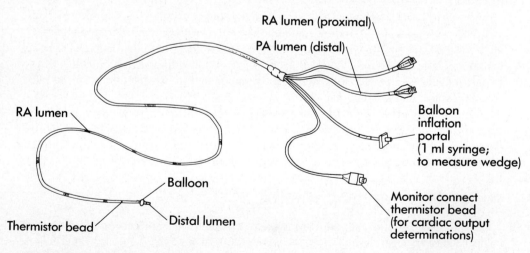

FIG. 6-1. Pulmonary artery catheter.

Pulmonary artery pressures are reflected by systolic and diastolic readings. The systolic value reflects right ventricular function, and the diastolic value reflects left atrial function or left ventricular end diastolic pressures. Pulmonary artery pressures are obtained by opening the distal lumen of the catheter to the transducer and monitor. Normal values for the pulmonary artery are 15-25/8-15 mm Hg. The pulmonary artery pressures may be elevated in cases of right and left ventricular failure, pulmonary hypertension and congestion, valvular stenosis, or tamponade. Pulmonary artery pressures may be low in cases of hypovolemia.

The intermittent monitoring capabilities of the pulmonary artery catheter allow for measurement of pulmonary artery (capillary) wedge pressures, cardiac output, cardiac index, and systemic and pulmonary vascular resistance. Each of these measurements contributes to an understanding of the status of the heart and vasculature.

Pulmonary artery wedge pressures (PAWP) reflect left atrial pressures and, theoretically, left ventricular end diastolic pressures (LVEDP). The pulmonary artery wedge pressure (PAWP) is also referred to as pulmonary capillary wedge pressure (PCWP) and the pulmonary artery occlusion pressure (PAOP). These descriptions are used interchangeably in the literature and clinically. In this text, the generic term "wedge" will be used to avoid confusion.

Ideally, the wedge pressure should be within 1 to 4 mm Hg of the pulmonary artery diastolic pressure (normal: 8 to 15 mm Hg). An elevated wedge may occur because of pulmonary congestion, left ventricular failure, mitral stenosis or regurgitation, or adult respiratory distress syndrome (ARDS). In cases of inadequate preload, the wedge may be low because of hypovolemia or obstruction to filling from the right side of the heart; these conditions might occur in cases of pulmonary embolism, pulmonic stenosis, or right ventricular failure.

The wedge pressure reading is obtained by inflating the catheter balloon with 1.5 cc of air and allowing the balloon to "float" into the pulmonary artery. The waveform tracing is monitored continuously until a dampened "wedge" tracing is noted. The value is recorded, and the syringe is detached, allowing the balloon to deflate passively. The PACU nurse should observe that the waveform has returned and that the balloon is no longer wedged.

The practice of wedging the balloon is not benign, for as the balloon is inflated into the "wedged" position, blood flow distal to the balloon is occluded. Therefore the PACU nurse should never leave the balloon inflated for more than 15 seconds. Prolonged wedging of the balloon may result in a pulmonary infarction or pulmonary artery rupture. No more than 1.5 cc of air should ever be injected into the balloon. A greater volume of air may result in a balloon rupture, causing air to be injected into central circulation (air embolism). If the balloon wedges with less than 1.5 cc of air, it may mean that the catheter is distally positioned or that a clot has formed at the end of the catheter. Nothing but air should ever be injected into the balloon.

Cardiac output (CO) measures may also be obtained from the catheter. Cardiac output is a measure of the volume of blood ejected from the ventricle each minute. It is a measure of flow. Cardiac outputs are obtained to diagnose function, evaluate ventricular performance, assess response to treatment, or obtain derived parameters such as cardiac index and vascular resistance.

Cardiac output measurements are obtained with a cardiac output computer, which uses the formula: stroke volume (SV) multiplied by heart rate (HR). The computer calculates cardiac output by thermodilution. The thermodilution method uses the theory of temperature changes as an indicator of circulating volume (stroke volume).

To obtain a cardiac output, the thermistor lead (temperature sensor) of the pulmonary artery catheter is connected to the cardiac output computer. Depending on institutional policy or protocol, a specified amount of a sterile solution (usually 3, 5, or 10 ml of normal saline or 5% dextrose) is injected into the proximal (CVP) port. The injection is timed to the cardiac output computer's command to inject. Because the injected solution is cooler than the blood into which it is injected, the change in temperature is sensed by the thermistor, located downstream from the right atrium in the pulmonary artery. A normal cardiac output (CO) is 4 to 8 L/min.

To determine if the cardiac output is adequate to meet the perfusion needs of a particular patient, a cardiac index (CI) can be calculated. The cardiac index provides a means to compare cardiac outputs from individuals of different sizes based on body surface area. A cardiac output of 5.2 L/min is not the same for a 92-pound, 5-foot female as it is for a 200-pound, 6-foot male.

Some cardiac output computers will calculate cardiac index automatically if the nurse enters the patient's height and weight into the computer's program. Otherwise, the nurse may manually calculate cardiac index by dividing the patient's cardiac output (CO) by his or her body surface area (BSA). BSA information can be obtained by using a body surface chart (Fig. 6-2). A normal cardiac index (CI) is 2.5 to 4.0 L/min/m^2. A cardiac index of less than 2 L/min/m^2 places the patient at risk for hypoperfusion of vital organs secondary to decreased myocardial function (left ventricular failure), dysrhythmias, or alterations in afterload.

The pulmonary artery catheter can also provide data from which to calculate systemic and pulmonary vascular resistance. Systemic vascular resistance (SVR) reflects left ventricular afterload or the resistance provided by systemic arteriolar circulation against left ventricular emptying. It is obtained by using a calculator and the formula:

$$SVR = \frac{\text{Mean arterial pressure} - CVP}{\text{Cardiac output}} \times 80$$

A normal systemic vascular reistance is 900 to 1400 dynes/sec/cm^{-5}.

Pulmonary vascular resistance (PVR) reflects right ventricular afterload or the resistance provided by the pulmonary vasculature to right ventricular emptying. It is obtained by using a calculator and the formula:

$$PVR = \frac{\text{Mean pulmonary artery pressure} - \text{Wedge}}{\text{Cardiac output}} \times 80$$

A normal pulmonary vascular resistance is 37 to 76 dynes/sec/cm^{-5}.

Increases in systemic and pulmonary vascular resistance may be caused by arterial

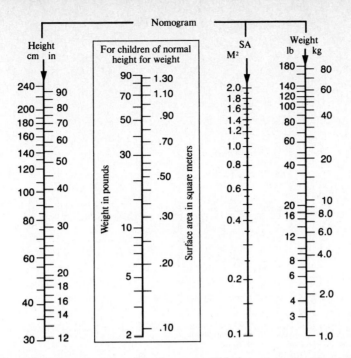

FIG. 6-2. Body surface area nomogram (also known as Dubois nomogram). If a straight edge is placed from the patient's height in the left column to his weight in the right column, the point of intersection in the surface area column indicates the body surface area. (Reproduced from Behrman RE and Vaughn VC (editors): Nelson's textbook of pediatrics, ed 12, Philadelphia, 1983, WB Saunders Co.)

constriction (secondary to hypothermia, vasopressor activity, or hypoperfusion) or by hypertension (idiopathic or pulmonary). To reduce elevated systemic and pulmonary vascular resistance, afterload must be reduced. Rewarming may be effective if the cause is hypothermia. Otherwise vasodilator therapy (sodium nitroprusside) may be indicated.

Decreases in systemic and pulmonary vascular resistance may be caused by arterial dilation (secondary to sepsis, anaphylaxis, or vasodilation therapy) or by hypotension (secondary to myocardial failure or hypovolemia). To improve vascular resistance, the cause of vasodilation should be corrected (for example, through the use of epinephrine to treat anaphylaxis). Volume should be given for hypovolemia. Vasopressors and inotropic medications may be indicated as well (ephedrine, phenylephrine, dopamine, dobutamine).

The monitoring capabilities of the pulmonary artery catheter are summarized in Table 6-1.

Table 6-1. Pulmonary artery catheter capabilities

Measuring capability	Reflects*	Calculated by	Normal values
Central venous pressure (CVP)	RA pressures	Opening proximal lumen to transducer and monitor	0-8 mm Hg
Pulmonary artery pressures (PA)	Systolic/RV function Diastolic/LA function	Opening distal lumen to transducer and monitor	Systolic 15-25 mm Hg Diastolic 8-15 mm Hg
Wedge pressure	LA pressures and LV end diastolic pressure (LVEDP)	Injecting 1.5 cc (max) air into catheter balloon Observe for wedge tracing	Equal to or within 1-4 mm Hg of PA diastolic pressure (8-15 mm Hg)
Cardiac output (CO)	Volume of blood ejected from ventricle in 1 minute	Thermodilution and cardiac output computer	4-8 L/min
Cardiac index (CI)	Cardiac output calculated to body size	CO ÷ BSA (Use Dubois nomogram to obtain BSA)	$2.5 - 4$ L/min/m^2
Systemic vascular resistance (SVR)	LV afterload	$\dfrac{\text{MAP}^\dagger - \text{CVP}}{\text{CO}} \times 80$	900-1400 dynes/sec/cm^{-5}
Pulmonary vascular resistance (PVR)	RV afterload	$\dfrac{\text{Mean PA} - \text{Wedge}}{\text{CO}} \times 80$	37-97 dynes/sec/cm^{-5}

*RA, right atrium; RV, right ventricle; LA, left atrium; LV, left ventricle
†MAP, mean arterial pressure.

Postoperative implications

On admission, the PACU nurse should obtain from the anesthesiologist the patient's history, which should suggest why the pulmonary artery catheter is needed. The catheter should be attached to the transducer and calibrated. A baseline set of readings should be obtained and compared with preoperative and intraoperative readings. All connections should be secured and taped to prevent disconnections. The balloon lumen should be locked into a closed position (Fig. 6-3). Precautions specific to the various measurements have already been discussed.

In addition to obtaining the readings, the PACU nurse should begin to investigate possible causes of readings above or below normal limits. One value in isolation provides little information. However, by examining all hemodynamic parameters, a determination of patient status can be made, and appropriate therapeutic interventions can be initiated. A framework for hemodynamic assessment and therapy is presented in Fig. 6-4.

Readings should be obtained and recorded as often as necessary. This may be as infrequently as every 4 hours in the stable patient who has had the catheter placed prophylactically; conversely, it may be several times an hour if medication, fluid, or balloon pump therapy is being titrated to patient data. The use of a flow sheet will facilitate the monitoring of data over time. (Fig. 6-5).

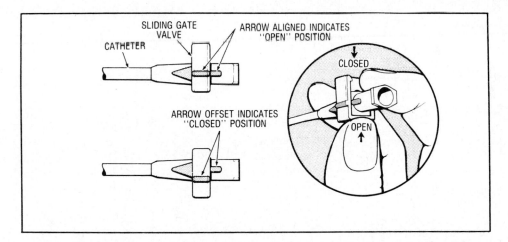

FIG. 6-3. Gate valve operation. (Copyright, Baxter Healthcare Corporation. Reprinted with permission.)

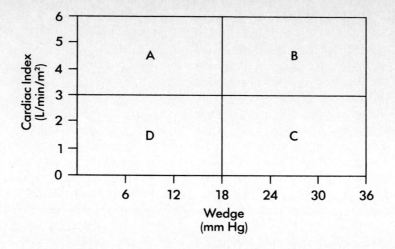

	Findings	Interpretation	Interventions
A	↑ CI Normal wedge	↑ Cardiac output to meet physiologic demand	None—reflects normal compensation
B	↑ CI ↑ Wedge	↑ Preload ↑ Systemic wall tension Hypervolemia	Diuretics Vasodilators Fluid restriction
C	↓ CI ↑ Wedge	↓ LV function ↑ Preload ↓ Afterload Pulmonary congestion	Vasodilators Inotropes Volume regulation
D	↓ CI ↓ Wedge	↓ Cardiac output Hypoperfusion Hypovolemia	Fluid therapy

FIG. 6-4. Hemodynamic assessment.

Date and Time													NORM
P R E S S U R E S	$\overline{AO}$													80—100
	$\overline{RA}$													1—5
	$\overline{PA}$													10—20
	PAd													5—12
	$\overline{PCWP}$													5—12
HR													80—110
CO													3.5—5.5
CI													2.8—4.2
SI													30—65
SVR													800—1500
PVR													50—250
Da—$\overline{v}O_2$													5cc/100ml
O_2 Deliv.													250cc/min.
Qs/Qt													$\leq$ 5%
STATUS													HT
Rx.:													WT
Initial													BSA

Rush-Presbyterian-St. Luke's Medical Center
Chicago, Illinois

**CARDIOVASCULAR PERFORMANCE RECORD
INTENSIVE THERAPY UNIT**

M/R FORM NO. 1985 REV. 3/83

FIG. 6-5. Hemodynamic monitoring flow sheet. (Reprinted with permission of Rush-Presbyterian-St. Luke's Medical Center, Chicago, Il.)

SUMMARY

Hemodynamic monitoring will be less intimidating for the PACU nurse and more beneficial for the patient if the rationale for monitoring, along with the capabilities of monitoring, are understood. Hemodynamic monitoring is not just for "the sick patient." It is indicated for any patient who has the potential for, or great likelihood of, physiologic instability because of pathology, surgery, or history.

REFERENCES

1. Barash P: Non-invasive cardiovascular monitoring, ASA Annual Refresher Course Lectures 411:1-7, 1988.
2. Birmingham P, Cheney F, and Ward R: Esophageal intubation: a review of detection techniques, Anesth Analg 65:886, 1986.
3. Blitt C (editor): Monitoring in anesthesia and critical care medicine, New York, 1985, Churchill-Livingstone.
4. Buell J: A practical, cost-effective, non-invasive system for cardiac output and hemodynamic analysis, Am Heart J 116:657-664, 1988.
5. Eichhorn J et al: Standards for patient monitoring during anesthesia at Harvard Medical School, JAMA 256:1017-1020, 1986.
6. Gaskey N and Berkebile P: Basic principles of cardiovascular monitoring: the Swan-Ganz catheter, Curr Rev Recov Room Nurses 4(13):99-103, 1982.
7. Gayes J: Transthoracic electrical bioimpedance: a non-invasive measurement of cardiac output, J Post Anesth Nurs 4(5):300-305, 1989.
8. Gondringer N and Cuddeford J: Monitoring in anesthesia: clinical application of monitoring central venous and pulmonary artery pressure, J Assoc Nurse Anesth 54(1):43-56, 1986.
9. Grundy B: EEG monitoring in the operating room and critical care unit: if, when and what machine, Anesthesiol Rev 12:73-80, 1985.
10. Kyff J: Invasive hemodynamic monitoring. Part 1: using the pulmonary artery catheter, J Post Anesth Nurs 4(5):287-295, 1989.
11. Kyff J: Invasive hemodyamic monitoring. Part II: hemodynamic formulas for use with the pulmonary artery catheter, J Post Anesth Nurs 4(5):296-299, 1989.
12. LaMantia K, Lehmann K, and Barash P: Echocardiography in the perioperative period, Acute Care 11:106-116, 1985.
13. Lowenstein E and Teplick R: To (PA) catheterize or not to (PA) catheterize—that is the question, Anesthesiol 53:361-363, 1980.
14. Nishimura R, Miller F, and Callahan M: Doppler echocardiography: theory, instrumentation, technique and application, Mayo Clin Proc 60:321-343, 1985.
15. Palmer P: Advanced hemodynamic assessment, Dimens Crit Care Nurs 1(3):139-144, 1982.
16. Reves J: Cardiac physiology and monitoring, Can Anaesth Soc J 32(3):S1-11, 1985.
17. Skoog R: Capnography in the postanesthesia care unit, J Post Anesth Nurs 4(3):147-155, 1989.
18. Smalhout B: A quick guide to capnography and its use in differential diagnosis, Andover, MA, 1986, Hewlett-Packard.
19. Spangler R: Hemodynamic monitoring: Using the pulmonary artery catheter, Cardiothoracic Nurse 5(3):3-5,10, 1987.
20. Standards for basic intraoperative monitoring. American Society of Anesthesiologists Newsletter. Chicago, Dec 1986, The Society.
21. Visalli F and Evans P: The Swan Ganz catheter: a program for teaching safe, effective use, Nursing '81 1:42-47, 1981.
22. Ward S: The capnogram: scope and limitations, Semin Anesth 1(3):216-228, 1987.

Review Questions

1. *Arterial pressure monitoring is used to provide* _____.
   a. Central venous filling pressure information
   b. Continuous direct arterial systolic, diastolic, and mean blood pressures
   c. Noninvasive blood pressure data
   d. Data about left ventricular function

2. *The average mean arterial pressure of* _____ *is required for adequate perfusion of vital organs.*
   a. 30 mm Hg
   b. 60 mm Hg
   c. 90 mm Hg
   d. 120 mm Hg

3. *A potential complication of arterial line monitoring is* _____.
   a. Pneumothorax
   b. Aortic laceration
   c. Carotid artery puncture
   d. Exsanguination

4. *Central venous pressure monitoring (CVP) is a measure of* _____.
   a. Systemic vascular resistance
   b. Peripheral vascular resistance
   c. Preload
   d. Afterload

5. *Measured with a manometer, a normal CVP is* _____.
   a. 0 to 6 cm H_2O
   b. 6 to 12 cm H_2O
   c. 12 to 18 cm H_2O
   d. 18 to 24 cm H_2O

6. *When obtaining a CVP reading, the ideal position for the patient is* _____.
   a. Head elevated 30 degrees
   b. Head elevated 90 degrees
   c. Supine
   d. Prone

7. *When obtaining a CVP reading from a pulmonary artery (Swan-Ganz) catheter, which port is open to the transducer?*
   a. Proximal
   b. Distal
   c. Thermodilution
   d. Thermistor

8. *Pulmonary artery systolic pressures reflect* _____.
   a. Left atrial function
   b. Left ventricular function
   c. Right atrial function
   d. Right ventricular function

9. *The normal wedge pressures should be equal to or within 1 to 4 mm Hg of* _____.
   a. The pulmonary artery systolic pressure
   b. The pulmonary artery diastolic pressure
   c. The central venous pressure
   d. The mean arterial pressure

10. *Pulmonary artery pressures may be high in all of the following cases EXCEPT:*
    a. Pulmonary hypertension
    b. Left ventricular failure
    c. Hypovolemia
    d. Tamponade

11. *A normal cardiac output is* _____.
    a. 0 to 4 L/min
    b. 4 to 8 L/min
    c. 8 to 12 L/min
    d. 12 to 16 L/min

12. *The cardiac index is used to* _____.
    a. Compare CVP with wedge pressures
    b. Evaluate mean arterial and pulmonary artery pressures
    c. Compare left and right ventricular function
    d. Compare cardiac outputs from individuals of different sizes

13. *The formula to calculate systemic vascular resistance is* _____.
    a. $\dfrac{MAP - CVP}{CO} \times 80$
    b. $Wedge - CVP$
    c. $\dfrac{CO - CI}{CVP} \times 80$
    d. $\dfrac{PA\ systolic - PA\ diastolic}{CO} \times 120$

14. *Use the following data to calculate the patient's pulmonary vascular resistance:*
    MAP 80   Wedge 13
    CVP 10   CO 4.12
    PA systolic/diastolic 23/12   CI 2.14
    PA mean 18
    a. PVR = 1359
    b. PVR = 1.21
    c. PVR = 694
    d. PVR = 97

15. *To reduce an elevated SVR, what must be reduced?*
    a. Preload
    b. Afterload
    c. Cardiac output
    d. Cardiac index

16. *A low SVR may be caused by* _____.
    a. Hypertension
    b. Volume overload
    c. Arterial dilation
    d. Peripheral vasoconstriction

17. *When obtaining a wedge pressure, the balloon should never be inflated for more than* ____.
    a. 15 seconds
    b. 30 seconds
    c. 90 seconds
    d. 120 seconds

18. *Cardiac output is a measure of* _____.
    a. Stroke volume × heart rate
    b. Left and right ventricular function
    c. Preload and afterload
    d. Vascular resistance

19. *The volume of air that should be used to obtain a wedge pressure is* _____.
    a. 0.5 cc
    b. 1.0 cc
    c. 1.5 cc
    d. 2.0 cc

20. *Cardiac index is calculated by the formula* _____.
    a. CVP − wedge
    b. CO × MAP
    c. BSA ÷ CO
    d. CO ÷ BSA

Answers

20. d	15. b	10. c	5. b
19. c	14. d	9. b	4. c
18. a	13. a	8. d	3. d
17. a	12. d	7. a	2. b
16. c	11. b	6. c	1. b

CHAPTER 7 _____

E_{very} day the PACU nurse will provide care to patients experiencing the common postoperative problems of pain, hypothermia, nausea and vomiting, and bleeding. Intraoperative positioning may also result in postoperative complications. This chapter will examine these problems with emphasis on assessment, diagnosis, identifying patients at risk, and nursing interventions for these problems.

COMMON POSTOPERATIVE PROBLEMS

Chapter Objectives

After reading this chapter, the reader should be able to take the postoperative problems of pain, hypothermia, nausea and vomiting, bleeding, and complications of positioning and

1. Identify their etiologies
2. Identify pathophysiologic changes that occur with each problem
3. Discuss assessment criteria for each problem
4. Describe treatment interventions for each postoperative problem

PAIN

Management of pain in the PACU is a challenging task, because the PACU nurse must use objective criteria to measure a subjective phenomenon. In addition, a myriad of factors are likely to influence a patient's perception of, and complaints about, pain. It is the role of the PACU nurse to assess patient responses to pain, with the goal of optimizing relief without compromising other organ systems.

Before any discussion of pain assessment, it is important for nurses to possess an operational definition of pain. "Pain is whatever the experiencing person says it is, existing whenever he or she says it does."[33]

This definition supports the subjective nature of pain and creates a challenge for the nurse who often relies on objective criteria to reinforce the decision to institute pain relief methods, especially narcotic administration.

Causes of postoperative pain

The most important factors influencing the occurrence, intensity, quality, and duration of postoperative pain include:

1. The site, nature, and duration of the surgery
2. The physiologic and psychologic make-up of the patient
3. The preoperative preparation of the patient
4. The presence of complications
5. The anesthetic management of the patient
6. Most important, *the quality of postoperative care*

Specific contributing factors to postoperative pain may be found in Table 7-1.

Assessment of pain

Although pain is a subjective experience, rarely do health care providers accept only a patient's report of the feeling of pain as the sole indicator of the need to institute intervention. Nurses may make a judgment as to whether the pain is "real" or not. *Subjective reports* might include statements such as, "My belly hurts," "I feel like something is sitting on my chest," or "I can't stand the pain anymore." Unfortunately, unless these statements are accompanied by physiologic (objective) data, interventions may be limited or withheld.

Objective signs of pain include manifestations of sympathetic stimulation, including tachycardia, hypertension, increased respiratory rate, dilated pupils, and increased muscular tension. The patient may be crying, moaning, or grimacing. Pain may also be suspected by guarding behaviors (protecting the surgical site), repositioning, or restlessness (in the absence of hypoxemia).

In addition to using subjective and objective measures of pain assessment, a number of pain assessment tools have been developed to quantify or qualify pain. Many are extremely detailed and too complex for the PACU patient immediately after surgery and anesthesia. However, several pain assessment tools, including the verbal rating and visual analog scales, have proved useful.

The *verbal rating scale* requires patients to rate their pain on a scale of 1 to 10, in which 1 represents no pain, and 10 represents the worst pain ever experienced. This

Table 7-1. Causes of postoperative pain

Incisional	Skin and subcutaneous tissue
Deep tissue	Cutting, coagulation, retraction, manipulation
Positional	On operating table, operative position, x-ray, traction
Respiratory tract	Endotracheal tube, sore throat
IV site	Needle trauma, extravasation, venous irritation
Ancillary	Casts, tight dressings, catheters, nasogastric tubes
Rehabilitation activity	Coughing, ambulating, voiding, deep breathing

scale provides the nurse with a number that may be reevaluated as comfort measures are instituted.

The *visual analog scale* (Fig. 7-1) requires patients to select the face that most represents how they are feeling. Again, there is a reference point to be used to evaluate comfort measures. Fig. 7-2 shows a visual analog scale especially designed for children, but readily and easily used with adults.

In addition to subjective, objective, and assessment scale data, it may be important for the PACU nurse to obtain some very specific information about the pain the patient

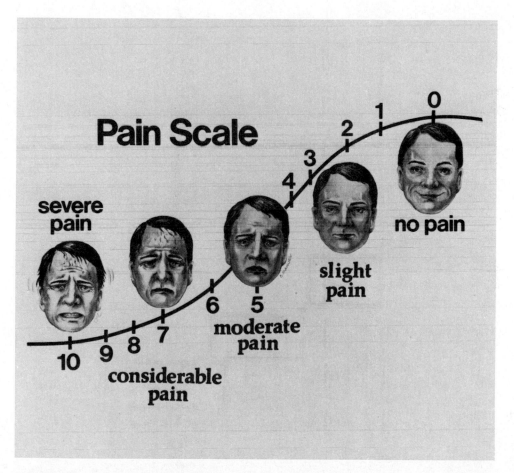

FIG. 7-1. Pain scale. (Reprinted with permission from the International Anesthesia Research Society, from Continuous epidural morphine for pain relief after throacic surgery: a new technique, by El-Baz N, Faber LP, and Jensik R, Anesthesia and Analgesia, vol 63, 1984, pp 757-764.)

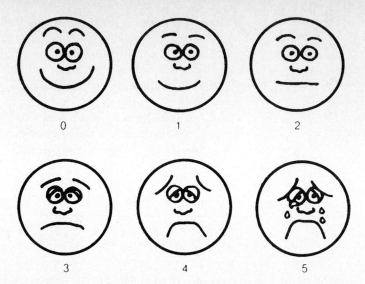

FIG. 7-2. Faces rating scale. Explain to the patient that each face is for a person who feels happy because he has no pain (hurt) or sad because he has some or a lot of pain. Face 0 is very happy because he doesn't hurt at all. Face 1 hurts just a little bit. Face 2 hurts a little more. Face 3 hurts even more. Face 4 hurts a whole lot, but Face 5 hurts as much as you can imagine, although you don't have to be crying to feel this bad. Ask the patient to choose the face that best describes how he is feeling. (From Whaley L and Wong D: Essentials in pediatric nursing, ed 2, St. Louis, 1985, The CV Mosby Co; research reported in Wong D and Baker C: Pain in children; comparison of assessment scales, Pediatr Nurs 14(1):9-17, 1988.)

is experiencing. Open-ended questions — such as those listed below — encourage the patient to detail the pain:

Where does it hurt? Show me.

What does the pain feel like?

Do you have any other symptoms?

These questions will help clarify the type of pain and may, therefore, guide interventions. A patient who is recovering from thoracotomy will be treated differently for complaints of chest pain along an incision line than for crushing chest pain accompanied by dyspnea and radiating arm pain. Assumptions about the cause of pain may result in ineffective treatment of the problem.

Treatment of pain

Ideally, the management of pain in the PACU will begin with a preventative approach, rather than solely a treatment approach. Attention of the anesthesia team to pain management begins preoperatively, with assessment of the patient in consideration of the surgery and expected postoperative management and problems. For example, a patient undergoing a total joint replacement might become a candidate for placement of an epidural catheter preoperatively for postoperative pain management.

Intraoperative attention to pain management includes verification of patient positioning, with attention to bony prominences. In addition, the administration of intravenous narcotics close to the end of the case, unless contraindicated, may allow the patient to awaken pain-free or with minimal discomfort. This is especially important for ambulatory surgical patients, who are expected to go home within hours of their surgery.

Postoperatively, the PACU nurse may employ both nonpharmacologic and pharmacologic interventions to increase patient comfort.

Nonpharmacologic interventions. These interventions include the use of verbal reassurance, touch, the relaxation techniques of imagery and controlled breathing, rewarming, and the use of the patient's support system, for example, a family member or significant other, or even a favorite toy. Nonpharmacologic comfort measures have the advantages of being introduced independently and easily by the nurses and of being cost-effective, readily available, and requiring no special equipment or monitoring. In fact, at times nonpharmacologic interventions may be the only interventions required, and they may be the only interventions that are safe to institute if the patient's physiologic stability is compromised.

The *transcutaneous electronic nerve stimulator* (TENS) is an additional nonpharmacologic intervention that may be used in the management of postoperative pain. The TENS unit is an electronic device used to transmit small electric impulses into the operative site through two to four electrodes placed around the incision area. The patient is able to control the intensity of the transmitted impulses via a control unit.

Two different mechanisms of action have been proposed for the pain management properties of the TENS. The first, the gate theory, was proposed in 1965 by Melzak and Wall. This theory proposed that the electrical stimulation of the large primary afferent neurons by the TENS unit would inhibit transmission of pain impulses to the brain.

The second theory is based on the concept of endogenous opiates. As the electrical impulses from the TENS unit stimulate cells within the spinal cord and brain, endogenous opiates (neurochemicals) are produced. These endogenous opiates act to modify pain sensation.

As a noninvasive, nonpharmacologic approach to pain management, TENS therapy may prove useful for patients recovering from caesarean section (who desire to breastfeed and do not want to pass narcotics via breast milk to the baby), for elderly patients (with decreased tolerance to medications), and for nonemergent surgeries (the trauma of unexpected surgery may interfere with patient instruction). The TENS has also been used for patients with phantom limb pain after an amputation, herpes zoster, and paralytic ileus (which could be further aggravated with narcotics). Ideally, the patient will receive instructions about TENS therapy preoperatively.

TENS therapy has been criticized as providing only weak analgesia with a 75% to 85% efficacy rate. However, TENS therapy may also be combined with conventional pharmacologic therapy to increase its effectiveness.

Pharmacologic interventions. Pharmacologic interventions may be ordered by the anesthesiologist or the surgeon for the management of pain. The physician must select not only a medication but also a route of administration. Pain medications that are commonly used in the PACU—including narcotics, agonists-antagonists, and nonnarcotics—are identified in the box below.

The administration of small, titrated doses of intravenously administered pain medication is the most common approach to pain management in the PACU. The PACU nurse titrates the medication incrementally, with the goal of optimizing pain relief without compromising physiologic stability. Intramuscular narcotics are still administered in some PACUs. The intramuscular route of administration precludes titration. Onset of action may also be unpredictable, particularly in the hypothermic patient.

To involve patients actively in their advancement toward wellness, patient-controlled analgesia provides an alternative to the traditional nurse-administered doses of intravenous narcotics. Patient-controlled analgesia (PCA) allows patients to self-administer preset doses of intravenous narcotics. The physician will determine the medication, dose, time interval between doses (lockout interval), and the maximum dosage that may be received in a specified time period. Patient-controlled analgesia pumps may be started immediately in the PACU.

Narcotics for pain relief may also be administered via epidural bolus or continuous infusion. Local anesthetics may be used for regional pain blocks as well. Regional anesthesia is discussed in detail in Chapter 4.

Evaluation of interventions. The decision to institute treatment for pain begins with an evaluation of the patient's physiologic status. The PACU nurse must not only evaluate complaints of pain, but must also evaluate the patient's neurologic, respiratory, and cardiovascular status. Is the patient responsive and able to communicate consistently, or does the patient complain of pain only when awake, but without stimulation falls asleep easily? The patient who is able to sleep without pharmacologic intervention for pain probably requires no such intervention.

PAIN MEDICATION IN THE PACU

Narcotics

Morphine sulfate
Meperidine (Demerol)
Codeine
Levorphanol (Levo-Dromoran)
Oxycodone
Hydromorphone (Dilaudid)
Oxymorphone (Numorphan)
Methadone (Dolophine)

Mixed agonists/antagonists

Pentazocine (Talwin)
Nalbuphine (Nubain
Butorphanol (Stadol)
Nonnarcotics
Acetaminophen (Tylenol)
Aspirin (A.S.A.)
Ibuprofen (Motrin, Advil, Nuprin)

The patient's respiratory status must also be evaluated. Because narcotics possess the inherent property of inducing respiratory depression, it is important for the PACU nurse to evaluate the patency of the patient's airway and the adequacy of ventilation prior to the administration of any narcotic. Pulse oximetry provides a useful diagnostic aid in the evaluation of ventilatory function.

Because narcotics, particularly morphine, may induce hypotension, it is important to ensure cardiovascular adequacy, including heart rate and blood pressure, before administering any narcotic.

Evaluation must also be directed toward ensuring that pain relief is adequate after an intervention has been instituted. Was the choice of intervention effective in the manner or quantity in which it was administered? Is additional intervention required? Has an intervention proved ineffective, requiring substitution of an alternative intervention? Is the narcotic causing physiologic instability? The evaluation of the efficacy of interventions should be documented on the PACU record.

Effective pain management is an integral part of the PACU care plan of patients. The achievement of optimal comfort is a goal of care and is discussed in greater detail in Chapter 5.

HYPOTHERMIA

Hypothermia is a condition characterized by an abnormally low core temperature of less than 96.8° F (36° C). Hypothermia occurs when systemic heat loss exceeds heat production. It has been estimated that 60% to 90% of all patients admitted to the PACU are hypothermic.[2,51] As hypothermia can prolong recovery and contributes significantly to postoperative morbidity, it is important for the PACU nurse to understand the mechanisms of heat loss, to identify patients at risk for hypothermia, to recognize the physiologic consequences of hypothermia, and to identify prevention and treatment interventions for the management of hypothermia.[28]

Mechanisms of heat loss

It is the patient's interaction with the environment that determines the degree of heat loss. There are four mechanisms of heat loss: radiation, convection, conduction, and evaporation.

Radiation. Radiant heat loss involves the loss of heat from a warm or hot surface (the body) to a cooler one (the operating room environment). In the operating room, it accounts for 40% to 60% of heat loss. Heat is transmitted to the environment as infrared radiation with 5 to 20 μm wavelengths at a rate of 50 kcal/hour when the patient is fully exposed and 10 kcal/hour when the patient is fully draped.[38]

Convection. Convection is heat loss to air currents, or the so-called wind-chill factor.[26] Heat loss depends on the existence of a temperature gradient between the body (i.e., skin and viscera) and the ambient or surrounding air. Twenty-five to thirty-five percent of intraoperative heat loss results from convective heat loss at a rate of 10 kcal/hour.[38]

Conduction. Conduction involves the loss of heat from a warm surface that comes in direct contact with a cooler one. In the operating room, the warm body (skin and tissues) comes in contact with and loses heat to the operating table, skin preparatory solutions, intravenous fluids, irrigants, cool sheets, and drapes. An additional source of conductive heat loss occurs from the body core to cooler and more peripheral tissues as anesthetic vasodilation commences. The rate of conductive heat loss to intravenous fluids at room temperature is 16 kcal/L. The rate of conductive heat loss to blood at 4° C is 30 kcal/L.[38]

Evaporation. Evaporation involves the transfer of heat on changing from a liquid to a gas. Evaporative heat loss occurs via perspiration and ventilation at a rate of 12 to 16 kcal/hour. Additional evaporative heat loss occurs as skin preparatory solutions evaporate and as exposed viscera and body cavities allow further extracellular fluid evaporation. Approximately 400 kcal/hour can be lost from exposed viscera.[28,38]

When losses from all four routes of heat loss are combined, patients may lose at least 90 kcal/hour in the operating room. Total heat production for a 70 kg man per hour during anesthesia with paralysis is an average of 40 kcal/hour. Heat loss (90 kcal) exceeds heat production (40 kcal), and hypothermia ensues.

Pathophysiology of hypothermia

In the anesthetized patient, hypothermia to 93° F (34° C) is generally well tolerated and, in fact, may prove to be protective as opposed to harmful. However, as hypothermia continues with temperatures of less than 92° F (33.9° C), urgency is required in maintaining body temperature and in correcting heat loss as progressive changes in cardiovascular function, renal function, hemoglobin function, coagulation function, and molecular function may prove to be detrimental to patient stability.

Hypothermia results in decreased oxygen availability by shifting the oxyhemoglobin dissociation curve to the left, binding oxygen more tightly to hemoglobin. Shivering associated with hypothermia increases oxygen demand by 400% to 500%. Vasoconstricted tissues contribute to the development of metabolic acidosis. Many critically ill, postsurgical patients are already experiencing oxygen deficits and acid-base abnormalities because of cardiac or respiratory insufficiencies.

Hypothermia slows metabolically dependent processes, and it may decrease drug biotransformation. Peripheral vasoconstriction makes subcutaneous and intramuscular medication administration unpredictable. Renal transport processes are also impaired, with a decrease in glomerular filtration rate. Gastrointestinal function is depressed and may result in the development of a paralytic ileus. Cardiac rate and rhythm disturbances may occur. Central nervous system depression may be profound and may present as coma. Hyperglycemia is common because of catecholamine and stress hormone release (cortisol). The physiologic consequences of hypothermia are summarized in the box on the right.

Clinical signs and symptoms

Generalized hypothermia occurs when core body temperature falls below 95° F (35° C). Patients will present with pallor and skin discoloration. Skin will be cool and dry to

_____ **PHYSIOLOGIC CONSEQUENCES OF HYPOTHERMIA**[18] _____

The Good

Reduced metabolism

Reduced oxygen demand (approximately 7% per 1° C drop)

Cerebral protection in the range of 34° to 36° C

Decreased minimum alveolar concentration

The Bad

Vasoconstriction: increased systemic vascular resistance, pulmonary vascular resistance, and central venous pressure; failure of pulse oximeter sensing

Loss of intravascular volume (serum but not proteins)

Bradycardia, decreased cardiac output, and eventually decreased blood pressure

Ventricular irritability

Cardiac conduction slowing and conduction blocks

Microvascular sludging and rouleaux formation

Decreased oxygen availability to tissue

Central nervous system depression and obtundation

Loss of respiratory carbon dioxide responsiveness

High sympathetic nervous system activity

Bronchospasm

Impaired renal tubular function, decreased glomerular filtration rate, decreased free water excretion, decreased drug elimination

Hyperglycemia

Coagulation defects, disseminated intravascular coagulation, platelet dysfunction

Decreased liver blood flow and drug metabolism

The Ugly

Shivering

Massive tissue oxygen demand and carbon dioxide production

Increased oxygen consumption by as much as 400% to 700%

Hypoxemia

Acidosis

Hypertension

Dysrhythmias

Tachycardia

Cardiac ischemia

Delayed emergence and delayed airway protection

Rewarming hypovolemia and hypotension

From Morrison, R: Hypothermia in the elderly, Int Anesthesiol Clin 26(2):124-133, 1988.

touch. It is not uncommon to find miotic pupils, bradycardia, and slow, shallow respiration. If hypothermia is severe or if it is allowed to continue, patients may become hypotensive, develop metabolic acidosis and ventricular dysrhythmias, and, most notably, develop ventricular fibrillation. Unconsciousness and death may ensue.

Identification of hypothermia

It would be remiss in a discussion of hypothermia not to include discussion of temperature monitoring. Temperature monitoring may reflect central (core) or noncentral (peripheral) temperature. Central temperature reflects the temperature of blood flowing by the temperature-sensitive center of the hypothalamus. Currently four sites are used to reflect central temperature: the tympanic membrane, the nasopharynx, the lower one third of the esophagus, and the pulmonary artery. The tympanic membrane and the nasopharynx reflect the blood temperature of the internal carotid artery and its branches. The lower esophagus reflects the blood temperature of the aorta. Pulmonary artery temperature monitoring is not the primary use of a Swan-Ganz catheter, but it is useful in ongoing measurement of central temperature.

Noncentral temperature monitoring may be done rectally, via the axilla, skin, or in the oropharynx. Each site has specific advantages and limitations that may apply in the critical care setting. Although noncentral temperature monitoring does not measure core temperature, it is useful to measure relative changes in body temperature. The advantages and disadvantages of temperature monitoring sites are identified in Table 7-2.

Table 7-2. **Advantages and disadvantages of various sites of temperature monitoring**

Site	Advantages	Disadvantages
Rectal	Good with intubated patients Good with confused patients Good with all ages	Requires lubrication Risk of infection ↓ after peritoneal lavage, cystoscopy, irrigation ↓ after replacement of bowel into abdomen ↓ with hypoperfused bowel Cannot use with GI bleed, diarrhea, hemorrhoids, rectal surgery Risk of perforation
Skin	Noninvasive Good with children Disposable sensors Approximates core temperature because forehead remains well perfused in hypothermic states	Temperature varies with subcutaneous blood flow Sensors costly Difficult with diaphoretic patients
Axilla	Noninvasive Good with intubated patients Useful with all ages Good with agitated patients	Temperature varies with blood flow and position ↓ with abduction ↓ with cold peripheral IV fluid
Oropharynx	Accepted well by patients Convenient Requires no position changes Approximates core temperature when obtained in posterior sublingual pocket	Reflects temperature of gases Not good for agitated patients Difficult after oral surgery Not used with infants
Aural	Relatively noninvasive Tolerated well by patients Reflects central temperature Rapid results	Difficult placement Potential for trauma Potential exacerbation of nausea via indirect stimulation of inner ear

Patients at risk

While all patients undergoing anesthesia and surgery are at risk for hypothermia, it is possible to identify patients at high risk for hypothermia and its physiologic sequellae.

The elderly patient is at risk of becoming hypothermic even with room temperatures of 60° F to 70° F. Given that the average operating room is 65° F (<20° C), most elderly patients will be hypothermic upon admission to the PACU. The elderly patient has a lower basal metabolic rate of heat production than a younger adult (about 10% less).[38]

The neonate is at risk for hypothermia because of an immature thermoregulatory center. In addition, infants have a small body mass (heat generator) and a large surface area (heat loser). The ratio of surface area to mass is 3 times that of the adult.[26]

Preexisting medical conditions may contribute to the development of hypothermia. Diseases of the thyroid, adrenal glands, diabetes mellitus, cardiac dysfunction, hepatic disease, and malnutrition reduce heat production. Peripheral vascular disease contributes to hypothermia because cool extremities preoperatively contribute to core cooling after anesthetic vasodilation.[28,38]

Burn victims have subcutaneous insulating tissue loss, high fluid requirements, and a high metabolic rate, all of which lead to rapid heat loss. Trauma patients are often severely hypothermic from environmental exposure and emergency fluid resuscitation. The intoxicated individual is at risk for hypothermia because of vasodilation and depression of the heat regulatory center.[26,28]

Medications can contribute to hypothermia. Patients on vasodilators, nonsteroidal antiinflammatory agents, and phenothiazines have alterations in thermoregulation because of either vasodilation or suppression of the thermoregulatory center. General anesthetics depress the thermoregulatory center. Narcotics and muscle relaxants depress voluntary shivering as a mechanism to generate heat. Regional anesthesia also contributes to hypothermia because flaccid muscles and vasodilation cause continued heat loss.

Any patient who has a body cavity entered is at risk for hypothermia via convective and evaporative heat loss. The use of irrigating solutions—as with patients undergoing transurethral resection of the prostate (TURP) or with cardioplegia in cardiac surgical patients—causes internal cooling. Because of evaporation, external cooling may occur in patients having lithotripsy.[28]

Prevention and treatment of hypothermia

The greatest heat loss occurs in the first hour of surgery, so heat conservation must begin as soon as the patient is brought into the operating room. Preventative measures will obviously be patient- and surgery-specific. For pediatric patients, prevention centers on increasing the ambient temperature in the operating room. The operating room should be heated to 27° C for premature infants or neonates, 26° C for infants to those 6 months of age, and 25° C for children 6 months to 2 years of age.[26]

Draping the patient on arrival will minimize exposure. Radiation and convection account for about 80% of all heat loss, and both can be greatly diminished if the patient is kept covered as much as possible. As much as 50% of the body's heat is lost from the scalp because scalp blood vessels are unable to vasoconstrict. Wrapping the head in drapes effectively prevents heat loss.[26]

Reflective mylar and aluminum blankets (Space Blankets, Thermadrape) have been used to prevent radiant and convective heat loss, but they are insufficient in preventing hypothermia unless 60% of the patient's body surface can be covered.[7]

The use of a heated humidifier is the best way to prevent and treat heat loss during the administration of anesthesia. Heated humidifiers spare the patient the energy cost of warming and humidifying dry gases and can actively transfer heat to the patient.[26]

Fluid warmers add major amounts of heat. Conductive heat loss will occur if cold fluids are infused in a warm patient. Administration of 1 L of room temperature (20° C) fluid will require the patient to expend 15 kcal to warm that fluid to 37° C. This represents about 20% of the patient's hourly caloric requirement. Blood products at 4° C will lower a patient's temperature by 0.5° C.[26,38] Fluid warmers are particularly useful in the operating room where high fluid volumes are administered. If blood loss and fluid replacement is to continue in the PACU, fluid warmers should be used there as well.

Rewarming in the PACU

Before rewarming interventions are initiated, oxygen therapy should be established. Hypothermia and shivering increase oxygen demand, creating additional physiologic demands.

Immediate care of the hypothermic patient includes passive rewarming. The goal of passive rewarming is to maximize basal heat production. Wet, cold sheets and gowns should be removed. Warm, dry gowns and blankets should be wrapped around the patient.[28] Active rewarming in the PACU usually consists of external rewarming techniques. The interventions vary in their efficacy.

Continuous fluid-circulating warming blankets have been shown in several studies to have no value in keeping adults warm because there is not enough highly perfused surface area in contact with the blanket.[17,37]

Radiant heat lamps are effective in rewarming some patients—especially pediatric patients. However, because the effectiveness of these lamps depends on exposure of large areas of body surface, their use is limited with adults.[24,52] The need to maintain modesty and privacy limits their use with adults. Infrared thermal ceilings are effective for rewarming, but they require total body exposure for maximum effect.[20] In addition, they are uncomfortable for PACU staff. Fluid and blood warmers are useful if high volumes of fluid are to be administered.

Heated humidifiers are extremely effective for both prevention of and correction of hypothermia. However, their usefulness is somewhat limited in extubated patients.[17] Warmed cotton blankets remain the mainstay of rewarming therapy in most PACUs. Warmed blankets provide a transient feeling of warmth for the patient.[52] Heating the skin limits the shivering response even if the core is cool.[38] Blankets must be changed frequently to maintain rewarming. A focused thermal environment (warm air therapy) is a new technology designed to provide a personalized microenvironment of moving warm air. The method is effective in rewarming patients because 70% of the body surface is in contact with heat. A focused thermal environment [Bair Hugger] unit is shown in Fig. 7-3.

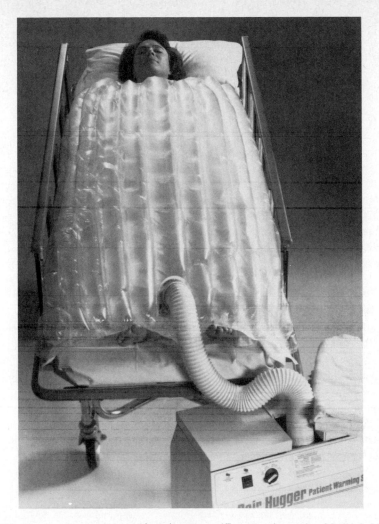

FIG. 7-3. Bair Hugger; Focused thermal environment. (Courtesy Augustine Medical, Minneapolis, Minn.)

Monitoring and rewarming during hypothermia

Obviously ongoing temperature monitoring is a must, particularly during active rewarming. Most PACUs have determined a minimum discharge temperature as a criterion for patient discharge, usually 96° F (or 36° to 36.5° C). Blood pressure and ECG monitoring is essential, as vasoconstricted vessels will present as hypertension and tachycardia. Oxygen demand is high. Pulse oximetry monitoring is useful to detect desaturation and hypoxemia.

In addition, as patients are actively rewarmed, peripheral vasodilation occurs; peripheral vasodilation may cause a paradoxical central cooling. Cooler blood that had been trapped in the periphery is suddenly released into central circulation. The myocardium becomes chilled, increasing the likelihood of dysrhythmias.

Hypothermia as a component of the PACU care plan is discussed in Chapter 5.

NAUSEA AND VOMITING

Postoperative nausea and vomiting has been reported in the medical literature for nearly 80 years. In 1914, the first journal devoted solely to the topic of anesthesia contained an article entitled, "Prophylaxis of Postanesthetic Vomiting."[8] Postoperative nausea and vomiting remains a leading cause of hospitalization among outpatients; it causes delays in recovery time, thereby increasing patient care costs; and it is responsible for increased morbidity and mortality in the postsurgical patient. The increase in morbidity and mortality is caused by aspiration of gastric contents with subsequent development of pneumonitis, destruction of lung tissue, pulmonary edema, and respiratory failure.

Physiology of nausea and vomiting*

Nausea is a subjective feeling of awareness of excitation of the medullary vomiting center. It is often a precursor to vomiting, which is the act of forcibly expelling gastric contents. The vomiting center may be stimulated by cortical afferents, including hypoxia, pain, increased intracranial pressure, sensory stimulation, and psychologic factors. The vomiting center may also be stimulated by visceral afferents, including diseases of the gastrointestinal tract, genitourinary tract, and the heart. Stimulation may be initiated externally to the vomiting center via the chemoreceptor trigger zone (CTZ), an area located at the base of the fourth ventricle. The chemoreceptor trigger zone may be stimulated by motion, drugs (such as morphine), radiation, and metabolic disturbances.

Stimulation of the vomiting center results in motor impulse transmission via cranial nerves V, VII, IX, X, and XII to the upper gastrointestinal tract and via spinal nerves to the diaphragm and abdominal muscles, causing the act of vomiting.[49] Fig. 7-4 is a schematic representation of the physiology of nausea and vomiting.

Risk factors

Numerous factors have been associated with postoperative nausea and vomiting, including anesthetic techniques, anesthetic agents, narcotics, age, gender, weight, type of surgical procedure, pain, and a history of prior nausea and vomiting or motion sickness.

Anesthetic technique. The use of positive-pressure ventilation by mask may affect the incidence of postoperative nausea and vomiting. Positive-pressure mask ventilation may be used to preoxygenate patients prior to induction. This type of ventilation may force air into the stomach, causing gastric distention and subsequent postoperative nau-

---

*Adapted from Litwack K and Parnass S: Practical points in the management of nausea and vomiting, JOPAN 3(4):275-277, 1988.

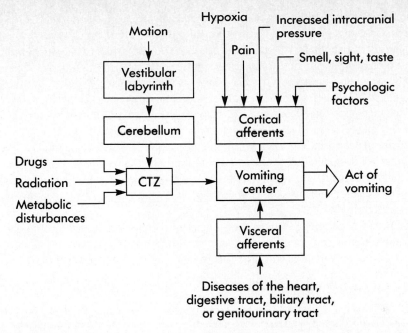

FIG. 7-4. Schematic view of some stimuli that may cause nausea and vomiting; the stimuli are organized by their afferent pathways. (From Orkin F and Copperman L; Complications in anesthesiology, Philadelphia, 1983, JB Lippincott Co.)

sea and vomiting. The length of anesthetic exposure time has also been associated with an increase in postoperative nausea and vomiting.[50]

Regional anesthetic techniques also may cause nausea and vomiting. Hypotension caused by sympathetic blockade during spinal anesthesia has been associated with medullary ischemia and resultant nausea and vomiting.

Anesthetic agents. The choice of anesthetic agent may influence the incidence of postoperative nausea and vomiting. Narcotic-based anesthesia—including the use of morphine, sufentanil, fentanyl, and alfentanil—increases the risk of postoperative nausea and vomiting. Narcotics directly stimulate the chemoreceptor trigger zone and ultimately the medullary vomiting center. Narcotics also act peripherally to slow gastric motility and to prolong gastric emptying time.[50]

The relationship between nitrous oxide and postoperative nausea and vomiting has been controversial in the literature. Experientially, enflurane (Ethrane) has shown promise as being the inhalation agent of choice, particularly with gynecologic outpatients, as it appears to be associated with less nausea and vomiting. However, no conclusive data has shown significant differences among the inhalation anesthetic agents.[41]

Patient variables. Swenson and Orkin[50] reported that women were 2 to 4 times more likely to experience postoperative nausea and vomiting than men. In addition, children and adolescents have an increased incidence of postoperative nausea and vomiting. The issue of weight has also been associated with postoperative nausea and vomiting. The obese patient may sequester drugs in fat compartments, slowing metabolism and elimination of anesthetics. Weight remains a controversial risk factor. Muir et al.[39] found no correlation between body mass index and postoperative nausea and vomiting. Obese patients are rarely candidates for positive-pressure mask ventilation because of airway management issues and concern for increasing the likelihood of gastric distention, which has been positively associated with nausea and vomiting.

Surgical procedure. The type of surgical procedure has also been cited as a contributing factor to postoperative nausea and vomiting. In the pediatric population, it has been clear that patients undergoing strabismus and orchiopexy surgery have a high incidence of postoperative nausea and vomiting, as do patients undergoing tonsillectomy and adenoidectomies.

In the adult population, Bonica et al. noted an increased frequency of postoperative nausea and vomiting in patients undergoing gastrointestinal procedures.[6] Diagnostic laparoscopic procedures involve filling the peritoneal cavity with carbon dioxide, which is very irritating and may increase the likelihood of postoperative nausea and vomiting. Smessaert et al.[46] and Haumann and Foster[19] reported a higher incidence of nausea and vomiting following otologic and ophthalmic procedures.[19,46] Postoperatively, gastrointestinal procedures requiring placement of a nasogastric (NG) tube may be associated with an increased incidence of nausea and vomiting secondary to dysfunction of effective intermittent suction.

Pain related to nausea and vomiting. The role of postoperative pain as a factor in postoperative nausea and vomiting has been well documented. Anderson and Krogh[5] found that complete pain relief without simultaneous relief of nausea was unusual. Of the 90% of their patients who had postoperative pain and nausea, half had both relieved after the first analgesic injection; the other half had both complaints relieved after the second dose. Only 10% of their patients complained of nausea without pain.

Preoperative history. Patients with a history of postoperative nausea and vomiting from previous surgeries and those patients with a history of motion sickness will have a significantly greater incidence of postoperative nausea and vomiting. It is important to obtain a good preoperative history, especially in the ambulatory surgical patient population (patients scheduled to return home the day of surgery).

Management of nausea and vomiting

Management of nausea and vomiting should ideally stem from a prophylactic as opposed to a therapeutic approach, particularly in patients identified to be at risk. Preventative therapy minimizes morbidity, increases and maintains patient comfort, and decreases the frustration often felt by nurses trying to manage the problem. Patient satisfaction is appreciably enhanced, particularly in the ambulatory surgical population.

Preoperative or intraoperative administration of antiemetics has been effective in decreasing the incidence of postoperative nausea and vomiting. Ideally, the anesthesia care team will anticipate the need for prophylactic therapy based on the identification of risk factors.[27]

Pharmacologic interventions

A number of pharmacologic interventions have been used in the treatment of post-operative nausea and vomiting. The most commonly prescribed medications used in the PACU are identified in the box on p. 166.

BLEEDING

Bleeding in the immediate postoperative period is cause for concern. It requires careful evaluation to determine if the bleeding is caused by loss of vascular integrity at the surgical site or by a coagulopathy. Treatment interventions will depend on the etiology. Immediate interventions can prevent significant blood loss, which will decrease circulatory volume, compromise perfusion and oxygenation, reduce cardiac output, and create physiologic instability.

Circulating blood volume in a normal, healthy adult is estimated at 75 ml/kg. A 20% loss of that normal volume can result in signs and symptoms of hypovolemic shock: decreased blood pressure, tachycardia, increased respiratory rate, cool skin, and pallor of the mucous membranes. As blood loss increases, signs and symptoms progress in severity.

The clinical signs of hypovolemic shock are identified in Table 7-3. The guidelines in the Table are based on the "three-in-one" rule. This rule derives from the empiric observation that most patients in hemorrhagic shock will require as much as 300 ml of electrolyte solution for each 100 ml of blood loss.

Circulating blood volume in the pediatric patient varies with age. A premature infant will average 95 to 100 ml/kg. A newborn will average 85 to 90 ml/kg. After 1 year of age, the child will approach the adult range of 75 ml/kg. Unlike in the adult, where a loss of 20% of the total circulating blood volume produces signs of hypovolemic shock, in the child, signs of hypovolemic shock are seen with a 10% to 15% loss of circulating volume. A loss of 20% to 25% of total circulating volume will drop the child's cardiac output and blood pressure by 50%. In children, a drop in blood pressure (if it is not caused by bradycardia or hypoxemia) is always attributed to a decreased blood volume until proven otherwise.

Loss of vascular integrity

The most common cause of bleeding in the PACU is loss of vascular integrity at the surgical site. As a result, the source and site of the bleeding is usually the surgical wound. Bleeding may be overt, noted in drains or on dressings, or it may be suspected because of physiologic instability of the patient as signs and symptoms of hypovolemic shock develop.

Whenever an overt bleed is detected, the source should be identified, with a determination made as to whether the loss is arterial or venous. Arterial blood loss occurs rapidly from high-flow, high-pressure vessels. Estimated blood loss should be determined, either by emptying a drain into a graduated measure or by "guestimating" the loss based on the number of gauze sponges saturated (that is, small, moderate, large).

ANTIEMETICS

Benzquinamide (Emete-Con)

Depresses chemoreceptor trigger zone
Contains antihistaminic, anticholinergic, and sedative properties
IM route preferred (best when given 15 minutes before emergence)
IM onset within 15 minutes, peaks within 30 minutes, duration 3 to 4 hours
IV route may cause hypertension, dysrhythmias, and ↑ respiratory rate
Dose—50 mg IM (if given IV 25 mg)
Metabolized in the liver
Not to be used with children

Droperidol (Inapsine)

Antiemetic, neuroleptic
Antagonizes emetic effects of morphine-like analgesics
Mild alpha-adrenergic blocking effects
Vasodilator→hypotension, tachycardia
May cause drowsiness
IV onset within 3 to 10 minutes, peaks within 30 minutes, duration 3 to 6 hours
IV dose 0.625 to 2.5 mg (IM dose 5 mg); pediatric dose 25 μg/kg
Metabolized by the liver

Metoclopramide hydrochloride (Reglan)

GI stimulant, dopamine antagonist, ↑ gastric emptying
Commonly used with outpatients as drug has few side effects in clinically used doses
Large ratio between therapeutic and toxic effects
IV onset 1 to 3 minutes, duration 1 to 2 hours; IV dose 10 mg
IM onset 10 to 15 minutes, duration 1 to 2 hours; IM dose 5 to 20 mg
Metabolized by the liver

Prochlorperazine (Compazine)

Antiemetic, antipsychotic, neuroleptic
Control of severe nausea and vomiting
Depresses cough reflex—patient must be watched to prevent aspiration
IM route preferred, IV route may cause hypotension
IM dose 5 to 10 mg; PR dose 25 mg
Pediatric dose 0.13 mg/kg IM or 0.4 mg/kg PR
Drug effects may last 12 hours

Trimethobenzamide hydrochloride (Tigan)

Depresses chemoreceptor trigger zone
Sedative, weak antihistaminic effects
IM route onset within 15 minutes, duration 2 to 3 hours
Important to restore hydration and electrolytes as adjunct to therapy
Patient should be monitored for hypotension
IM and PR dose 200 mg
Pediatric dose 4 mg/kg

From Litwack K and Parnass S: Practical points in the management of postoperative nausea and vomiting, Post Anesth Nurs 3(4):275-277, 1988.

Table 7-3. **Estimated fluid and blood requirements***

	Class I	Class II	Class III	Class IV
Blood loss (ml)	Up to 750	750-1500	1500-2000	2000 or more
Blood loss (%BV)	Up to 15%	15%-30%	30%-40%	40% or more
Pulse rate	<100	>100	>120	140 or higher
Blood pressure	Normal	Normal	Decreased	Decreased
Pulse pressure (mm Hg)	Normal or increased	Decreased	Decreased	Decreased
Capillary refill test	Normal	Positive	Positive	Positive
Respiratory rate	14-20	20-30	30-40	>35
Urine output (ml/hr)	30 or more	20-30	5-15	Negligible
CNS—mental status	Slightly anxious	Mildly anxious	Anxious and confused	Confused or lethargic
Fluid replacement (3:1 rule)	Crystalloid	Crystalloid	Crystalloid + blood	Crystalloid + blood

From American College of Surgeons, Committee on Trauma: Advanced Trauma Life Support Student Manual, Chicago, 1984, The College.
*These guidelines are based on the initial presentation of a 70 kg male and on the "three-for-one" rule. This rule derives from the empiric observation that most patients in hemorrhagic shock will require as much as 300 ml of electrolyte solution for each 100 ml of blood loss.

The PACU nurse always has the option of saving saturated sponges for the physician to make an independent judgment.

When evaluating blood loss, the difficulty is in the determination of how much blood is too much blood. The decision to return a patient to the operating room for surgical repair of bleeding vessels will depend on knowledge of the procedure and expected postoperative blood loss, the amount of blood loss actually occurring, the rate of blood loss (steady or tapering off), the patient's stability, and the likelihood of a successful outcome. For example, a "status post coronary artery bypass graft" patient who is steadily bleeding 400 to 500 ml per hour for 3 hours and who has a blood pressure of 80 is likely to be returned to the operating room. A patient who is saturating 2 to 3 gauze sponges per hour after a difficult cleft lip repair might not be returned to the operating room, because further exploration of the lip might result in such swelling that the surgeon feels reclosure of the lip might not be possible. Hemostasis is instead achieved with external pressure and ice (vasoconstriction).

In addition to surgical repair of bleeding vessels, treatment of symptomatic blood loss will include fluid (volume) replacement. A hemoglobin of less than 10 g/dl is considered to be the "transfusion trigger" used by most physicians. Patients may be transfused with whole blood or packed red blood cells.

Whole blood is indicated for patients in hypovolemic shock who require volume replacement. Whole blood provides patients with red blood cells, white blood cells, and plasma. If the unit has not been stored in the blood bank for more than 2 days, it will also contain platelets and clotting factors. The usual unit of whole blood provides approximately 500 ml of volume and a hematocrit of 35% to 40%.

Most transfusions given today are in the form of packed red blood cells. Packed red blood cells contain the same amount of hemoglobin as whole blood, but because the plasma has been removed, the volume is lower. Packed red blood cells are indicated to correct red blood cell deficiencies (anemias) and to improve the oxygen-carrying capacity of blood. The use of packed red blood cells also reduces the potential hazard of circulatory overload and excessive electrolyte and metabolic loads (that is, increased potassium and ammonium from stored blood). Packed red blood cells increase volume by 250 to 300 ml.

Bleeding from the surgical site is seldom fatal if the culprit vessels are appropriately repaired and volume losses are promptly replaced.

Blood transfusions are not benign events, despite the frequency with which they are administered. Complications associated with transfusion therapy include transfusion reactions, metabolic abnormalities, transmission of disease, and infusion of microaggregates. The cause, symptoms, incidence, and treatment of transfusion reactions are highlighted in the box below.

Metabolic abnormalities that occur after blood administration are related to changes that occur during the storage of blood. Hydrogen ions, carbon dioxide, and potassium increase; erythrocyte concentrations of 2,3-diphosphoglycerate decrease. (The reader is reminded that 2,3-diphosphoglycerate influences oxyhemoglobin binding and dissociation). The citrate used as a preservative may contribute to the development of metabolic alkalosis as citrate binds to calcium.

TRANSFUSION REACTIONS

Allergic	Caused by reaction to incompatible plasma proteins in correctly typed and crossmatched blood
	Manifested by pruritis, erythema, urticaria, and laryngospasm if severe
	Occurs in 3% of patients
	Treatment—diphenhydramine (Benadryl); stop transfusion
Febrile	Caused by interaction of recipient antibodies to donor antigens on leukocytes or platelets
	Manifested by increased temperature, headache, nausea, and vomiting
	Occurs in 0.5% to 10% of all transfusions
	Treatment—slow transfusions, acetaminophen (Tylenol); stop transfusion if severe
Hemolytic	Caused by tranfusion of incompatible blood (mismatched)
	Manifested by chest or back pain, fever, dyspnea, hypotension, and evidence of hemolysis
	Most common cause of transfusion reactions
	Treatment—stop transfusion, maintain renal function with fluids and diuretics, send patient and donor blood samples to blood bank

Transmission of viral diseases, specifically hepatitis and human immunodeficiency virus (AIDS), is a major hazard of transfusion therapy. Other viruses, including cytomegalovirus (CMV) and Epstein-Barr virus (EBV), can also be transmitted via blood products. This fear of disease transmission has contributed to blood shortages, to an increase in autologous and designated donor donations, and to the institution of universal body fluid precautions.

Blood shortages are occurring because of a mistaken perception that people can get hepatitis or AIDS from donating blood. Public information campaigns are underway to confront this misconception. Patients are also donating blood for themselves to guarantee blood availability and to avoid the risk of disease transmission (autologous donation).

Autologous donation of blood eliminates the risk of disease transmission and of sensitivity reactions. It is the safest form of transfusion. Patients may donate one unit of blood every 3 to 7 days, up to 72 hours before surgery. Because of the frequency of donation, patients are usually given ferrous sulfate (iron) supplementation.

Designated donors are usually friends or relatives who donate a unit of blood for a patient. Ideally the person is known (or believed) to be free of disease, although there is no evidence available that supports the efficacy of designated donation in reducing the risk of disease transmission.

Health care providers who administer blood products should take care to protect themselves from contact with those products. The implementation of universal body fluid precautions applies to the patient receiving the blood and to contact with donor blood products. The wearing of gloves is mandatory when administering blood products.

The infusion of microaggregates is also of concern. During storage of blood, platelets and leukocytes form microaggregates. The number of microaggregates becomes significant after 3 to 5 days. For example, one unit of blood stored for 21 days may have anywhere from 50 to 100 million microaggregates, ranging in size from 10 to 170 μ. Microaggregates can cause pulmonary vascular obstruction, pulmonary edema, and disseminated intravascular coagulation. As a result, blood products are usually administered through a microaggregate or micropore filter.

Bleeding resulting from alterations in coagulation

If surgical integrity is intact, an alteration in coagulation should be suspected. Understanding normal clotting mechanisms facilitates the management of patients with defects in coagulation.

The process of coagulation is considered to consist of three interrelated phases: vascular spasm, platelet aggregation, and coagulation. When a blood vessel is severed, hemostasis is achieved via the interaction of each phase of coagulation.

Vascular phase. The vascular phase in coagulation is characterized by vasoconstriction in the area of the break in the vessel. Vasoconstriction occurs as a result of sympathetic stimulation and spasm of vascular smooth muscle. If the vessel broken is small, vasoconstriction alone may be sufficient to achieve hemostasis.

Platelet aggregation. The platelet phase of coagulation is initiated when circulating platelets are exposed to endothelial tissue on the wall of the broken blood vessel. Platelets adhere to collagen within the vessel's walls, coalescing to form a platelet plug. This platelet plug contributes to hemostasis and to clot formation.

Platelet aggregation depends on normal platelet levels (a mean value of $250,000/mm^3$). Platelet levels will be decreased in patients who have received multiple transfusions, who are on aspirin or nonsteroidal antiinflammatory therapy, or who have leukemias. Patients with too few platelets (thrombocytopenia) or with platelets that function poorly may have oozing from surgical and venipuncture sites.

Although patients may receive platelets when they receive a transfusion of fresh, whole blood, platelet concentrate is an additional component that may be administered. Platelets are indicated in patients with thrombocytopenia, to treat bleeding associated with abnormally functioning platelets, or they may be given prophylactically to patients with rapidly falling or low platelet levels (less than $25,000$ mm^3). One unit of platelets is required to raise a platelet count by 5000 to $10,000$ mm^3. Usually six to ten units are given. Platelet administration is associated with a high incidence of febrile transfusion reactions, and, as a result, patients are usually premedicated with antihistamines (diphenhydramine) and acetaminophen prior to transfusion.

Coagulation. Coagulation is a biochemical process whereby fibrinogen is converted to fibrin, the end product of coagulation. The formation of a fibrin clot is the third mechanism of hemostasis. Coagulation, or the "clotting cascade," can be initiated by either the intrinsic or extrinsic pathway. The intrinsic pathway is stimulated as a result of endothelial injury, whereby collagen in the vascular wall is exposed to clotting factors within blood. The extrinsic pathway is stimulated when blood comes in contact with a damaged vascular wall or extravascular tissue. Roman numerals are used to represent the clotting factors in the coagulation process (Fig. 7-5).

Deficiencies in the clotting factors result in disruption of the clotting mechanism and present clinically as hemophilia. Coagulation disorders in the PACU are usually caused by the patient's exposure to heparin or warfarin (Coumadin).

Heparin is an anticoagulant that may be given to patients preoperatively and postoperatively as prophylaxis against deep venous thrombosis and pulmonary embolism, particularly in obese and bedridden patients. Heparin may also be given intraoperatively to provide anticoagulation during operative procedures, particularly vascular surgeries. Heparin neutralizes thrombin activity, preventing the conversion of fibrinogen to fibrin.

The clinical effects of heparin are monitored by the partial thromboplastin time (PTT) and the activated clotting time (ACT), both of which are tests of the intrinsic pathway of coagulation. The anticoagulant effects of heparin may be antagonized by the administration of protamine. Protamine combines with heparin to form a complex devoid of anticoagulant activity.

Warfarin (Coumadin) is an oral anticoagulant that may be given to patients to reduce the incidence of thromboembolism associated with artificial heart valves and to prevent deep vein thrombus formation. Warfarin interferes with vitamin K–dependent clotting

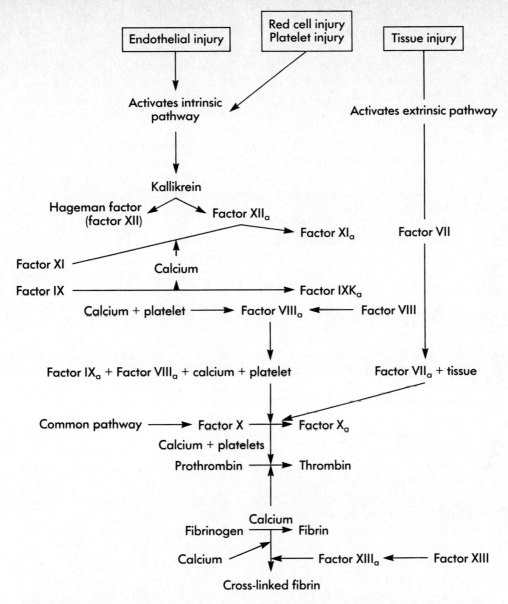

FIG. 7-5. Diagram of the coagulation cascade. Roman numerals with the subscript letter *a* indicate the activated factors. (From Abels L; Critical care nursing: a physiologic approach, St. Louis, 1986, The CV Mosby Co.)

factors in the liver (specifically factors II, VII, IX, and X). The clinical effects of warfarin therapy are monitored by the prothrombin time (PT), a test of the extrinsic pathway of coagulation.

For major surgical procedures, oral anticoagulants are generally discontinued for 1 to 3 days preoperatively to allow coagulation times to approach normal. In an emergent situation where this is not possible, intravenous administration of vitamin K, fresh whole blood, or fresh, frozen plasma may be effective in counteracting the anticoagulant effect of warfarin.

Vitamin K is administered to treat deficiencies in plasma concentrations of prothrombin and related clotting factors. Fresh whole blood contains clotting factors. Fresh, frozen plasma (FFP) is the liquid component of whole blood, separated and frozen within 6 hours of collection. Fresh, frozen plasma contains albumin, globulins, coagulation factors, water, and electrolytes. It is a source of plasma proteins, coagulation factors, and fibrinogen. Usually two to four units of fresh, frozen plasma are given to restore depressed coagulation factors or platelets; a rule of thumb is that for every four to five units of blood given, one unit of fresh, frozen plasma will be given to replace coagulation factors. For every 10 units of blood given, 10 to 12 units of platelets will be given.

Disseminated intravascular coagulation

Disseminated intravascular coagulation (DIC) is a common cause of an acquired bleeding tendency, characterized by widespread activation of the coagulation process. DIC usually occurs as a complication of a surgical, obstetric, or traumatic event that allows thromboembolic materials to enter the circulation. These events include generalized sepsis with release of bacterial endotoxins, hemolytic transfusion reactions, amniotic fluid embolism, and tissue necrosis (for example, burns).

As thromboembolic materials are released, the normal physiologic processes of coagulation are initiated, and generalized fibrin deposits develop (the end product of coagulation). After 24 to 48 hours, normal processes of clot resolution are initiated via the conversion of plasminogen to plasmin. Plasmin causes fibrinolysis by enzymatically breaking down fibrin into fibrin split products (FSP). The fibrin split products interfere with platelet aggregation, thereby exerting an anticoagulant effect.

With DIC there is an uncontrolled and excessive formation of thrombin, causing diffuse intravascular coagulation, particularly within microcirculation. Coagulation proteins and platelets are consumed, resulting in severe depletion of factors VIII and V, platelets, and fibrinogen. Spontaneous hemorrhage is common.

Unfortunately, because DIC usually occurs in a state of circulatory failure, shock, hypovolemia, and/or increased vascular permeability, management is difficult. The most effective therapy must be directed toward correction of the initiating event, ongoing cardiovascular support, and administration of platelet concentrates and fresh, frozen plasma. Morbidity and mortality remain high.

COMPLICATIONS OF POSITIONING

The positioning of a patient during surgery is designed to maximize accessibility of the surgical site. Unfortunately, the positioning of the patient may compromise physiologic stability intraoperatively and may influence postoperative care in the PACU. It is the purpose of this section to identify the most commonly used positions, their indications for use, and their impact on intraoperative management and postoperative care. Each position causes a redistribution of body weight and alterations in circulation tissue perfusion and alveolar ventilation. The goals of positioning a patient include the following:

1. Maximizing exposure to the operative site
2. Maintaining patient accessibility for induction
3. Minimizing circulatory compromise
4. Protecting the patient from nerve injury
5. Maintaining maximum respiratory function
6. Providing the patient with minimum exposure

Supine position

In the supine position (Fig. 7-6), patients are placed flat on their back, with their arms at their sides and their palms down; their legs are straight and their feet are slightly separated. This position is commonly used for abdominal, mediastinal, and cardiac surgery.

Modifications of this position include a contoured supine position (back flat, thighs flexed 15 degrees on the trunk, knees flexed 15 degrees in the opposite direction), scultetus position (10 to 15 degrees Trendelenburg), sitting position (upright), and lithotomy position. The sitting position and lithotomy position are described in the next section.

The supine position offers the greatest degree of patient stability, surgical accessibility, and patient safety of all positions. However, there are potential intraoperative and postoperative complications that may result.

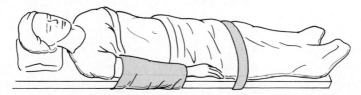

FIG. 7-6. Supine position. (From Phipps W et al: Medical-surgical nursing: concepts and clinical practice, St. Louis, 1987, The CV Mosby Co.)

Intraoperatively. Although most patients will tolerate this position with little cardiac or respiratory compromise, the obese patient or any patient with an intraabdominal growth (tumor, developing fetus) may have supine occlusion of the inferior vena cava, causing hypotension. Placement of a towel roll under the right lower back and hip will cause a left lateral displacement and correct caval occlusion.

Obese patients and patients with large intraabdominal masses may have respiratory difficulties as the weight of abdominal contents forces the diaphragm upward, limiting respiratory excursion and reducing functional residual capacity (FRC). The patient will probably require controlled ventilation to maximize oxygenation and gas exchange. Elevating the head of the operating table will help to displace abdominal contents from the thorax; however, surgical accessibility may be compromised.

Postoperatively. Complications reported from problems with supine positioning include postural hypotension, pressure alopecia, pressure point compression, nerve injuries, and backache. Although these complications are the direct result of positioning difficulties, they are often not detected until the patient awakens in the PACU.

Postural hypotension. Although the horizontal supine position is associated with little alteration in vascular tone, elevations of the head (reverse Trendelenburg, sitting position), may result in venous pooling and inadequate central perfusion. A mean arterial pressure of 60 mm Hg is required to maintain central perfusion. In the presence of hypovolemia, fluid therapy may be all that is indicated to treat the hypotension. If the hypotension is more severe, vasopressors may be required. If problems with hypotension occurred intraoperatively, the PACU should monitor vital signs and assess neurologic functioning as an indicator of perfusion. Awareness of the problem may help to explain higher than expected intraoperative fluid totals and use of the vasopressors ephedrine and phenylephrine (Neo-Synephrine).

Pressure alopecia. Prolonged compression secondary to impaired perfusion of hair follicles may produce hair loss (alopecia). Rarely detected in the PACU, alopecia usually becomes apparent between the third and twenty-eighth postoperative day. Hair growth usually recurs by 3 months. Use of a padded head support intraoperatively and postoperatively can decrease the risk of pressure-related alopecia.

Pressure point compression. Unless proper padding is applied to bony prominences (elbows, shoulders, heels, sacrum), ischemic necrosis of compromised tissues may occur. Protection of bony prominences is especially important if the patient is extremely thin or if the surgery is expected to take several hours. The PACU nurse should inspect pressure points on admission to the PACU, maintaining protection of these sites as indicated and documenting any areas of redness, tenderness, or edema.

Nerve injuries. Unless care is taken in positioning the extremities, damage may occur to nerves. In some cases, nerve damage caused by intraoperative positioning results in permanent injury. Attention should be given to both restraint and support of the extremities. It is important for intraoperative care-givers to maintain anatomic alignment of the extremities, avoiding extremes in abduction, adduction, flexion, and extension. Damage has been documented to the brachial plexus (from tight shoulder braces), subclavian neurovascular bundle (from nerve compression between the clavicle and first rib), axillary neurovascular bundle (from excessive abduction of the arm), radial nerve (from excessive pressure against the lateral arm), and ulnar nerve (from extreme elbow flexion with the forearm across the trunk).

Postoperatively, any report of extremity paresthesia (numbness), loss of sensation, and impaired mobility (wrist drop) should be promptly reported to the anesthesiologist and documented.

Backache. Placing a patient in a horizontal supine position alters the normal curvature of the lumbar spine. Placing a towel roll or several folded towels under the lumbar spine will help to restore the normal curvature. Postoperatively, complaints of backache will be treated symptomatically, with repositioning, support, medications, and heat.

Lithotomy

The lithotomy position (Fig. 7-7) is a modification of the supine position. In the lithotomy position, the patient lies on his or her back with the buttocks at the end of the table. The thighs and legs are flexed simultaneously into stirrups. The arms are crossed across the abdomen or extended laterally on arm boards. This position is used for gynecologic, urologic, perineal, and perianal surgeries.

Intraoperatively. As the legs are flexed back against the abdomen, intraabdominal contents are forced against the diaphragm by the thighs. Intrathoracic pressure is increased, with a decrease in functional residual capacity. Ventilation is usually controlled.

Hypotension may occur after surgery when the patient's legs are lowered to the table. To decrease sudden hypotension as the vascular volume returns to the lower extremities, the legs should first be returned to the sagittal plane and then slowly lowered to baseline.

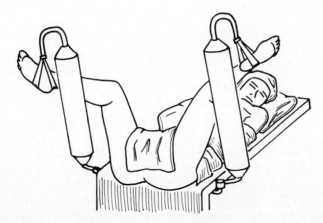

FIG. 7-7. Lithotomy position. (From Phipps W et al: Medical-surgical nursing: concepts and clinical practice, St. Louis, 1987, The CV Mosby Co.)

Postoperatively. Postoperative complications of the lithotomy position include those of the supine position plus lumbar distress. Because of the pressure placed against the lumbar spine in positioning the patient in lithotomy, the patient may complain of lower back pain. Treatment is usually symptomatic.

Sitting position

The sitting position is most commonly used for neurosurgery and exists as a variation of the supine position. In this position the patient may be sitting upright or semireclining with the legs elevated to the level of the heart. The head is secured ventrally on the neck by a face rest or a skull-fixation frame.

Intraoperatively. Hypotension is perhaps the major sequelae of the sitting position as blood shifts downward from the upper body. Cardiac output may decrease 20% to 40%. Compensatory tachycardia may result in a 30% increase in heart rate. Systemic vascular resistance increases 30% to 60% as the body attempts to maintain a mean arterial pressure of greater than 60 mm Hg.

Respiratory effort is maximally enhanced by this position, as respiratory excursion remains uncompromised by any abdominal pressure.

Postoperatively. Complications that have been reported from the use of the sitting position include postural hypotension, air embolism, facial edema, and airway edema.

Postural hypotension. The occurrence of intraoperative hypotension may be treated with fluids, vasopressors, and reduction of anesthetic concentration. The PACU nurse should inquire about the occurrence of intraoperative hypotension and of any interventions required. Once normal positioning is restored, blood pressure should stabilize, requiring no further intervention.

Air embolism. Whenever an open vein exists above the level of the heart (as occurs in the sitting position), the potential for air to enter the vessel exists. If air gets into circulation, (1) it may move through the heart, causing irritability, and (2) it may ultimately enter the pulmonary vasculature, compromising gas exchange. Air embolization is potentially fatal.

To prevent and protect against air embolization, care must be taken by the neurosurgeons to prevent air entrainment. Monitoring by the anesthesia team will include observing and auscultating for a cardiac murmur, change in heart sounds via Doppler, dysrhythmias, hypotension, and a decrease in end tidal carbon dioxide levels. Venous air embolism may be treated by causing vein "bleed-back" to evacuate the air, by applying positive end expiratory pressure (PEEP), or by the use of fluid and vasopressors to increase cardiac output.

If the occurrence of a venous air embolism is suspected to have occurred, the patient should be monitored postoperatively for any changes in neurologic and pulmonary function. Most neurosurgeons and anesthesiologists prefer to have their patients awake and extubated at the end of the case to evaluate neurologic functioning. Inability to extubate because of pulmonary dysfunction will require careful attention on the part of the PACU nurse to the patient's oxygenation and ventilation (breath sounds, arterial blood gases, oxygen saturation).

Facial and airway edema. When the patient is in the sitting position, the neck is forced into flexion onto the chest. Postoperatively, there have been reports of edema of the face, tongue, and neck from venous and lymphatic obstruction.[31] The PACU nurse should be alert for any airway swelling or respiratory compromise that may occur after extubation. In extreme cases a tracheostomy is required to provide airway access.[13]

Prone position

In the prone position (Fig. 7-8), the patient lies on his or her abdomen with the face turned toward one side. The arms are positioned at the sides, and the palms are up; the elbows are slightly flexed, and the feet are elevated slightly on a pillow to prevent plantar flexion. The prone position is most commonly used for procedures of the back, spine, and rectal area.

Modifications of this position include a prone jackknife (where the thighs are flexed on the trunk) and the kneeling position (where the patient is flexed at the hips and knees and supported on a kneeling frame).

Intraoperatively. The primary intraoperative alteration is chest and abdominal compression from the body weight of the anesthetized patient. Respiratory excursion is reduced as is movement of the diaphragm. Ventilation must be controlled.

If the prone position is modified to the kneeling position, venous pooling in the legs can become significant. The weight of the body also causes a fall in stroke volume and cardiac index. Because of the increased vascular resistance, little change is noted in the mean arterial pressure, central venous pressure, or pulmonary artery pressure.

Postoperatively. Complications reported to result from problems with prone positioning include eye abrasion, ear compression, neck pain, nerve injuries, and joint damage. Although these complications are the direct result of positioning difficulties, they are frequently not diagnosed or detected until the patient is admitted to the PACU.

Eye abrasion. When the patient is in the prone position, it is important for the eyes to be lubricated and covered to protect them from accidental abrasion. It is also important to confirm that ECG leads and intravenous tubing are not lying under or near the eye. Postoperatively, the patient may complain of eye pain, and the eye may be red and weepy. The anesthesiologist should be notified, and the patient should be evaluated for a corneal abrasion. This usually involves an ophthalmology consult, the use of fluorescein dye, and an ophthalmoscope. If present, a corneal abrasion is usually treated with topical antibiotics and a sterile dressing.

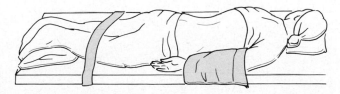

FIG. 7-8. Prone position. (From Phipps W et al: Medical-surgical nursing: concepts and clinical practice, St. Louis, 1987, The CV Mosby Co.)

Ear compression. When the patient is moved into the prone position, soft padding should be placed around the dependent ear, and the placement of the ear should be carefully checked. If the ear lies unprotected or bent, cartilaginous injury may occur.

Neck pain. Positioning a patient in the prone position with the head rotated laterally can stretch skeletal muscles and ligaments, injuring cervical articulations. Postoperatively, the patient may complain of neck pain and limitation of motion. Treatment is usually symptomatic.

Nerve injury. Damage has been reported to the brachial plexus (secondary to stretch injury of the nerve roots) and to the subclavian vessels (thoracic outlet syndrome as the nerves are compressed near the first rib). Patients may complain of arm pain, paresthesias, and compromised mobility.

Joint damage. Care must be taken when positioning patients in the prone position. Patients are anesthetized in the supine position and turned prone. The spine must be adequately supported during turning to avoid sudden shifts of posture. If the patient is also placed in a kneeling position, care should be taken to protect the knees with padding, particularly if the patient is obese.

Lateral position

In the lateral position (Fig. 7-9), the patient is positioned on his or her side. This position is usually used for renal surgery (nephrectomy).

Intraoperatively. The major problems with the lateral position include venous pooling of the dependent extremities and ventilation-perfusion mismatch (V-Q). These problems occur because the dependent lung is well perfused but poorly ventilated and the upper lung is well ventilated but not as well perfused. Venous pooling can be prevented with the use of compression stockings. Ventilation problems may be minimized with the use of controlled, positive pressure ventilation.

Postoperatively. Complications associated with this position include eye abrasion, ear compression, neck pain, nerve injury, and atelectasis. The mechanisms causing eye

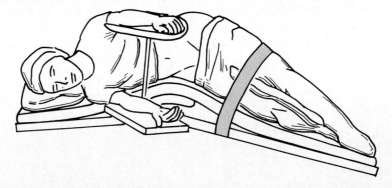

FIG. 7-9. Lateral position. (From Phipps W et al: Medical-surgical nursing: concepts and clinical practice, St. Louis, 1987, The CV Mosby Co.)

abrasion, ear compression, and neck pain are similar to those occurring in the prone position.

Nerve injuries center on the suprascapular nerve. The positioning of the dependent shoulder can result in a stretching of the suprascapular nerve. Postoperatively, patients may complain of diffuse, dull shoulder pain. Prevention calls for placing a pad under the thorax, with the goal of raising the chest off of the shoulder. Treatment may require surgery to decompress the nerve.

Atelectasis is the result of the inability of the dependent lung to expand. It is not a complication of lateral positioning, but an expected outcome. Postoperatively, the PACU nurse should carefully auscultate breath sounds bilaterally, comparing the dependent lung with the operative-side lung. Deep breathing should be promoted to encourage expansion.

SUMMARY

Although the PACU nurse has no control over patient positioning in the operating room, the complications of surgical positioning may not be diagnosed or suspected until the patient awakens in the PACU. Knowledge of potential complications associated with the various surgical positions (Table 7-4) will allow the PACU nurse to expand the postoperative surgical assessment to evaluate for the presence of these complications and to understand the rationale for intraoperative actions (for example, medications and fluid therapy).

Table 7-4.   **Complications of surgical positioning**

Position	Common complications
Supine	Postural hypotension
	Pressure alopecia
	Pressure joint compression
	Nerve injuries
	Backache
Lithotomy (exaggerated supine)	Lumbar distress
Sitting (head elevated)	Postural hypotension
Prone	Eye abrasion
	Ear compression
	Neck pain
	Nerve injury
	Joint damage
Lateral	Eye abrasion
	Ear compression
	Neck pain
	Nerve injury
	Atelectasis

REFERENCES

1. Abels L: Critical care nursing: a physiologic approach, St Louis, 1986, The CV Mosby Co.
2. Ackley RE: A comparison of the incidence of perioperative hypothermia and postoperative confusion in the elderly and younger perioperative patients, Masters Degree Thesis, University of Kansas, School of Nursing 1985.
3. Altsberger D and Shrewsbury P: Postoperative pain management: the PACU nurse's challenge, J Post Anesth Nurs 3(6):399-403, 1988.
4. American College of Surgeons: Advanced trauma life support manual, Chicago, 1984, The College.
5. Anderson R and Krogh K: Pain as a major source of postoperative nausea, Can Anaesth Soc J 23:366, 1976.
6. Bonica JJ et al: Postoperative nausea, retching and vomiting, Anesthesiol 19:532-540, 1958.
7. Bourke D, Wurm H, Rosenberge M, and Russell S: Intraoperative heat conservation using a reflective blanket, Anesthesiol 60:151-154, 1984.
8. Buckler HW: Prophylaxis of postanesthetic vomiting, Am J Surg Q (Anesth Analg suppl) Oct 1914, p 13.
9. Chernow B and Lake C: The pharmacologic approach to the critically ill patient, Baltimore, 1983, Williams & Wilkins.
10. Committee on Component Therapy: Circular of information for use of blood and blood components, Washington, DC, 1986, American Association of Blood Banks.
11. Cousins M and Phillips G: Acute pain management, New York, 1986, Churchill-Livingstone.
12. Dodson M: The management of postoperative pain, London, 1985, Edward Arnold Publishers.
13. Ellis S, Bryan-Brown C, and Hyderally H: Massive swelling of the head and neck, Anesthesiology 42:102, 1975.
14. Estafanous F: Opioids in anesthesia, Boston, 1984, Butterworth Publishers.
15. Glass D: Blood coagulation, coagulopathies and anticoagulation therapy, ASA Refresher Course Lectures pp 1-6, 1985.
16. Greig J: Intraoperative nursing. In Phipps W, Long B, and Woods N (editors): Medical-surgical nursing, ed 3, St Louis, 1987, The CV Mosby Co, pp 463-487.
17. Hardy EB, Cirillo BL, and Gutzeit MN: Rewarming patients in the PACU: can we make a difference? J Post Anesth Nurs 3:313-316, 1988.
18. Harmer M, Rosen M, and Vickers M: Patient-controlled analgesia, Oxford, 1985, Blackwell-Scientific.
19. Haumann J and Foster P: The antiemetic effect of halothane, Br J Anaesth 35:114-117, 1963.
20. Henneberg S et al: Effects of a thermal ceiling on postoperative hypothermia, Acta Anesth Scand 29:602-606, 1985.
21. Hill C and Fields W (editors): Advances in pain research and therapy, New York, 1989, Raven Press.
22. Holahan JR: Coagulopathies. In Decision-making in anesthesiology, Philadelphia, 1987, Decker, pp 236-237.
23. Kirby R: Current concepts in hemorrhagic shock, Curr Rev Recov Room Nurse 8(6):42-47, 1986.
24. Kucha DH, Nichols GA, Christ NM, and Bynum JW: The warming of postoperative patients, Milit Med 139:388-390, 1974.
25. Laws H: Assessment and management of postoperative hemorrhage, Curr Rev Recov Room Nurse 1(22):171-175, 1980.
26. Lilly R: Inadvertent hypothermia: a real problem, ASA Refresher Courses in Anesthesiol 15(8):93-107, 1987.
27. Litwack K and Parnass S: Practical points in the management of postoperative nausea and vomiting, J Post Anesth Nurs 3:275-277, 1988.

28. Litwack K: Practical points in the management of hypothermia, J Post Anesth Nurs 3(5):339-341, 1988.
29. Litwack, K: Practical points for transfusion therapy, J Post Anesth Nurs 2(4):257-261, 1987.
30. Martin J: Positioning in anesthesia and surgery, Philadelphia, 1987, WB Saunders Co.
31. McAllister R: Macroglossia-A positional complication, Anesthesiology 40:199, 1974.
32. McCaffery M and Beebe A: Pain: clinical manual for nursing practice, St Louis, 1989, The CV Mosby Co.
33. McCaffery M: Nursing management of the patient with pain, ed 2, Philadelphia, 1979, JB Lippincott Co.
34. McNiece WL: Disorders of coagulation. In Anesthesia and Co-existing Disease, New York, 1983, Churchill-Livingstone, pp 541-551.
35. Meinhart N and McCaffery M: Pain: a nursing approach to assessment and analysis, Norwalk, Conn, 1983, Appleton-Century-Crofts.
36. Merskey C: DIC: identification and management, Hosp Pract 17(12):83-94, 1982.
37. Morris RH and Kumar A: The effect of warming blankets on maintenance of body temperature of the anesthetized, paralyzed adult patient, Anesthesiol 36:408-411, 1972.
38. Morrison R: Hypothermia in the elderly, Int Anesthesiol Clin 26(2):124-133, 1988..
39. Muir JJ, Warner MA, and Offord K: Role of nitrous oxide and other factors in postoperative nausea and vomiting: a randomized and blinded prospective study, Anesthesiol 66:513-518, 1987.
40. Ordog G, Wasserberger J, and Balasubramanium S: Coagulation abnormalities in traumatic shock, Ann Emerg Med 14(3):650-655, 1985.
41. Parnass S: Nausea and vomiting in the PACU, Curr Rev Post Anesth Care Nurse 10(20):155-159, 1988.
42. Perry S: The undermedication of pain, Psychiatr Ann 14:11, 1984.
43. Puntillo K: The phenomenon of pain and critical care nursing, Heart Lung 17(3):262-271, 1988.
44. Quimby C and Bailey M: Anesthesia recovery care, New York, 1986, Igaku-Shoin Medical Publishers, Inc.
45. Siskind J: Handling hemorrage wisely, Nursing '84 14(1):34-41, 1984.
46. Smessaert A, Schehr C, and Artusio J: Nausea and vomiting in the immediate postanesthetic period, JAMA 170:2072-2076, 1959.
47. Stoelting R: Blood components and substitutes. In Pharmacology and physiology in anesthetic practice, Philadelphia, 1987, JB Lippincott Co, pp 546-554.
48. Stoelting R: Hemostasis and blood coagulation. In Pharmacology and physiology in anesthetic practice, Philadelphia, 1987, JB Lippincott Co, pp 814-818.
49. Stoelting R: Pharmacology and physiology in anesthesia practice, Philadelphia, 1987, JB Lippincott Co.
50. Swenson E and Orkin F: Postoperative nausea and vomiting. In Orkin F and Cooperman L (editors): Complications in anesthesiology, Philadelphia, 1983, JB Lippincott Co, pp 429-435.
51. Vaughan MS, Vaughan RW, and Cork RC: Postoperative hypothermia in adults: relationship of age, anesthesia and shivering to rewarming, Anesth Analg 60:746-751, 1981.
52. Vaughn MS: Shivering in the recovery room, Curr Rev RR Nurse 6:2-7, 1984.
53. Watchler B: Anesthesia for ambulatory surgery, Philadelphia, 1985, JB Lippincott Co.

Review Questions

1. *Pain is operationally defined as* _____.
   a. Behavioral signs of crying and restlessness
   b. Whatever the experiencing person says it is
   c. Objective displays of discomfort
   d. Psychosomatic manifestations of distress
2. *Which of the following is a subjective assessment criteria of pain?*
   a. Tears
   b. Guarding behavior
   c. Splinting
   d. Patient report of pain
3. *Pain assessment tools* _____.
   a. Are too complex to use in the immediate postoperative period
   b. Should only be used by advanced pain management specialists
   c. Require patients to be awake, alert, and verbal
   d. Provide objective confirmation of a subjective phenomenon
4. *An example of a nonpharmacologic intervention for pain is* _____.
   a. Relaxation breathing
   b. Morphine sulfate
   c. Acetaminophen with codeine
   d. Ibuprofen
5. *The patient most likely to benefit from TENS therapy is* _____.
   a. A 4-year-old boy recovering from circumcision
   b. An 80-year-old woman with organic brain syndrome recovering from total hip arthroplasty
   c. A 28-year-old woman who has just had a caesarean section
   d. A 27-year-old man admitted through the emergency room for multiple fracture repairs
6. *Which of the following is an example of an agonist-antagonist used to treat pain?*
   a. Acetaminophen (Tylenol)
   b. Butorphanol (Stadol)
   c. Methadone (Dolophine)
   d. Hydromorphone (Dilaudid)
7. *A warm surface losing heat via direct contact to a cooler surface is an example of* _____.
   a. Conduction
   b. Evaporation
   c. Radiation
   d. Convection
8. *Which of the following statements is FALSE?*
   a. Hypothermia develops when heat loss exceeds heat production
   b. Hypothermia causes the oxyhemoglobin curve to shift to the left
   c. Hypothermia is never desirable
   d. Hypothermia slows metabolically-dependent processes

9. *Hypothermia is defined as a core body temperature of less than* _____.
    a. 36° C
    b. 35° C
    c. 34° C
    d. 33° C

10. *Which of the following is not a site that reflects central (core) temperature?*
    a. Tympanic membrane
    b. Nasopharynx
    c. Pulmonary artery
    d. Rectum

11. *The intoxicated individual is likely to be* _____.
    a. Hyperthermic because of vasodilation
    b. Hypothermic because of vasodilation
    c. Hyperthermic because of vasoconstriction
    d. Hypothermic because of vasoconstriction

12. *The goal of passive rewarming is to* _____.
    a. Maximize basal heat production
    b. Apply external rewarming techniques
    c. Prevent shivering
    d. Increase oxygen demand

13. *Paradoxical central cooling occurs* _____.
    a. When abdominal viscera are exposed to air
    b. When irrigating solutions are instilled in a body cavity
    c. When cool blood in the periphery is released into central circulation
    d. When active rewarming techniques are ineffective

14. *An example of visceral afferent stimulation that may cause nausea and vomiting is*
    _____.
    a. Hypoxia
    b. Pain
    c. Increased intracranial pressure
    d. Gastrointestinal disease

15. *Narcotics contribute to postoperative nausea and vomiting by* _____.
    a. Inducing sympathetic blockade and medullary ischemia
    b. Causing gastric distention
    c. Directly stimulating the chemoreceptor trigger zone
    d. Increasing anesthesia exposure time

16. *Droperidol (Inapsine) works by* _____.
    a. Increasing gastric emptying
    b. Antagonizing the emetic effects of morphine-like analgesics
    c. Depressing the chemoreceptor trigger zone
    d. Increasing gastric pH

17. *Metoclopramide hydrochloride (Reglan) works by* _____.
    a. Increasing gastric emptying
    b. Antagonizing the emetic effects of morphine-like analgesics
    c. Depressing the chemoreceptor trigger zone
    d. Blocking the stimulation of the vomiting center

18. *A blood loss of* _____ *can produce signs and symptoms of hypovolemic shock in the adult patient.*
    a. 20%
    b. 30%
    c. 40%
    d. 50%

19. *Circulating blood volume in the adult is estimated at* _____.
    a. 15 ml/kg
    b. 45 ml/kg
    c. 75 ml/kg
    d. 95 ml/kg

20. *The most common cause of bleeding in the PACU is* _____.
    a. Heparinization
    b. Alterations in coagulation
    c. Thrombocytopenia
    d. Loss of vascular integrity at the surgical site

21. *The vascular phase of coagulation is characterized by* _____.
    a. Platelet aggregation to the vascular wall
    b. Disruption of vascular integrity
    c. Vasoconstriction in the area of vascular damage
    d. Clot formation at the site of injury

22. *Thrombocytopenia is defined as* _____.
    a. A hemoglobin of less than 10 gm/dl
    b. A platelet deficiency
    c. A hematocrit of 28%
    d. Elevated prothrombin times

23. *The most common type of transfusion reaction is* _____.
    a. Hemolytic
    b. Febrile
    c. Viral
    d. Allergic

24. *The clinical effects of heparin are monitored via the* _____.
    a. Partial thromboplastin time (PTT)
    b. Prothrombin time (PT)
    c. Platelet count
    d. Hemoglobin count

25. *Warfarin (Coumadin) works by* _____.
    a. Neutralizing thrombin activity
    b. Interfering with vitamin K–dependent clotting factors
    c. Blocking platelet formation
    d. Destroying preformed thrombi
26. *Which of the following statements about disseminated intravascular coagulation (DIC) is TRUE?*
    a. The morbidity and mortality associated with DIC is low
    b. DIC occurs when clotting factors are conserved and finally overwhelm the circulatory system
    c. Systemic hypercoagulation ultimately becomes systemic hypocoagulation
    d. DIC can be instantly reversed with protamine administration
27. *In the supine position, the patient is positioned* _____.
    a. Flat on the back
    b. Face down
    c. Flat with thighs and hips flexed into stirrups
    d. Semireclining
28. *Air embolism is a potential complication of which position:*
    a. Lateral
    b. Lithotomy
    c. Prone
    d. Sitting
29. *Atelectasis is a potential complication of which position?*
    a. Prone
    b. Supine
    c. Lithotomy
    d. Lateral
30. *Pressure alopecia is a potential complication of which position?*
    a. Prone
    b. Supine
    c. Sitting
    d. Lateral

Answers

1. b	6. b	11. b	16. b	21. c	26. c
2. d	7. a	12. a	17. a	22. b	27. a
3. d	8. c	13. c	18. a	23. a	28. d
4. a	9. b	14. d	19. c	24. a	29. d
5. c	10. d	15. c	20. d	25. b	30. b

CHAPTER 8

ASPAN has made the statement, "Some must watch while others sleep." The credo stems from the underlying concern that the patient undergoing surgery and experiencing anesthesia is at risk for postoperative and postanesthetic complications. If undetected or unrecognized, the complication can become life threatening.

Common postanesthetic and postoperative emergencies are identified and discussed in this chapter. The discussion of each emergency includes identification of patients at risk, signs and symptoms, treatment, and preventative interventions.

POSTOPERATIVE AND POSTANESTHETIC EMERGENCIES

Chapter Objectives

After reading this chapter, the reader should be able to:

1. Identify common postanesthetic and postoperative emergencies.
2. Identify patients at risk for postoperative and postanesthetic emergencies.
3. Identify clinical signs and symptoms indicative of patient distress.
4. Discuss appropriate treatment interventions for emergency situations.
5. Identify ways to prevent patient emergencies in the PACU.

PULMONARY EMERGENCIES

The first priority in the care of any patient in the PACU is the assessment and establishment of an adequate airway and ventilation. Failure to do so immediately places the PACU patient at risk for an acute airway emergency. Pulmonary emergencies fall into one of three categories: patients may initially be seen with or develop *obstruction, hypoxemia,* or *hypoventilation.*

Obstruction

Tongue obstruction. As is learned in cardiopulmonary resuscitation (CPR) certification, the tongue is always considered the primary cause of upper airway (pharyngeal) obstruction. In the postanesthetic patient the tongue causes the majority of airway obstructions. Airway obstructions occur when the tongue falls back into a position in which it occludes the pharynx, blocking the flow of air in and out of the lungs.

Patients at risk. Patients may be at risk for tongue obstruction for reasons of anatomy, poor muscle tone, or swelling. Anatomic reasons for a tongue obstruction include obesity, a very large neck (bull neck), or an unusually short neck ("no neck"). Patients with Down's syndrome are also at risk, because their tongues are significantly larger than normal. A postoperative lack of muscle tone is usually caused by residual anesthetics (that is, narcotics or muscle relaxants). Respiratory fatigue may contribute to poor tone. Tongue swelling may be caused by pressure on the tongue as a result of an endotracheal tube or instrumentation (that is, bronchoscope or surgical instrumentation used during ear, nose, and throat surgery; plastic surgery; or neurologic surgical procedures). Infections and radiation treatment for head and neck cancers can cause soft tissue swelling as well. Anaphylaxis can also result in tongue swelling.

Signs and symptoms. Patients with tongue obstructions are usually somnolent and often snoring. People rarely develop tongue obstructions while they are awake. As the patient attempts to generate a negative inspiratory pressure strong enough to draw in air, accessory muscles will be used. Activation of these accessory muscles is demonstrated by nasal flaring, intercostal and suprasternal retractions, and "paradoxical" respirations (diaphragmatic breathing).

Treatment. Treatment of a tongue obstruction is based on a series of interventions. If the first is unsuccessful, the second intervention must be implemented. The goal in treating a tongue obstruction is to achieve a patent airway. Therefore the first step is to open the airway. This may be as simple as stimulating the patient to take deep breaths, or it may require the nurse to open the airway by a chin lift or jaw thrust. To achieve a chin lift, the nurse should lift the chin gently with one hand while pushing down on the forehead with the other hand to tilt the head back.

To achieve a jaw thrust, the nurse should displace the temporomandibular joint forward bilaterally. Treatment may also necessitate the placement of an artificial airway. Either an oral or a nasal airway may be used because both maintain airway patency and are within the scope of the PACU nurse's ability to place. The nasal airway is indicated in patients who are arousable or awake; the placement of an oral airway in these patients may result in gagging, vomiting, or aspiration. Oral airways are indicated for unresponsive patients and small infants (mouth-breathers).

The correct placement of oral and nasal airways is depicted in Fig. 8-1.

If the artificial airway in insufficient (that is, if the patient is still heavily narcotized or paralyzed), intubation or ventilation may be required. Finally, if the patient's tongue swells, making airway placement is impossible, a tracheotomy may be the only option. All PACUs should have a tracheotomy set available on the unit.

Prevention. Prevention of tongue obstructions begins in the operating room with good anesthetic and surgical management. Postoperatively, the PACU nurse continues preventative interventions by assessing airway patency on admission, encouraging the patient to awaken and take deep breaths, and judiciously administering pain medications. Prevention also includes ensuring the ready availability of oral and nasal airways, reintubation equipment, suction equipment, a ventilator, and a tracheotomy set.

Laryngeal Obstruction. Most PACU nurses might be more comfortable referring to laryngeal obstruction as laryngospasm. Whatever the terminology, the outcome remains the same. The muscles of the larynx close down and obstruct the flow of air in and out of the lungs. Laryngeal obstruction is an acute airway emergency, for the patient is unable to ventilate and will rapidly become hypoxemic.

Patients at risk. Recognizing patients at risk begins with the recognition that laryn-

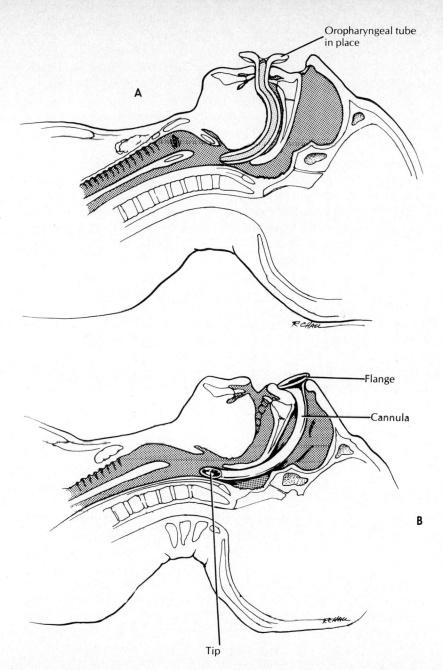

FIG. 8-1. A, Oral airway; **B,** nasal airway. Airways are positioned to relieve upper airway obstruction. (From Eubanks DH and Bone RC: Comprehensive respiratory care: a learning system, ed 2, St Louis, 1990, Mosby–Year Book, Inc.)

geal obstruction (laryngospasm) is the result of an irritable airway. The airway irritability may begin preoperatively, intraoperatively, or postoperatively. Preoperative causes of airway irritability include a history of asthma, COPD, or smoking. An airway may be irritated intraoperatively by an endotracheal tube or by multiple attempts at intubation or surgical airway manipulation. Postoperative causes of airway irritability include coughing, bucking on an endotracheal tube, or repeated suctioning or secretions (for example, bleeding after procedures such as tonsillectomy, submucous resection, and uvulopalatoplasty.)

Signs and symptoms. Patients experiencing laryngeal obstruction (laryngospasm) are awake and usually agitated for they are experiencing a feeling of suffocation. They are unable to get air and will respond by nodding their head when asked if they are having trouble "getting air." These patients are in acute respiratory distress, experiencing dyspnea, hypoxemia, and hypoventilation. Chest wall movement is an unreliable indicator of airway adequacy. By auscultating the lungs bilaterally, the nurse will rapidly detect the absence of breath sounds.

Treatment. Treatment of laryngospasm must be immediate, for hypoxemia and hypercarbia are immediate consequences. Positive pressure ventilation with an Ambu-bag mask and oxygen is the initial treatment. This may be difficult if the patient is awake and fighting for air, because having a mask placed over the face will contribute to his or her feeling of suffocation. Patients may have to be sedated to be successfully ventilated. Ideally, narcotics should not be used for sedation, because they will further depress respiratory drive. If manual ventilation of the patient is ineffective, succinylcholine (Anectine, 0.1 mg/kg IV) may be given with the goal of relaxing laryngeal musculature. If laryngospasm is caused by fluid or foreign bodies, succinylcholine will cause the irritating substance to pass into the lungs. Obviously, involvement and the immediate presence of an anesthesiologist are mandatory. Two additional medications may be used in the management of laryngeal obstruction: lidocaine and steroids. Lidocaine (1 mg/kg IV) is useful in decreasing airway irritation after successful resolution of the obstruction. Steroids may be used to decrease airway swelling. Ideally, reintubation is unnecessary if laryngeal obstruction is successfully treated. The airway is already irritated, and manipulation with a laryngoscope and endotracheal tube would cause further irritation. The patient should receive supplemental humidified oxygen via nasal cannula or mask until vital signs return to normal. Nursing responsibilities also include carefully evaluating the cause and treatment of the airway irritability.

Prevention. Prevention of laryngeal obstruction (laryngospasm) begins intraoperatively. Muscle relaxants are added to the patient's anesthetic regimen to prevent intermittent laryngospasm. As soon as the patient regains protective airway reflexes and is adequately exchanging air without ventilatory assistance, he or she is extubated to prevent straining and bucking. Although its use is somewhat controversial, lidocaine (1 mg/kg intravenously) may be given to prevent coughing and decrease the potential for laryngospasm.

On admission to the PACU, patients are given humidified oxygen to decrease airway irritation and to improve oxygenation. Unresponsive patients are often placed on their side, enabling secretions to run from the mouth as opposed to entering the airway.

Hypoxemia

Hypoxemia, in its strictest definition, is a Pao_2 (partial pressure of oxygen in blood) of less than 60 mm Hg. The term *hypoxemia* is often used synonymously with *hypoxia* (oxygen deficit at the tissue level). Although tissue hypoxia cannot be measured clinically, hypoxemia is measurable. The presence of hypoxemia is accepted as evidence that hypoxia is present. Postoperative hypoxemia is a common occurrence, mandating the ability of the PACU nurse to anticipate the problem.

Patients at risk. Patients are at risk for postanesthetic hypoxemia for a number of reasons. Every patient receiving a general anesthetic experiences some degree of respiratory depression or ventilation/perfusion imbalance. In addition, most patients are routinely transferred from the OR to the PACU without supplemental oxygen. Tyler et al[26] monitored healthy physical status I and II patients postoperatively during transport to the PACU. On arrival, 35% were found to be hypoxemic ($Sao_2 < 90\%$; $Pao_2 < 58$ mm Hg). Some centers have begun to routinely put supplemental oxygen in place when transporting a patient to the PACU, particularly if the patient is intubated, critically ill, or unstable.

The routine of most PACUs is to provide supplemental oxygen to the postanesthetic patient on admission, either via humidified nasal cannula, face mask, or face tent. The standard 2 to 4 L or 40% may be insufficient in a patient with great demands for oxygen (for example, because of metabolic or physiologic stress).

Patients may also be at risk for hypoxemia because of residual anesthetics, (inhalation agents, narcotics, barbiturates, muscle relaxants) and subsequent hypoventilation. Hypoventilation remains the most common cause of postanesthetic hypoxemia. Shivering and hypothermia decrease tissue perfusion, and may increase the demand for oxygen by 400% to 500%. Aspiration compromises gas exchange, as does pulmonary edema, by increasing the thickness of the alveolar-capillary membrane. Low hemoglobin levels decrease the oxygen-carrying capacity of blood. Pulmonary embolism compromises pulmonary circulation. Pneumothorax/hemothorax prevents gas exchange. Respiratory or cardiac arrest results in no ventilation or perfusion.

Signs and symptoms. Recognition of hypoxemia is difficult, and confirmation depends on an arterial blood gas assessment. However, clinical signs may aid in the diagnosis. Patients may be somnolent from decreased cerebral perfusion, or they may be agitated. The most common cause of postoperative agitation is hypoxemia; furthermore, the cause of postoperative agitation is *always* assumed to be hypoxemia until proven otherwise. Tachycardia may be present as a compensatory mechanism designed to enhance cardiac output and oxygen availability. Bradycardia will be present if cardiac work is found to be overwhelming. For this reason, children respond to hypoxemia with bradycardia. Blood pressure may likewise be elevated to increase perfusion and oxygen availability, or it may fall in the presence of prolonged hypoxemia. Color is an unreliable indicator of hypoxemia. Cyanosis may be a sign of hypoxemia, hypothermia, or cardiac problems.

Technology has provided another diagnostic aid in the diagnosis of hypoxemia: pulse oximetry. A standard of care now, pulse oximetry provides a noninvasive means to evaluate oxygenation. Pulse oximeters measure oxygen saturation of arterial hemoglobin (Sao_2). The relationship between Sao_2 and Pao_2 can be determined by use of the oxyhemoglobin dissociation curve. Sao_2 and Pao_2 are related because the pressure of oxygen gas drives oxygen molecules onto hemoglobin molecules. Fig. 8-2 shows, for a healthy adult under standard conditions, the oxygen saturation of arterial hemoglobin at any Pao_2. Standard conditions are defined as a body temperature of 37° C, blood pH of 7.4, a normal 2,3-diphosphoglycerate (2,3-DPG) level, and a Pco_2 of 40. Diphosphoglycerate is a chemical present in the red blood cell. It regulates the affinity of hemoglobin for oxygen. Lower concentrations of 2,3-DPG are found in bank blood stored in acid-citrate-dextrose (ACD) medium. In the normal oxyhemoglobin dissociation curve, Sao_2 increases as Pao_2 increases.

In the PACU, not all patients exist under "standard conditions." If the patient becomes alkalotic, hypothermic, has a low 2,3-DPG, or is hyperventilating (a PACU patient in pain), the normal curve of the oxyhemoglobin dissociation curve shifts to the left, reflecting a greater affinity of oxygen to hemoglobin. This means that oxygen binds more tightly to hemoglobin, and it is not released as readily in the tissues. If the patient becomes acidotic, febrile, has an increased 2,3-DPG, or is hypoventilating (a septic patient), the curve shifts to the right, reflecting a decreased affinity of oxygen to hemoglobin. This means that oxygen is readily released from hemoglobin to meet the increasing metabolic demands at the tissue level. Figs. 8-3 and 8-4 summarize the curve changes.

Treatment. Treatment of hypoxemia, simply stated, involves treating both the cause of hypoxemia and the symptom. The symptom is a low Pao_2 (less than 60 mm Hg), so the treatment always involves oxygen. If oxygen is already being supplied, it is then necessary to reevaluate the oxygen delivery system. For example, an endotracheal tube

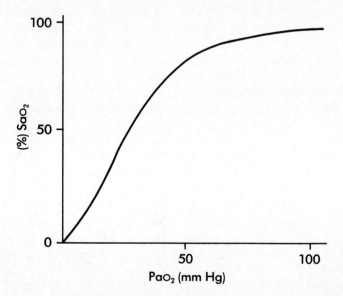

FIG. 8-2. Oxyhemoglobin dissociation curve. (From Nellcor, Inc, Haywood, Calif.)

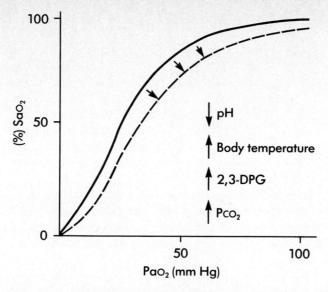

FIG. 8-3. Right shift of the oxyhemoglobin dissociation curve (decreased oxygen affinity of hemoglobin is caused by decreased pH, increased body temperature, increased 2,3-DPG, or elevated CO_2). (From Nellcor, Inc, Haywood, Calif.)

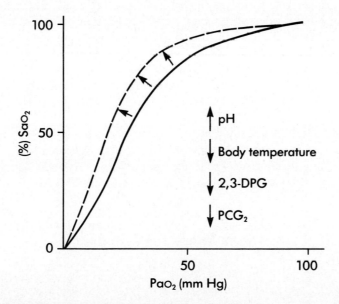

FIG. 8-4. Left shift of the oxyhemoglobin dissociation curve (increased oxygen affinity of hemoglobin is caused by increased pH, decreased body temperature, or decreased 2,3-DPG, or abnormally low CO_2). (From Nellcor, Inc, Haywood, Calif.)

may be found to have slipped into the right mainstem bronchus. In addition, the cause must be treated.

Residual narcotics and muscle relaxants may need reversal. Shivering and hypothermia should be treated by rewarming (see Chapter 7). Treatment of aspiration requires aggressive pulmonary hygiene, antibiotics, and continued monitoring after discharge from the PACU. Treatment of pulmonary edema requires diuretics, cardiac stimulants, fluid restriction, positive pressure ventilation (PEEP), and possible hemodynamic monitoring. Anemia may require transfusion. Pneumothorax and hemothorax necessitate the placement of a chest tube. Respiratory arrest and cardiac arrest will require artificial ventilation and chest compression. If the cause cannot be determined or corrected, reintubation and ventilation are indicated.

Prevention. Prevention of hypoxemia begins preoperatively with a pulmonary history and physical examination of every patient. Critically ill patients and patients scheduled for cardiothoracic procedures should have a baseline arterial Pao_2 obtained before surgery to assess the degree of existing hypoxemia and to guide pulmonary care postoperatively.

Prevention also begins with the recognition that postanesthetic hypoxemia is a common postoperative problem. Hypoxemia may develop because of inadequate oxygen availability, impaired alveolar-capillary gas exchange, inadequate perfusion, or excessive oxygen use by tissues.[10]

The initial assessment of the patient on admission to the PACU begins with an evaluation of ventilation and perfusion, including respiratory rate, presence of bilateral breath sounds, and evaluation of respiratory effort and neurologic status, heart rate, and blood pressure. Oxygen therapy is instituted immediately on admission, often before the patient assessment is initiated.

Continuous pulse oximetry monitoring should be instituted, particularly in patients at risk for hypoxemia. Patients who are at risk for hypoxemia—and who are, therefore, ideal candidates for pulse oximetry monitoring—are identified in the box below.

Hypoventilation

Hypoxemia is frequently accompanied by hypercarbia (retention of carbon dioxide) secondary to hypoventilation and inadequate oxygenation. Hypoventilation (hypercarbia) is defined as a $Paco_2$ of greater than 45 mm Hg. However, its degree of significance

---

PATIENTS AT RISK FOR HYPOXEMIA

Neonates	Smokers	Physical status III and IV
Elderly	Unresponsive	Cardiac surgery
Intubated	Agitated	Thoracic surgery
Obese	Sickle cell	COPD

is clearly dependent on the patient's preoperative baseline, for patients with COPD may run chronically high $Paco_2$ (45 to 50 mm Hg). It is important to know the patient's history.

Patients at risk. Patients experiencing residual effects of anesthetics have a greater risk for hypoventilation than any other patients in the PACU. Other patients at risk include those who are shivering and unable to take deep breaths and those with suboptimal ventilatory mechanics, including patients with large thoracic or abdominal incisions, patients who are in pain, pregnant patients, and obese patients; the risk of hypoventilation increases when these patients are placed supine on carts. Poor circulatory perfusion will also contribute to high CO_2 levels, because cells become increasingly hypoxic.

Signs and symptoms. Clinical signs and symptoms of hypoventilation are only slightly more specific than those for hypoxemia. Patients tend to be sedated or extremely somnolent as opposed to agitated. Heart rates and blood pressures may be elevated or depressed, varying with the degree of hypoxemia, hypoventilation, and physiologic fatigue. A low (for age) respiratory rate, accompanied by shallow respirations, is often the only confirming sign of hypoventilation. Capnography is an emerging technology designed to measure end-tidal carbon dioxide. An arterial blood gas level with a $Paco_2$ of greater than 45 mm Hg is another sign of hypoventilation.

Treatment. Treatment of hypoventilation, as with hypoxemia, involves managing both the cause and the symptoms of hypercarbia. The symptom is a high $Paco_2$, so the patient will be stimulated to take deep breaths postoperatively. If the patient is unable to take deep breaths because of narcotics or residual muscle relaxants, pharmacologic reversal is indicated. If the cause is splinting because of pain from an incision, the treatment may include an intercostal nerve block, placement of an epidural catheter, or judiciously administered pain medication.

The patient may have be to repositioned: for example, a pregnant woman may need to be placed on her left side, or an obese patient may need to be moved from a cart to a bed. Elevating the head of the cart or bed increases tidal volume and vital capacity significantly, especially in the morbidly obese patient. If the cause of hypoventilation is related to poor circulatory perfusion, the patient must be treated for hypotension. If the nurse is unable to detect the cause or to intervene, the patient will have to be intubated and ventilated, allowing the ventilator to "blow off" carbon dioxide.

Prevention. Prevention of hypoventilation begins intraoperatively with careful anesthetic management, particularly in the use of drugs capable of interfering with or depressing ventilation, including narcotics, barbiturates, inhalation agents, and muscle relaxants. Ideally, unless contraindicated by the patient's history or surgery, patients should arrive in the PACU extubated and arousable. The PACU nurse will perform an admission assessment, institute pulse oximetry monitoring, administer oxygen, and repeatedly encourage the patient to awaken and to take deep breaths. Careful administration of pain medications is also preventative; and nurses must remember that narcotics are central respiratory depressants. Patients at risk for pulmonary emergencies are identified in Table 8-1.

Table 8-1. **Patients at risk for pulmonary emergencies**

Specialty	Mechanism
Plastic/reconstructive	
Face lift	Restricted positioning makes it difficult to maintain airway
Rhinoplasty	Nose is packed, and oropharynx can be obstructed by blood and material
Otolaryngologic	
Myringotomy	Drainage from ear finds way to throat and causes laryngospasm
Tonsillectomy, adenoidectomy	Airway obstruction with material, laryngospasm from cord irritation
Ophthalmologic	
Open eye surgery such as corneal transplant, cataract	Very deep anesthesia, and patient is extubated "deep" so as not to stimulate coughing with an endotracheal tube
Head and neck	
Tracheostomy	Tube occlusion or displacement, aspiration of secretions or blood, pneumothorax
Thyroidectomy	Aspiration of secretions because of cord paralysis (a complication)
Radical neck dissection	Obstruction from secretions and edema of the neck of the airway
Urologic	
Nephrectomy	Pneumothorax because of the close proximity of the operative site to the diaphragm

From Nellcor, Inc, Haywood, Calif.

cont'd on p. 197

CARDIOVASCULAR EMERGENCIES

Second only to the need for airway and ventilation in the postanesthetic patient is the need to ensure circulatory adequacy and perfusion. Patients in the PACU may develop one or more of three cardiovascular emergencies: *hypotension, hypertension,* and *dysrhythmias.*

Hypotension

Classically, hypotension has been defined as a blood pressure of less than 20% of the baseline or preoperative blood pressure. This definition is problematic, however, because in many patients only one preoperative reading may have been obtained. The patient may have been in pain or anxious (especially true with an unscheduled admission)

Table 8-1—cont'd.   **Patients at risk for pulmonary emergencies**

Specialty	Mechanism
Orthopedic	
Long bone fractures	Fat emboli can lodge in the lung and cause pulmonary infarction
Spinal	V/Q mismatch resulting from hours of being prone on the operating room table
General	
Abdominal	Profound muscular relaxation is required—deep anesthesia; pain is also a strong reason for hypoventilation; reanesthetization from narcotics for pain control is a danger
Pediatric	
Generally	Laryngospasm is seen more frequently with cord irritation; edema and obstruction can occur from the endotracheal tube; respiratory reserve is very small
Neurologic	
Intracranial	Brain tolerates swelling poorly; brain swelling can impair respiratory centers, and hypoxia can be the result of brain swelling
Thoracic	
General	Pneumothorax from a violated thoracic cavity; pain; paralyzed diaphragm

or may have been an outpatient who spent the morning rearranging his or her schedule, not eating, finding the ambulatory admitting office, and having lab tests drawn. In both instances, the baseline blood pressure will be elevated and will exceed the patient's resting baseline. As a result, the PACU nurse will find the clinical signs and symptoms of hypotension a more reliable indicator of hypotension and inadequate perfusion.

Patients at risk. Remembering that blood pressure is derived from cardiac output and vascular resistance, it becomes possible to identify patients at risk for hypotension using these two indicators. Fig. 8-5 provides a guiding framework for identifying patients at risk for hypotension.

Patients are at risk for hypotension if cardiac dysfunction is present. In primary cardiac dysfunction—as in the case with a myocardial infarction, tamponade, or embolism—the heart is no longer an effective pump and is incapable of either filling or emp-

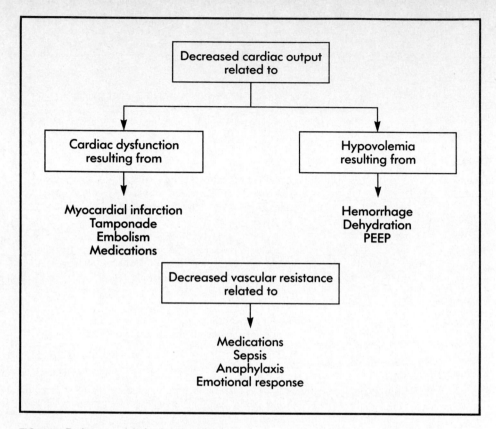

FIG. 8-5. Patients at risk for hypotension.

tying to its capacity. In secondary cardiac dysfunction, medications may exert a negative inotropic or negative chronotropic effect on myocardial tissue. Halothane (Fluothane) is a myocardial depressant, as is sufentanil (Sufenta).

Hypovolemia also reduces cardiac output and may be caused by hemorrhage or insufficient volume replacement. Positive end-expiratory pressure (PEEP) is not a true hypovolemia, but it can accentuate existing low volume states. With PEEP, intrathoracic pressure is increased. As a result, venous return to the heart is reduced, causing a fall in cardiac output.

Low vascular resistance may contribute to hypotension as well. A number of anesthetic agents cause histamine release with subsequent vasodilation (for example, barbiturates, morphine, succinylcholine, *d*-tubocurarine, and meperidine), and many anesthetic agents cause vasodilation by directly relaxing smooth muscle (for example, enflurane, isoflurane, and local anesthetics used to produce spinal anesthesia).

If sepsis is present, it will be accompanied by vasodilation caused by the endotoxins released from (most commonly) gram-negative bacteria. Anaphylaxis is a rapidly developing, severe antigen-antibody reaction that results in the release of large amounts of histamine, increasing capillary permeability and causing arteriolar and capillary vasodilation.

Emotions can trigger low-resistance states as well. Examples include fainting in response to strong emotion and the reaction produced by overwhelming fear, grief, or pain.

Signs and symptoms. As previously mentioned, the absolute reading of a blood pressure may be limited as an indicator of hypotension. The clinical signs and symptoms of hypotension are unequivocal. Pale, cool, clammy skin reflects cutaneous vasoconstriction, a compensatory mechanism designed to shunt blood from the periphery into central circulation. Compensatory tachycardia occurs with the goal of boosting cardiac output and perfusion. Urine output falls to less than 30 ml/hour. Restlessness, disorientation, and anxiety are signs of cerebral hypoxia. Respirations become rapid and shallow, also as a compensatory mechanism designed to correct acidosis, which occurs as a result of decreased perfusion. Prompt intervention is necessary to prevent prolonged circulatory insufficiency to vital organs.

Treatment. Treatment of hypotension requires prompt recognition of the problem and correction of its cause. If the cause is low cardiac output secondary to myocardial depression, the treatment interventions may include oxygenation, cardiac stimulants (epinephrine, atropine, dopamine, dobutamine), and possibly CPR.

Hypovolemia is treated with fluids or blood replacement or both. If hemorrhage is the cause, the patient will likely be returned to the operating room for surgical repair. The patient can be evaluated for hemorrhage by obtaining hematocrit and hemoglobin levels and by observing the surgical site and drains.

Peripheral vasodilation may be treated with fluids, vasopressors (ephedrine, dopamine, epinephrine), and elevation of the patient's legs, thereby increasing core circulation. Anaphylactic reactions are treated with epinephrine and antihistamines (diphenhydramine [Benadryl]).

Debate exists as to the use of the Trendelenburg position to correct hypotension. In its favor, the Trendelenburg position does provide an "autotransfusion" of 500 to 1000 ml of blood instantaneously, ensuring coronary and cerebral circulation and perfusion. Opponents of the Trendelenburg position cite the occurrence of rebound hypotension as baroreceptors sense the increased flow.

Prevention. Prevention of hypotension begins in the operating room with ongoing evaluation of the patient's response to anesthetic agents and to the surgery. In addition, it is the responsibility of the anesthesiologist or anesthetist to maintain fluid balance.

In the PACU, the nurse will monitor blood pressure frequently (usually every 15 minutes), will monitor intake and output, will assess for bleeding, and will notify the anesthesiologist promptly in the event of hypotension.

Attempts at prevention also involve communication between the surgeon, anesthesiologist, and the PACU nurse. Knowledge of intraoperative problems, specifically bleeding or a difficult repair, will alert the PACU nurse to potential problems.

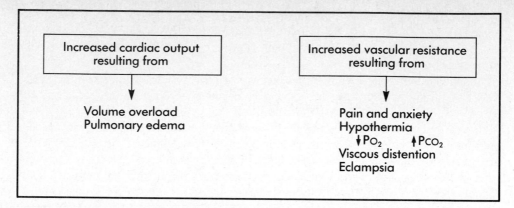

FIG. 8-6. Patients at risk for hypertension.

Hypertension

Although hypertension is a common occurrence in the PACU, careful investigation of its causes is always required. This patient problem is clearly one in which the cause will be the key to treatment.

Patients at risk. As with hypotension, it is important to recognize that alterations in cardiac output and peripheral vascular resistance can cause hypertension. Fig. 8-6 provides a framework for identifying patients at risk for hypertension.

Patients may present with high cardiac outputs secondary to volume overload or pulmonary edema or both. This is to be suspected in patients in whom fluid resuscitation was used (for example, in trauma patients).

Pain and anxiety stimulate the sympathetic nervous system, causing release of catecholamines, specifically epinephrine and norepinephrine. Both are vasoconstrictive. Hypothermia also results in peripheral vasoconstriction as a mechanism to shunt warm blood into central circulation. Hypoxemia and hypercarbia result in vasoconstriction as the body attempts to improve central perfusion and gas exchange.

Viscous distention, in particular, a full bladder, may contribute to hypertension via sympathetic stimulation. A history of hypertension may cause a patient to present with an elevated blood pressure postoperatively, particularly if the patient is extremely dependent on medications for management and is overdue for his or her next dose. Patients who are eclamptic release vasoactive substances from the placenta, causing direct vasoconstriction.

Signs and symptoms. Unfortunately there are no clinical signs and symptoms of hypertension other than the actual reading of systolic and diastolic values. Although the American Heart Association defines hypertension as a blood pressure of greater than 140/90, most PACU personnel do not consider treating hypertension until systolic values approach or exceed 180 and diastolic values approach or exceed 100. Diastolic hypertension is more hazardous than systolic hypertension. Obviously, there are instances when aggressive therapy for hypertension will be initiated much earlier, especially after carotid, coronary, or neurosurgical procedures.

Treatment. Treatment of postoperative hypertension involves treatment of the cause. Volume overload and pulmonary edema require diuretics, hemodynamic monitoring, and fluid restriction. Patients in pain need pain medication; conveniently, morphine sulfate not only treats pain but also causes the release of histamine, which is a vasodilator. Hypothermia is treated with rewarming. Hypoxemia and hypercarbia are treated with improved ventilation. Viscous distention is treated with catheterization. Patients should be restarted on preoperative antihypertensive medications as soon as possible.

Obviously, there are times when pharmacologic intervention will be required to manage postoperative hypertension. Commonly used antihypertensives and their mechanisms of action are identified in Table 8-2.

Table 8-2. **Antihypertensive therapy**

Drugs	Route of administration	Action	Important information
Nitroglycerin (Tridil; Nitrostat; Nitrodur; Nitropaste)	Sublingual Dermal Intravenous infusion	Relaxation of vascular smooth muscle Coronary vasodilation Decrease in venous return Decrease in ventricular filling	Intravenous infusion necessitates infusion pump, arterial line monitoring, and glass bottle and tubing
Sodium nitroprusside (Nipride)	Intravenous infusion	Direct peripheral vasodilator Afterload reduction	Requires infusion pump and arterial line monitoring; infusate must be protected from light
Hydralazine (Apresoline)	IV bolus	Relaxation of vascular smooth muscle Preferential relaxation of arterioles Maintains cardiac output	
Labetalol hydrochloride (Normodyne, Trandate)	IV bolus	Alpha-blocker—peripheral vasodilation Beta-blocker—decreases heart rate	Do not administer if patient is bradycardic
Enalapril maleate (Vasotec)	IV bolus	Suppression of renin-angiotensin-aldosterone system	Avoid with diuretics or volume depletion; onset occurs in 15 minutes; peak of action usually within 1 hour but occasionally up to 4 hours
Nifedipine (Procardia)	Oral Sublingual	Calcium channel blocker Relaxes coronary artery smooth muscle Dilates peripheral arteries	Capsule can be opened for liquid to be given sublingually

Prevention. Prevention of postoperative hypertension begins intraoperatively with carefully monitored and maintained fluid balance. In addition, anticipating the need for pain management and administering a narcotic intraoperatively help to minimize immediate postoperative discomfort. When possible, the patient should be covered to prevent hypothermia. Fluids can be warmed as well. Pain management and hypothermia is discussed in greater detail in Chapter 7. Urinary catheterization is warranted for long surgeries with anticipated fluid balance problems, such as blood loss or third spacing, and for monitoring of hourly urine outputs.

Dysrhythmias

Postoperative dysrhythmias fall into one of two categories: the common (including sinus tachycardia, sinus bradycardia, and premature ventricular contractions) and the uncommon (including asystole, ventricular fibrillation, and ventricular tachycardia).

Sinus tachycardia. Sinus tachycardia is defined as rapid heart rate (greater than 100 beats per minute in an adult), with a regular rhythm, and P-waves present. The most common causes of sinus tachycardia in the immediate postoperative period include pain, hypoxemia, and hypovolemia. Treatment interventions are directed toward the cause and include pain medication, oxygen, and fluid therapy. Rarely, but occasionally, it is necessary to consider agents such as propranolol (Inderal) or verapamil (Isoptin). Fig. 8-7 shows an example of sinus tachycardia on an ECG tracing.

Sinus bradycardia. Sinus bradycardia is defined as a slowed heart rate (in the adult less than 60 beats per minute) with a regular rhythm and P-waves present. The most common causes of sinus bradycardia in the immediate postoperative period include hypoxemia, hypothermia (especially in children), and a high-spinal anesthetic level. Treatment of bradycardia is unnecessary unless hypotension or ventricular ectopy are present. If indicated, atropine, 0.5 mg to 1.0 mg intravenously, is the drug of choice. Fig. 8-8 shows an example of sinus bradycardia on ECG tracing.

Premature ventricular complexes. Premature ventricular complexes (PVCs) are defined as a depolarization that arises in the ventricle prematurely. On ECG, PVCs are represented by wide (0.12 seconds or greater) and bizarre-looking QRS complexes. In the immediate postoperative period, the most common causes of PVCs include hypoxemia and hypokalemia. In the absence of cardiac disease or hypotension, treatment of PVCs is often unnecessary. When intervention is necessary, lidocaine (1 mg/kg intravenously) is the drug of choice. Fig. 8-9 shows an example of PVCs on an ECG tracing.

Asystole. Ventricular asystole is a rare event in the postanesthetic or postoperative patient. It is characterized by a complete absence of ventricular electrical activity. Because it is a rare event, it is impossible to identify patients at risk for asystole. Treatment includes prompt recognition of the dysrhythmia and initiation of CPR and ACLS protocols. Fig. 8-10 shows an example of asystole on an ECG tracing. The ACLS algorithm for asystole is reproduced in Fig 8-11.

Ventricular fibrillation. Ventricular fibrillation is also a rare dysrhythmia; it is characterized by chaotic electrical activity and no cardiac output. As with asystole, it is impossible to identify patients at risk for ventricular fibrillation. Treatment includes prompt

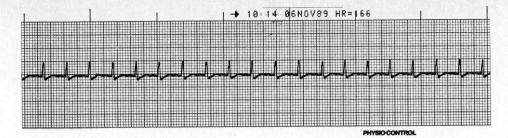

→ 10:14 06NOV89 HR=166

FIG. 8-7. Sinus tachycardia.

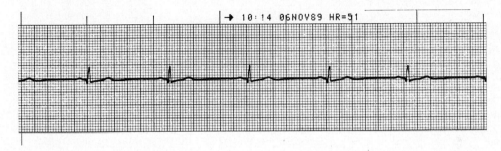

→ 10:14 06NOV89 HR=51

FIG. 8-8. Sinus bradycardia.

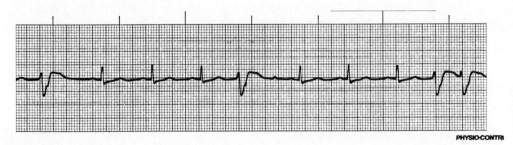

FIG. 8-9. Premature ventricular complexes.

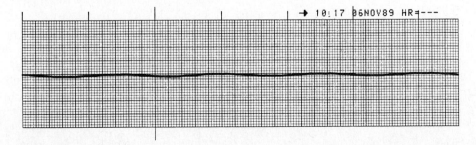

→ 10:17 06NOV89 HR=---

FIG. 8-10. Asystole.

**If Rhythm Is Unclear and Possibly Ventricular
Fibrillation, Defibrillate as for VF. If Asystole is Present**[a]
↓
Continue CPR
↓
Establish IV Access
↓
Epinephrine, 1:10,000, 0.5—1.0 mg IV Push[b]
↓
Intubate When Possible[c]
↓
Atropine, 1.0 mg IV Push (Repeated in 5 min)
↓
(Consider Bicarbonate)[d]
↓
Consider Pacing

Asystole (cardiac standstill). This sequence was developed to assist in teaching how to treat a broad range of patients with asystole. Some patients may require care not specified herein. This algorithm should not be construed to prohibit such flexibility. Flow of algorithm presumes asystole is continuing. VF indicates ventricular fibrillation; IV, intravenous.

[a]Asystole should be confirmed in two leads.

[b]Epinephrine should be repeated every 5 minutes.

[c]Intubation is preferable; if it can be accomplished simultaneously with other techniques, then the earlier the better. However, cardiopulmonary resuscitation (CPR) and use of epinephrine are more important initially if patient can be ventilated without intubation. (Endotracheal epinephrine may be used.)

[d]Value of sodium bicarbonate is questionable during cardiac arrest, and it is not recommended for the routine cardiac arrest sequence. Consideration of its use in a dose of 1 mEq/kg is appropriate at this point. Half of original dose may be repeated every 10 minutes if it is used.

FIG. 8-11. Algorithm for asystole. (Reproduced with permission from the American Heart Association, Textbook of advanced cardiac life support, Dallas, TX, 1987, The Association.)

recognition of the dysrhythmia and initiation of CPR and defibrillation. ACLS protocols should be instituted. The ACLS algorithm for ventricular fibrillation is reproduced in Fig. 8-12. Fig. 8-13 shows an example of ventricular fibrillation on an ECG tracing.

Ventricular tachycardia. Ventricular tachycardia is the last of the uncommon dysrhythmias. It is characterized by a rate of greater than 100, a regular rhythm, absent P-waves, and wide, bizarre QRS complexes. As with the other uncommon dysrhyth-

```
      Witnessed Arrest                          Unwitnessed Arrest
  Check Pulse—If No Pulse                    Check Pulse—If No Pulse
              │                                          │
       Precordial Thump                                  │
              │                                          │
  Check Pulse—If No Pulse                                │
              │                                          │
              └──────────────────────┬───────────────────┘
                                     │
              CPR Until a Defibrillator Is Available
                                     │
              Check Monitor for Rhythm—if VF or VT
                                     │
                  Defibrillate, 200 Joules[b]
                                     │
                Defibrillate, 200-300 Joules[b]
                                     │
             Defibrillate With up to 360 Joules[b]
                                     │
                        CPR If No Pulse
                                     │
                    Establish IV Access
                                     │
         Epinephrine, 1:10,000, 0.5-1.0 mg IV Push[c]
                                     │
                    Intubate If Possible[d]
                                     │
             Defibrillate With up to 360 Joules[b]
                                     │
                 Lidocaine, 1 mg/kg IV Push
                                     │
             Defibrillate With up to 360 Joules[b]
                                     │
                 Bretylium, 5 mg/kg IV Push[e]
                                     │
                  (Consider Bicarbonate)[f]
                                     │
             Defibrillate With up to 360 Joules[b]
                                     │
                 Bretylium, 10 mg/kg IV Push[e]
                                     │
             Defibrillate With up to 360 Joules[b]
                                     │
                Repeat Lidocaine or Bretylium
                                     │
             Defibrillate With up to 360 Joules[b]
```

Ventricular fibrillation (and pulseless ventricular tachycardia).[a] This sequence was developed to assist in teaching how to treat a broad range of patients with ventricular fibrillation (VF) or pulseless ventricular tachycardia (VT). Some patients may require care not specified herein. This algorithm should not be construed as prohibiting such flexibility. Flow of algorithm presumes that VF is continuing. CPR indicates cardiopulmonary resuscitation.

[a]Pulseless VT should be treated identically to VF.

[b]Check pulse and rhythm after each shock. If VF recurs after transiently converting (rather than persists without ever converting), use whatever energy level has previously been successful for defibrillation.

[c]Epinephrine should be repeated every 5 minutes.

[d]Intubation is preferable. If it can be accompanied simultaneously with other techniques, then the earlier the better. However, defibrillation and epinephrine are more important initially if the patient can be ventilated without intubation.

[e]Some may prefer repeated doses of lidocaine, which may be given in 0.5 mg/kg boluses every 8 minutes to a total dosage of 3 mg/kg.

[f]Value of sodium bicarbonate is questionable during cardiac arrest, and it is not recommended for routine cardiac arrest sequence. Consideration of its use in a dose of 1 mEq/kg is appropriate at this point. Half of original dose may be repeated every 10 minutes if it is used.

FIG. 8-12. Algorithm for ventricular fibrillation. (Reproduced with permission from the American Heart Association, Textbook of advanced cardiac life support, Dallas, TX, 1987, The Association.)

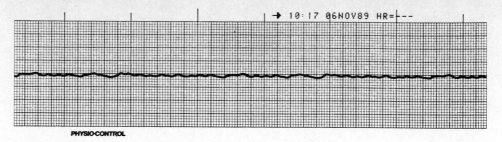

FIG. 8-13. Ventricular fibrillation.

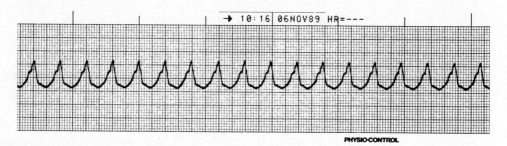

FIG. 8-14. Ventricular tachycardia.

mias, the goal is treatment, not identification of patients at risk. In the hemodynamically stable patient, treatment involves lidocaine (1 mg/kg intravenously). If the patient is hemodynamically unstable, treatment involves cardioversion and lidocaine. Fig. 8-14 shows an example of ventricular tachycardia on an ECG tracing. The ACLS algorithm for ventricular tachycardia is reproduced in Fig. 8-15.

EMERGENCE DELIRIUM

Emergence delirium is a term used to describe either responsive or unresponsive agitation. Although it is not a life-threatening emergency, emergence delirium has the potential to greatly interfere with the ability of the PACU nurse to provide care for the patient. In addition, there are emergencies, most notably hypoxemia, which may first appear as emergence delirium and which do require immediate attention.

Patients at risk

Although it is not possible to identify every patient who will develop emergence delirium, it is possible to identify patients at risk. As previously mentioned, the "number one" cause of postoperative agitation is hypoxemia; and the cause of postoperative agi-

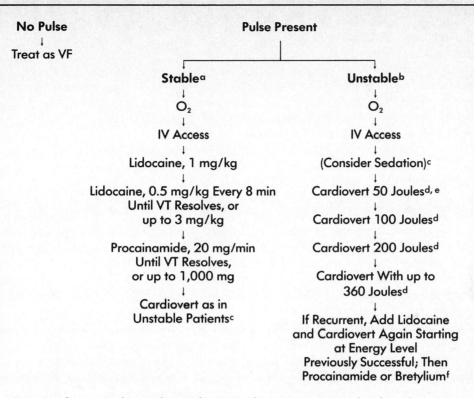

No Pulse	Pulse Present	
↓		
Treat as VF		

Stable[a]

↓

O₂

↓

IV Access

↓

Lidocaine, 1 mg/kg

↓

Lidocaine, 0.5 mg/kg Every 8 min
Until VT Resolves, or
up to 3 mg/kg

↓

Procainamide, 20 mg/min
Until VT Resolves,
or up to 1,000 mg

↓

Cardiovert as in
Unstable Patients[c]

Unstable[b]

↓

O₂

↓

IV Access

↓

(Consider Sedation)[c]

↓

Cardiovert 50 Joules[d, e]

↓

Cardiovert 100 Joules[d]

↓

Cardiovert 200 Joules[d]

↓

Cardiovert With up to
360 Joules[d]

↓

If Recurrent, Add Lidocaine
and Cardiovert Again Starting
at Energy Level
Previously Successful; Then
Procainamide or Bretylium[f]

Sustained ventricular tachycardia (VT). This sequence was developed to assist in teaching how to treat a broad range of patients with sustained VT. Some patients may require care not specified herein. This algorithm should not be construed as prohibiting such flexibility. Flow of algorithm presumes that VT is continuing. VF indicates ventricular fibrillation.

[a]If patient becomes unstable (see footnote b for definition) at any time, move to "Unstable" arm of algorithm.

[b]Unstable indicates symptoms (e.g., chest pain or dyspnea), hypotension (systolic blood pressure <90 mm Hg), congestive heart failure, ischemia, or infarction.

[c]Sedation should be considered for all patients, including those defined in footnote b as unstable, except those who are hemodynamically unstable (e.g., hypotensive, in pulmonary edema, or unconscious).

[d]If hypotension, pulmonary edema, or unconsciousness is present, unsynchronized cardioversion should be done to avoid delay associated with synchronization.

[e]In the absence of hypotension, pulmonary edema, or unconsciousness, a precordial thump may be employed prior to cardioversion.

[f]Once VT has resolved, begin intravenous (IV) infusion of antiarrhythmic agent that has aided resolution of VT. If hypotension, pulmonary edema, or unconsciousness is present, use lidocaine if cardioversion alone is unsuccessful, followed by bretylium. In all other patients, recommended order of therapy is lidocaine, procainamide, and then bretylium.

FIG. 8-15. Algorithm for ventricular tachycardia. (Reproduced with permission from the American Heart Association, Textbook of advanced cardiac life support, Dallas, TX, 1987, The Association.)

tation should be assumed to be hypoxemia until proven otherwise. Emergence delirium has also been associated with the anesthetic agents including ketamine (a phencyclidine derivative), atropine (an anticholinergic), and scopolamine (another anticholinergic). Patients in pain and those with full bladders may present with emergence delirium. Patients with extreme preoperative anxiety or those whom the anesthesiologist reports "went to sleep with a fight" often wake up the same way. Substance abusers also tend to demonstrate difficulties with emergence. Children demonstrate emergence delirium far more frequently than adults (15% to 20% incidence).

Signs and symptoms. *Emergence delirium* is a term used to describe either responsive or unresponsive agitation. Patients may appear with strong, nonpurposeful movements, crying, verbalizing, or moaning and are unable to follow commands. Likewise, the term may describe aggressive, purposeful movements, such as trying to get out of bed. If hypoxemia is a contributing factor, pulse oximetry will confirm a low saturation.

Treatment. Treatment of emergence delirium involves treatment of the cause and the maintenance of staff and patient safety. If the cause is hypoxemia, treatment is centered on improving oxygenation. If the cause is a full bladder, treatment is catheterization or encouraging the patient to void. If the cause is atropine or scopolamine, the treatment is physostigmine (Antilirium). Other patients, including substance abusers, extremely anxious patients, and patients who have received ketamine, frequently require sedation with benzodiazepines (midazolam). Because midazolam can produce respiratory depression, it should be administered with caution and with pulse oximetry monitoring in place. Children are rarely treated pharmacologically, and their emergence delirium usually resolves with time. Children respond well when parents are made an integral part of PACU postoperative care.

In addition, patient and staff safety must be maintained. Side rails and restraints are useful in keeping patients in bed, intravenous lines protected, and endotracheal tubes in place. The nurse should be on the alert for scratching, grabbing, kicking, and biting. An attack is rarely personal; and once the emergence delirium is resolved, most patients return to their preoperative status with no recollection of their uncontrolled behaviors.

Prevention. Prevention of emergence delirium begins with recognition that little can be done to predict who will wake up delirious or to prevent the delirium. Patients who have received ketamine are allowed to wake up on their own, bypassing the PACU verbal and tactile postoperative stir-up routine. Intubated patients are restrained on admission. Airway patency and oxygenation is evaluated and secured. Warnings by anesthesia personnel about patient idiosyncracies can sometimes allow the nurse to anticipate the potential for emergence delirium.

MALIGNANT HYPERTHERMIA

The defect that causes malignant hyperthermia (MH) appears to be in skeletal muscle and is associated with a biochemical defect in intracellular homeostasis.[1] Before detailing the alterations that occur in malignant hypothermia, it is important to briefly review normal cell physiology and the role of calcium.

In cells, calcium plays a central role in the cell's energy-producing functions. In normal cells, calcium is released from its storage site in the sarcoplasmic reticulum in response to neuronal stimulation. Calcium concentrations increase, triggering phosphorylase (an enzyme) to mediate the breakdown of glycogen into lactic acid, carbon dioxide, and heat, providing energy for intracellular activities.

As calcium concentrations continue to increase, another enzyme, myosin ATP-ase, is activated. It acts on adenosine triphosphate (ATP), causing the release of heat and free energy. This energy activates another enzyme, which promotes the crossbridge linking of contractile proteins actin and myosin, causing muscle fibers to contract.

When the neuronal signal subsides, cellular membrane channels open, and an ionic pump forces calcium back into the sarcoplasmic reticulum. Intracellular calcium levels fall, actin and myosin separate, and the muscle fiber relaxes.

In malignant hyperthermia, triggering agents (anesthetic agents) somehow interfere with calcium's reentry into the sarcoplasmic reticulum. Therefore with each neuronal stimulus, more calcium is released, forcing the cell into a state of hypermetabolism.[3]

Patients at risk. As mentioned, exposure to anesthetic agents can "trigger" the development of malignant hyperthermia. Those agents most frequently associated with malignant hyperthermia include halothane, enflurane, isoflurane, succinylcholine, and ketamine. Malignant hyperthermia also carries with it a genetic predisposition via autosomal dominant transmission.

Malignant hyperthermia has been described in all racial groups. Male and female children are affected equally until puberty, after which malignant hyperthermia is more common in males. In children, malignant hyperthermia has been reported to occur once per 7000 to 14,000 administrations of anesthetics. In adults, the incidence ranges from 1:50,000 to 1:200,000. It occurs most commonly in patients between 3 and 30 years of age.[2]

Signs and symptoms. Sympathetic hyperactivity (tachycardia, sweating, hypertension) is frequently the first sign of the hypermetabolism associated with malignant hyperthermia. Stores of oxygen are readily depleted, resulting in a respiratory and metabolic acidosis. As ATP (energy) levels fall, cellular functions are disrupted, causing a leak of potassium, magnesium, phosphate, and myoglobin into plasma.[3] These biochemical alterations lead to disturbances in many organ systems.

The increase in potassium contributes to ventricular dysrhythmias, cardiac instability, falling cardiac output, and ultimately to cardiac arrest. Myoglobin blocks the renal tubules, resulting in renal failure and acute tubular necrosis (ATN). The chemical imbalance leads to a collapse of the coagulation system. Levels of factor VIII and fibrinogen fall, resulting in widespread bleeding.

Ongoing muscle contractions produce skeletal rigidity. As contractions remain sustained, body temperature rises as much as 1° C every 5 minutes. The increase in temperature, increase in potassium, and progressive hypoxia contribute to central nervous system effects that include acute cerebral edema and intracranial hypertension; these effects present as coma, areflexia, unresponsiveness, and fixed, dilated pupils.[9]

Treatment. Treatment of malignant hyperthermia depends on recognition of clinical

Table 8-3.   **Treatment of malignant hyperthermia**

Interventions	Rationale
Discontinue all anesthetic agents	Remove all triggers
Hyperventilate with 100% oxygen	Correct hypoxemia and acidosis
Administer dantrolene sodium (2 mg/kg IV to maximum 10 mg/kg, every 5-8 hours × 3 doses)	Inhibits release of calcium from sarcoplasmic reticulum
Administer bicarbonate (2-4 mEq/kg IV)	Correct acidosis
Initiate active cooling	Reduce fever and decrease oxygen demand
Monitor urine output	Evaluate for acute tubular necrosis and myo-globulinuria
Further treatment is guided by dysrhythmias, blood gases, temperature, muscle tone, and urine output as indicated	Individualize therapy to patient needs
Monitor laboratory values—including electro-lytes, liver enzymes, renal function, CBC, and coagulation profiles	Assess organ system and physiologic function-ing

For additional information about malignant hyperthermia emergencies, the Malignant Hyperthermia Associa-tion of the United States (MHAUS) has established a 24-hour emergency hotline at (209) 634-4817.

signs and symptoms, including sympathetic stimulation, hypercarbia, metabolic acido-sis, and increasing temperature. Treatment interventions and their rationales are summa-rized in Table 8-3. Because of prompt recognition of the clinical signs and the advent of dantrolene sodium, the mortality associated with malignant hyperthermia has decreased to 7%.[16]

Prevention. Prevention of malignant hyperthermia begins with preoperative evalua-tions that are focused to detect any personal or family history of problems with anesthe-sia. Individuals identified to be "at risk" for malignant hyperthermia will be given dan-trolene sodium (2 mg/kg intravenously) before induction. Anesthesia will consist of ni-trous oxide, barbiturates, opiates, tranquilizers, and nondepolarizing relaxants (nontrig-ger agents). Regional anesthesia is safe and may be preferred for certain procedures in susceptible patients.[9]

EMERGENCIES ASSOCIATED WITH SPECIFIC SURGICAL PROCEDURES

A specific postoperative emergency is associated with many surgical procedures: for example, malignant hypertension is associated with carotid endarterectomy; tamponade is associated with cardiac surgery; loss of pulses may occur after vascular bypass sur-gery; and an acute change in neurologic functioning may occur after an intracranial pro-cedure. It is beyond the scope of a book of this nature to discuss all of the postsurgical emergencies that may occur in the PACU. However, it is important for the nurse practicing in the PACU to be aware of the cause and management of potential emergencies associated with the types of surgical procedures with which they are likely to be dealing. This type of information should be included during PACU orientation and reviewed periodically as necessary to keep the management strategies familiar.

EMERGENCY READINESS

Inherent in the prevention and treatment of emergency situations is unit readiness, including the availability of equipment and medications. Medications and equipment that should be included on the PACU emergency cart are identified in the boxes that follow. The equipment should be regularly inspected for safety and performance and outdatedness and to ensure that it is there. Medication carts should be checked monthly to ensure the presence of the drugs and to check expiration dates.

EMERGENCY CART DRUG CHECKLIST

Aminophylline	Dopamine	Phenylephrine
Atropine sulfate	Ephedrine	Phenytoin
Bretylium tosylate	Epinephrine	Procainamide
Calcium chloride	Furosemide	Propranolol
Dextrose 50%	Lidocaine	Sodium bicarbonate
Digoxin	Magnesium sulfate	Sodium nitroprusside
Diphenhydramine	Naloxone	Verapamil
Dobutamine	Nitroglycerin	

EMERGENCY CART EQUIPMENT CHECKLIST

Intracaths—8 inch and 24 inch	Wire cutter
Angiocaths 14 G and 16 G	Sterile scissors
Tourniquet	Sterile hemostat
Alcohol preps	Blood pump (pressure bag)
Tape	Flashlight
Syringes (3, 5, 10, 20, 50 ml)	Cardiac needles (20 G × 6 inch)
IV labels	Trocar (chest tube) kit (12 F and 28 F)
Arterial line kit	Pleurovac
Arterial blood gas kit	Tracheostomy set
Needles (18 G and 20 G)	Cut down tray
CVP manometer	Minor surgery tray
Blood tubing	Backboard (for CPR)
Infusion pump	Defibrillator

**REINTUBATION EQUIPMENT (MAY BE PART OF EMERGENCY CART OR
SEPARATE REINTUBATION TRAY OR BOX)**

Laryngoscope blades (straight 2, 3, 4; curved 2, 3, 4)	Lubricant Lidocaine spray
Endotracheal tubes (pediatric and adult)	Nasal airways (6-9 mm) Oral airways (5-10 mm)
Magill forceps	5 ml syringes
Stylet wire	Tape
Ambu-bag	Face masks (pediatric and adult)
	Extra batteries and bulbs

In addition to equipment and medications, all staff should be recertified annually in CPR, should know the whereabouts of all emergency equipment, and should know the mechanism for summoning emergency assistance when necessary. Some PACUs have gone so far as to mandate ACLS certification of staff.

CONCLUSION

It is clear that the patient in the PACU is at risk for a number of postoperative or postanesthetic emergencies. Vigilance on the part of the PACU nurse is mandatory, as is awareness of potential emergencies, patients at risk, and treatment and prevention strategies.

REFERENCES

1. Benca J and Rockoff M: Malignant hyperthermia. In Stoelting R, Barash P, and Gallagher T (editors): Advances in anesthesia, vol 5, Chicago, 1988, Year Book Medical Publishers, Inc, pp 237-259.
2. Britt B: Malignant hyperthermia, Can Anesth Soc J 32:666-667, 1985.
3. Britt B: Malignant hyperthermia: a nightmare for anesthesiologists and patients, JAMA 255(6):709-715, 1986.
4. Brown S: Pulmonary aspiration in the postanesthetic period, J Post Anesth Nurs 1(2):87-91, 1986.
5. Carlson C and Thorton S: Hypertensive crisis in the PACU, J Post Anesth Nurs 1(3):157-160, 1986.
6. Easton C and MacKenzie F: Sensory-perceptual alterations: delirium in the intensive care unit, Heart Lung 17(3):229-235, 1988.
7. Glazener C and Motoyama E: Hypoxemia in children following general anesthesia, Anesthesiology 61(3A):A416, 1984.
8. Greany D and Brown M: Malignant hyperthermia: a concern for critical care nurses, Focus Crit Care 13(2):52-57, 1986.
9. Gribert G: Malignant hyperthermia. In Miller R (editor): Anesthesia, New York, 1986, Churchill Livingstone, Inc, pp 1871-1994.
10. Julien R: Understanding anesthesia, Menlo Park, Calif, 1984, Wesley.
11. Leicht P, Wisborg T, and Chraemmer-Jorgensen, B: Does IV lidocaine prevent laryngospasm after extubation in children? Anesth Analg 64:1193-1196, 1985.
12. Litwack K and Gulczynski B: Practical points in the care of patients with ventricular ectopy, J Post Anesth Nurs 4(3):165-169, 1989.
13. Litwack K and Zeplin K: Practical points in the management of laryngospasm, J Post Anesth Nurs 4(1):36-39, 1989.
14. Malignant Hyperthermia Association of the United States: Understanding malignant hyperthermia, The Association, 1986, Darien, Conn.
15. Meagher T: The incidence of emergence excitement: a descriptive study, J Post Anesth Nurs 3(4):247-253, 1988.
16. Mitchell M: Malignant hyperthermia, Curr Rev Recov Room Nurses 10(9):78-83, 1987.
17. Murray D and Tinker J: Profound hypotension and hypertension, Curr Rev Recov Room Nurses 95-100, 1983.
18. Nellcor, Inc. Pulse oximetry note number 3, Hayward, Calif, 1987, Nellcor, Inc.
19. Orkin F and Cooperman L (editors): Complications in anesthesiology, Philadelphia, 1983, JB Lippincott Co.
20. Orkin F and Cooperman L (editors): Complications in anesthesiology, Philadelphia, 1983, JB Lippincott Co.
21. Salem MR: Laryngospasm and bronchospasm, Curr Rev Recov Room Nurses 7:66-71, 1985.
22. Shapiro B, Harrison R, and Trout C: Clinical application of respiratory care, Chicago, 1985, Year Book Medical Publishers, Inc.
23. Standards and guidelines for cardiopulmonary resuscitation (CPR) and emergency cardiac care, JAMA 255:2905-2992, 1986.
24. Thomas S: Malignant hyperthermia, Crit Care Nurse 9(6):58-59, 1989.
25. Toledo L: Pulse oximetry: clinical implications in the PACU, J Post Anesth Nurs 2(1):12-17, 1987.
26. Tyler I, Tantisira B, Winter P, and Motoyama E: Arterial oxygen saturation during transfer to the recovery room, Anesthesiology 63(suppl 3A):A524, 1985.
27. Zeller F, Klamerus, K, and Brundage B: Cardiac support drugs in the surgical intensive care unit, Probl Gen Surg 4(4):441-454, 1987.

Review Questions

1. *The most common cause of upper airway obstruction is* _____.
   a. An incorrectly placed oral airway
   b. An endotracheal tube
   c. The tongue
   d. Laryngospasm

2. *The first action to be taken to relieve an upper airway obstruction is* _____.
   a. Immediate placement of an oral or nasal airway
   b. To notify the anesthesiologist to reintubate the patient
   c. To perform a tracheotomy to open the airway
   d. To open the airway with a jaw thrust or chin lift

3. *Observing chest movement is a reliable indicator of respiratory adequacy.*
   a. True
   b. False

4. *The first action to be taken to treat laryngospasm is* _____.
   a. Elevating the head of the bed 45 degrees
   b. Reintubation and ventilation
   c. Administration of succinylcholine
   d. Positive pressure ventilation with an Ambu-bag and mask

5. *Lidocaine may be given to prevent or to treat laryngospasm. Lidocaine works to* _____.
   a. Decrease airway irritability
   b. Induce bronchoconstriction
   c. Decrease airway swelling
   d. Enhance protective airway reflexes

6. *Hypoxemia is defined as a Pao_2 of less than* _____.
   a. 90 mm Hg
   b. 80 mm Hg
   c. 70 mm Hg
   d. 60 mm Hg

7. *Assuming adequate ventilation, normothermia, and a pH of 7.4, a pulse oximetry saturation of 90% is equal to a Pao_2 of* _____.
   a. 90-100 mm Hg
   b. 80-90 mm Hg
   c. 70-80 mm Hg
   d. 60-70 mm Hg

8. *Hypothermia, hyperventilation, and alkalosis cause the oxyhemoglobin curve to shift to the* _____, _____ *availability of oxygen to tissues.*
   a. Left, decreasing
   b. Left, increasing
   c. Right, decreasing
   d. Right, increasing

9. *Acidosis, hypoventilation, and hyperthermia cause the oxyhemoglobin curve to shift to the* _____, _____ *the availability of oxygen to tissues.*
   a. Left, decreasing
   b. Left, increasing
   c. Right, decreasing
   d. Right, increasing
10. *Capnography is designed to measure* _____.
    a. Oxygen saturation
    b. End-tidal carbon dioxide
    c. The oxygen content of blood
    d. The $Paco_2$ of blood
11. *Hypotension is best defined by* _____.
    a. Clinical signs of hypoperfusion
    b. A blood pressure of less than 20% of baseline
    c. Any pressure less than 100/60
    d. A blood pressure of less than 120/80
12. *Positive end expiratory pressure (PEEP) causes hypotension by* _____.
    a. Inducing pneumothorax
    b. Promoting vascular hemorrhage
    c. Increasing intrathoracic pressure, thereby decreasing venous return to the heart
    d. Potentiating inhalation anesthetics
13. *Viscous distention may cause hypertension because of* _____.
    a. An increase in cardiac output
    b. Sympathetic stimulation of the bladder
    c. Vasodilation
    d. Discomfort causing catecholamine blockade
14. *Sodium nitroprusside (Nipride) reduces blood pressure by which action?*
    a. Suppression of the renin-angiotensin-aldosterone system
    b. Peripheral vasodilation
    c. Inhibition of intracellular calcium release
    d. Beta-blockade
15. *Enalapril maleate (Vasotec) reduces blood pressure by which action?*
    a. Suppression of the renin-angiotensin-aldosterone system
    b. Peripheral vasodilation
    c. Inhibition of intracellular calcium release
    d. Beta-blockade
16. *The most common cause of postoperative dysrhythmias is* _____.
    a. Hyperkalemia
    b. Pain
    c. Hypoxemia
    d. Medication toxicity

17. *The treatment for ventricular fibrillation is* _____.
    a. Synchronized cardioversion
    b. Immediate fluid resuscitation
    c. 1.0 mg of intracardiac epinephrine
    d. Defibrillation
18. *The most common cause of postoperative agitation is* _____.
    a. Pain
    b. Hypoxemia
    c. Ketamine
    d. A history of substance abuse
19. *If midazolam (Versed) is used to sedate an agitated patient, the PACU nurse should monitor the patient for* _____.
    a. Respiratory depression
    b. Excessive salivation
    c. Orthostatic hypotension
    d. Tachycardia and hypertension
20. *Malignant hyperthermia* _____.
    a. Occurs when patients are rewarmed too quickly
    b. Is an acute anesthetic emergency requiring prompt intervention
    c. Is caused by the release of intracellular potassium
    d. Does not occur with the newer inhalation anesthetics
21. *One of the first signs of malignant hyperthermia is* _____.
    a. An increase in temperature
    b. Ventricular ectopy
    c. Sympathetic hyperactivity
    d. Myoglobinuria
22. *The key to emergency readiness is* _____.
    a. Vigilance
    b. Preparation
    c. Knowledge
    d. All of the above

Answers

1. c	9. d	17. d
2. d	10. b	18. b
3. b	11. a	19. a
4. d	12. c	20. b
5. a	13. b	21. c
6. d	14. b	22. d
7. d	15. a	
8. a	16. c	

CHAPTER 9

Every patient admitted to the PACU requires post anesthesia and postsurgical care. However, several patient groups, specifically, geriatric, pediatric, and ambulatory surgical patients, have additional special needs.

Geriatric and pediatric patients have unique needs because of age-related physiologic alterations. It is interesting to note that while the pediatric patient is in the process of maturing physiologically and the elderly patient is experiencing physiologic decline, the two patient groups have many similar needs.

Ambulatory surgical patients have unique needs as well. Because they will be discharged to home instead of being admitted to an inpatient facility, it is important for patients to be physiologically stable. Pre-screening and patient selection factors are important considerations. As the anesthesiologist begins to administer the anesthetic agent, he or she should assist the patient to anticipate the "waking up" phase. The patient must be as functional as possible after surgery to ensure an uncomplicated recovery period at home.

It is the purpose of this chapter to discuss these special patients. Nursing care priorities will be presented with attention to "special needs." Geriatric, pediatric, and ambulatory surgical patients will require highly individualized care, which is the goal of post anesthesia nursing.

PATIENTS WITH SPECIAL NEEDS

Chapter Objectives

After reading this chapter, the reader should be able to:

1. Identify the physiologic changes that occur with aging.
2. Identify disease processes commonly found in elderly patients that may increase intraoperative risk.
3. Discuss the importance of the preoperative assessment for the geriatric patient.
4. Identify anesthetic considerations for the geriatric patient.
5. Discuss postoperative priorities for the geriatric patient.
6. Identify the physiologic differences in the pediatric patient.
7. Discuss the importance of the preoperative assessment for the pediatric patient.
8. Identify anesthetic considerations for the pediatric patient.
9. Discuss postoperative priorities for the pediatric patient and family.
10. Identify the rationale supporting ambulatory surgery.
11. Specify patient criteria for ambulatory surgery.
12. Specify procedural criteria for ambulatory surgery.
13. Discuss the importance of the preoperative assessment for the ambulatory surgical patient.
14. Identify anesthetic considerations for the ambulatory surgical patient.
15. Discuss postoperative priorities for the ambulatory surgical patient.

ELDERLY PATIENTS

The elderly represent the fastest growing segment of our society, with more than 11% of our population over the age of 65. Longevity continues to increase, as the overall health of our society improves through access to medical care, vaccinations, antibiotics, clean water, and technology.

The risks associated with anesthesia and surgery are increased in elderly patients. As a result, the elderly patient in the PACU will require extra care. When planning patient

219

care, the PACU nurse must consider the age of the patient.

In this section, physiologic and pharmacologic changes associated with aging will be presented. The importance of a preoperative assessment with the goal of reducing intraoperative and postoperative risks will be emphasized. Postoperative priorities for the PACU nurse in caring for the elderly patient will also be presented.

Physiologic changes associated with aging

In identifying physiologic changes associated with aging, it is important to remember that these are normal, physiologic changes. These changes occur independently from any pathophysiologic process that may occur as a result of injury or disease. The rate and degree of change is highly individualized, but averages a 1% decline per year in organ system deterioration.

Cardiovascular changes. Perhaps the biggest change in the cardiovascular system is the loss of large artery elasticity, secondary to arteriosclerotic changes in all major vessels. Because of this loss of elasticity, organ perfusion and compensatory regulation in all body systems will be decreased.

Myocardial changes include an increase in myocardial irritability and myocardial hypertrophy. Cardiac reserve and the heart's effectiveness as a pump decline. As a result of the anatomic changes within the myocardium and within vessels, hemodynamic alterations occur, including a decrease in cardiac output and an increase in blood pressure. Cardiac output declines about 1% per year after age 30. The decrease in cardiac output slows circulation time and may slow the onset of action of drugs, including the inhalation agents.

Orthostatic hypotension occurs as blood vessel tone decreases. Baroreceptors within the carotid body and aortic arch fail with age. In addition, the elderly patient may be taking medications that contribute to, or have the side effect of, orthostatic hypotension; such medications include antihypertensives, diuretics, and tricyclic antidepressants.

Respiratory changes. Anatomic changes that occur within the respiratory system include an increase in anterior-posterior (A-P) diameter of the chest, a progressive flattening of the diaphragm, an increase in chest wall rigidity, and reduction in alveolar surface. Total lung capacity is reduced by approximately 10%. Loss in skeletal muscle mass results in intercostal muscle wasting.

As a result of these anatomic changes, physiologic changes are many. There is a generalized reduction in pulmonary elasticity and chest wall mobility. Pulmonary compliance declines, increasing airway resistance and air-trapping. Ventilation-perfusion (V-Q) alterations develop, including declining tidal volume and vital capacity, altered oxygen and carbon dioxide exchange, and decreased aerobic capacity. The oxygen content of blood (Pao_2) normally decreases with age, reflected by the following equation:

$$Pao_2 = 100 - (0.4 \times age\ [yr]) = mm\ Hg$$

For example, in an 80-year-old adult,

$$Pao_2 = 100 - (0.4 \times 80) = 68\ mm\ Hg$$

as opposed to the normal value of 100 mm Hg.

Central nervous system changes. An important central nervous system change associated with aging is the decrease in nerve conduction, secondary to neurogenic atrophy and loss of peripheral nerve fibers. Reflexes are slowed. Perhaps more important, there is a decline in the sympathetic response. When we remember that sympathetic stimulation results in the release of catecholamines (epinephrine and norepinephrine) and a heightened physiologic ability of the body to face stressors, it becomes clear that a fall in sympathetic response contributes to a fall in cardiac reserve and responsiveness. Thermoregulation is also compromised.

Secondary to arteriosclerotic changes within the cardiovascular system are higher incidences of chronic brain syndrome, cerebrovascular accidents (strokes), and multiinfarct dementia. Cerebral blood flow and central nervous system activity is decreased. An acute decline in mental function is more commonly caused by malnutrition, medication intolerance, depression, or dehydration than by the results of aging. These acute disturbances are usually physiologic in nature and reversible, and therefore they should be closely evaluated.

Gastrointestinal changes. Gastrointestinal changes include a decrease in salivation and peristalsis. As a result, gastric emptying is delayed, and the risk of aspiration increases. Perhaps the most significant change is a decline in hepatic blood flow, secondary to the arteriosclerotic changes with the cardiovascular system and decreasing cardiac output. As a result, drugs metabolized and excreted via the liver (such as fentanyl and vecuronium) will remain present and active for a prolonged period of time. There is also a decreased absorption of orally administered drugs and nutrients, particularly ferrous sulfate (iron) and calcium.

Renal changes. Anatomic changes within the renal system include a decrease in bladder capacity, muscle tone, and weakening of sphincters. More important, there is a decrease in the glomerular filtration rate secondary to decreased renal blood flow (related to arteriosclerotic changes within the cardiovascular system). Glomerular filtration decreases by 1% to 1.5% per year. As a result, there is decreased renal metabolism and clearance of medications, including pancuronium, antibiotics, and digoxin.

The response time required to correct fluid and electrolyte imbalances is increased. In addition, urine concentrating ability is reduced. The inability to conserve sodium may result in hyponatremia. A decrease in renin activity and plasma aldosterone may result in hyperkalemia.

Orthopedic changes. The most significant change within the skeletal system is *osteoporosis:* a decline or decrease in the bone matrix, which compromises skeletal support. In osteoporosis, bone resorption increases the rate of bone formation. The elderly patient is at an increased risk for pathologic fractures, pain, and skeletal deformities. Fractures are commonly seen in the lower thoracic and lumbar vertebral bodies.

Endocrine changes. With increasing age, there is a progressive impairment in the body's ability to metabolize glucose, resulting in glucose intolerance. Pancreatic function declines, and the incidence of adult onset diabetes mellitus increases with age. Plasma renin concentration and activity decline by 30% to 50%, decreasing the plasma concentration of aldosterone and increasing the risk of hyperkalemia.

Dermatologic changes. An anatomic change with important physiologic sequelae is the decline in subcutaneous fat. Temperature regulation and maintenance is compromised, putting the elderly patient at risk for hypothermia. In addition, the decline in the number and efficacy of sweat glands compromises the elderly person's ability to lose heat when hyperthermic. Finally, there is a decline in skin pigmentation, making pallor an unreliable indicator of anemia and respiratory or cardiac distress.

With aging, the epidermis begins to atrophy, and collagen is lost. As a result, the elderly patient is at an increased risk for skin breakdown and decubitus ulcers. Careful positioning is essential. In addition, good skin care requires caution in placing and removing adhesive tape.

Sensory changes. Sensory changes resulting from a reduction in afferent innervation cause alterations in all forms of perception, including vision, hearing, and sensation. Visual changes include a decrease in visual acuity and peripheral vision. Auditory changes center on a decreased sensitivity to sound, especially to high-pitched tones. The senses of smell and taste are altered. There is also a decrease in tactile sensation and response to pain.

Pharmacologic alterations in aging

Because of alterations in the organs responsible for drug metabolism and clearance—including the lungs, kidneys, and liver—elderly patients experience alterations in pharmacodynamics. Elderly patients are more susceptible to prolonged action and elimination of drugs. As a result, doses of anesthetics must be reduced in the elderly.

In addition, because of the delayed elimination of drugs, the elderly patient is prone to cumulative drug effects and adverse drug interactions. Careful monitoring to assess individual patient differences is essential both intraoperatively and in the PACU.

Pathophysiologic conditions in the elderly

To this point, discussion has centered on the normal physiologic and pharmacologic changes associated with aging. But it must be recognized that there is an increase in system dysfunction with aging. Hypertension, atherosclerosis, and renal disease are common findings in the aging population. There is also an increased incidence of diabetes mellitus, anemia, and malignancy.

This increase in concomitant diseases is significant, because the mortality rate associated with anesthesia and surgery in patients with concomitant disease is 10 to 30 times greater than the 0.5% mortality rate for patients without preexisting conditions.[9] In addition, the number of associated medical conditions increases the rate and risk of perioperative complications. The American Society of Anesthesiologists classifies the physical status of patients by medical conditions, not age. This is based on the recognition that disease—rather than age itself—increases perioperative risk.

In addition to the increased hazards associated with concomitant diseases, the medications used in the management and treatment of these diseases, as well as alterations in liver and kidney function, may further contribute to perioperative complications. Diuretics may predispose the patient to hypokalemia and hypovolemia. Antihypertensives may decrease functioning of the autonomic nervous system. Beta adrenergic antagonists may also decrease autonomic functioning and contribute to the development of bronchospasm and bradycardia. Antibiotic therapy may increase the duration of action of muscle relaxants.

Preoperative assessment

Given the normal physiologic changes that occur with aging, combined with the pathophysiologic changes associated with disease or injury, it becomes of major importance to conduct a preoperative assessment. The primary purpose of the preoperative assessment is to obtain a precise preoperative baseline. A complete physical examination targeted to systems and patient history should be obtained and documented. Information about preexisting disease, including medication history, is also obtained at this time, so that preoperative physical status can be improved. The elderly patient should be questioned about the regular use of over-the-counter medications in addition to prescription medications. The preoperative period is the ideal time to obtain a baseline neurologic assessment.

By involving nurses preoperatively in patient assessment, it becomes possible to identify special patient needs and to anticipate postoperative sequelae. For example, it may be found that the patient wears bilateral hearing aids and is unable to hear without them. The nurse may then be able to make arrangements to either have the patient go into surgery with the hearing aids in place or to have them available on return to the PACU. A language barrier may be identified, and the nurse can arrange for a family member to be present in the PACU postoperatively for translation.

The preoperative assessment also is the ideal time to begin patient teaching with both the patient and family. Teaching may be about preoperative routines, intraoperative plans, or postoperative recovery and discharge.

Anesthetic options in the elderly patient

The geriatric patient is a potential candidate for general, regional, and intravenous sedation anesthesia. Each technique and each medication that is used will offer specific advantages and disadvantages. Ideally, the anesthesiologist, in cooperation with the patient and in consideration of the procedure to be performed, will select the technique best suited for each individual patient.

General anesthesia. General anesthesia is often the technique of choice for the elderly patient because of the smooth induction and generally rapid recovery. It should be remembered, however, that there are anatomic and physiologic changes associated with aging that will affect the anesthetic requirements of the elderly patient.

Minimum alveolar concentration (MAC) decreases at the rate of 4% per decade after the age of 40. As a result, the inhalation requirements for the elderly will be less. In addition, because hepatorenal function declines with age, drug metabolism and clearance of anesthetic agents will be delayed. The intravenous anesthetics, including the barbiturates, benzodiazepines, and opioids, must be given in decreased doses. Because the clearance of all anesthetic agents is decreased, the PACU nurse may see remaining pharmacologic drug effects in the PACU.

It is also important to note the relationship between general anesthesia and intraoperative hypothermia. General anesthesia compromises thermoregulation, prevents shivering, and increases peripheral vasodilation. Because intraoperative heat loss exceeds heat production, hypothermia is a frequent finding in the PACU.

Finally, the elderly patient may be edentulous and difficult to ventilate by mask. Arthritis, particularly cervicospinal, may make positioning for intubation difficult.

Regional anesthesia. Regional anesthesia may prove beneficial to the elderly patient, primarily because it is associated with minimal physiologic alterations. There are decreased incidences of cardiac and pulmonary complications and of postoperative confusion. Anesthesia is limited to the site or region of surgery. In addition, the patient is awake, decreasing the need for invasive monitoring. The patient can provide data as to physical status. Finally, regional anesthesia provides for postoperative analgesia, minimizing the need for the administration of additional narcotics in the PACU.

Spinal anesthesia. Spinal anesthesia is a useful technique for procedures of the lower abdomen and lower extremities in cooperative, alert patients. It is important to note that duration of spinal anesthesia will be prolonged in the elderly. Spinal anesthetics are absorbed and eliminated from pia and arachnoid circulation. Because circulatory time is slowed in the elderly, the injectate requires a longer time to dissipate, and the blockade is prolonged. Hypotension may be problematic in the elderly patient receiving spinal anesthesia. Hypotension occurs secondary to the sympathetic blockade. The elderly patient is at further risk for hypotension because of decreased catecholamines, baroreceptor failure, and decreased myocardial reserve. Small doses of intravenous ephedrine may be effective in correcting the hypotension.

Epidural anesthesia. Epidural anesthesia has the advantage of requiring a smaller dose of local anesthetic than is required with spinal anesthesia. However, epidural spread of the injectate is increased in the elderly because of anatomic changes in the intervertebral foramina. Therefore the dose of anesthetic should be decreased by 25% to 50%.

Again, the choice of anesthetic should be determined by the patient's condition, the surgical requirement, and the skill of the anesthesiologist.

Postoperative priorities

The goal in providing care to any patient in the PACU is the reduction of morbidity and mortality associated with surgery and anesthesia. For the elderly patient, this becomes increasingly important in consideration of all of the physiologic changes associated with aging. Nursing priorities exist in the areas of ventilation, fluid balance, activity stir-up, and comfort.

Ventilation. If we remember the age-related anatomic and physiologic changes in the respiratory system—especially the increases in ventilation/perfusion mismatch that result in hypoxemia—it becomes possible to identify three nursing care goals related to ventilation in elderly patients. The goals are (1) to promote optimal gas exchange, (2) to prevent respiratory infections, and (3) to monitor compromised function.

The first goal, *to promote optimal gas exchange,* mandates several interventions for the PACU nurse. To fulfill this goal, the nurse must perform a thorough respiratory assessment, provide high-humidity oxygen, elevate the head of the bed unless contraindicated by surgery, and encourage the patient to take deep breaths.

The second goal, *to prevent respiratory infections,* requires that the PACU nurse use sterile technique when suctioning an endotracheal tube, protect the patient against aspiration, and, again, encourage the patient to take deep breaths.

Finally, the third goal, *to monitor compromised function,* requires that the PACU nurse evaluate the patient for residual anesthetics, consider preexisting disease and health history (for example, smoking history), maintain artificial airways, and stimulate the patient to breathe deeply. Pulse oximetry monitoring is useful to detect hypoxemia. (For additional nursing interventions related to ventilation see Chapter 5.)

Fluid balance. Fluid balance is the second postoperative priority for the elderly patient. The first goal is to *correct preoperative dehydration.* The patient has been NPO since midnight, may be on diuretic therapy, or may have had a preoperative problem with nausea and vomiting. In correcting dehydration, the PACU nurse should *prevent fluid overload.* Nursing interventions include maintaining intake/output records and monitoring intravenous rates, breath sounds, and blood pressure. *Monitoring urine output* is also a priority, given the decreased bladder capacity and sphincter tone of the elderly patient. Because there are decreases in renal blood flow and glomerular filtration rate with aging, the elderly patient will require a longer response time to correct fluid and electrolyte imbalances. Medication clearance will be prolonged.

Activity stir-up routine. When we remember all of the age-related anatomic and physiologic changes within the cardiovascular, respiratory, and central nervous systems, the importance of an aggressive postoperative activity stir-up routine becomes apparent. The stimulation of the patient to awaken, breathe deeply, and follow commands *promotes circulation and ventilation.* This routine also allows the nurse to *assess neurologic functioning.* This includes evaluating the patient's ability to move all extremities, to follow commands, and to be oriented to place. Finally, the activity stir-up routine *promotes thermoregulation.* Achievement of normothermia promotes cardiovascular stability and patient comfort and decreases myocardial oxygen demands.

Comfort. When we remember all of the age-related anatomic and physiologic changes within the cardiovascular, central nervous, gastrointestinal, renal, orthopedic, and dermatologic systems, we become aware of how many possibilities for discomfort there are in an elderly patient. Implementing comfort measures is a priority. One goal is to take *care in positioning the patient.* Repositioning the patient should be accomplished with sufficient patient support to prevent tugging on extremities or shearing the patient across the sheets. Bony prominences should be padded, and side rails can be covered with blankets. *Skin care* is also a priority. If the elderly patient is found to be lying on wet sheets on admission to the PACU, the sheets should be changed and the skin dried. Care should be taken in applying tape to friable skin. Even noninvasive automatic blood pressure cuffs have caused bruising. The PACU nurse should be careful when removing ECG leads and tape. *Pain management* is also a priority. Because the elderly patient has a decreased response to pain and delayed hepatic and renal metabolism of drugs, pain medications should be judiciously administered, with attention to ventilation and airway management. Another step in the implementation of comfort measures is *to provide psychologic support,* which includes reorienting the patient and using clear communication and touch. Information should be simply stated and repeated as necessary.

The elderly patient does have unique needs that warrant special attention. By recognizing the physiologic changes that occur with aging, taking the time to complete a preoperative assessment, and establishing clear postoperative priorities, the PACU nurse can provide the best possible care for the elderly patient.

PEDIATRIC PATIENTS

Although most practitioners would agree that the pediatric patient is not just a "miniature adult," children do resemble adults physiologically. Psychologic development, to be sure, takes years. The purpose of this section is to highlight physiologic differences in the neonate and infant. Developmental issues related to surgery, hospitalization, and response to pain in all pediatric patients will also be presented.

Cardiovascular system

In the neonate and infant, the myocardium is less compliant than in the adult, resulting in a decreased stroke volume. As a result, infants depend on heart rate and adequate circulating blood volume to maintain cardiac output. In addition, the infant and neonate have immature sympathetic nervous systems, which allow only limited catecholamine stores, decreasing myocardial reserve. It is important to remember that many anesthetic agents are associated with myocardial depression. Neonates, in particular, are especially sensitive to negative inotropes.

Although the sympathetic nervous system is underdeveloped, the parasympathetic nervous system is mature at birth. As a result, vagal bradycardia occurs during stress (for example, during intubation). Therefore, children are usually premedicated with an anticholinergic (for example, atropine or scopolamine).

By the age of 2 years, assuming no pathology, the pediatric cardiovascular system achieves adult functioning. Normal values for blood pressure and pulse in pediatric patients are identified in Table 9-1.

Respiratory system

Anatomically, the infant has a disproportionately large head and a short neck. The infant's tongue is large, and the glottis is high and narrow, making laryngoscopy and intubation more difficult. The infant also tends to have an increased anterior-posterior chest diameter and may appear barrel-chested.

Breathing patterns are generally diaphragmatic, and periods of apnea may occur in the very young (premature especially). As the child matures, the functional work of the intercostal muscles improves, decreasing the work of breathing.

It should be remembered that the pediatric patient has a high basal metabolic rate, creating a high demand for oxygen. While tidal volumes in the infant are the same as for

Table 9-1. **Normal pediatric blood pressure and pulse values**

Age	Approximate systolic blood pressure (mm Hg)	Approximate pulse rate per minute
2 hr	60	120-160
5 days	80	120-160
6 mo	90	110-130
6 yr	100	100
10 yr	110	90
15 yr	120	80

From Dripps R, Eckenhoff J, and Vandam L: Introduction to anesthesia, Philadelphia, 1988, WB Saunders Co.

the adult (1 ml/kg), oxygen demand is 3 times greater, requiring a respiratory rate approximately 3 times that of the normal adult (40 to 60 breaths per minute as opposed to 12 to 16 breaths per minute).

Protective responses to hypercarbia (increased $Paco_2$) and hypoxemia (decreased Pao_2) are limited. Unlike what occurs in the adult, in whom respiratory compromise is usually compensated by tachycardia, in the infant bradycardia is always a sign of hypoxemia until proven otherwise.

Central nervous system

Perhaps no other organ system shows greater development throughout infancy and childhood than does the central nervous system, as evidenced by an increase in motor, sensory, and intellectual functioning with maturation.

The neonatal central nervous system is immature. Sympathetic nervous system responsiveness is not yet developed, manifested by decreased catecholamine stores. Physiologic stress is poorly tolerated. Responsiveness to states of hypoxemia, hypercarbia, and hypothermia is slow.

Gastrointestinal system

For the first month of life, there is a relative state of hepatic immaturity. Liver enzyme function and hepatic blood flow are diminished, contributing to a decrease in metabolism of any drug that requires hepatic biotransformation. After the first month of life, hepatic action assumes adult levels of functioning.

A gastrointestinal finding that continues throughout infancy is children's increased level of salivation. The anticholinergic given preoperatively to prevent intraoperative induction bradycardia is useful in controlling salivation.

Genitourinary system

In the early months of life, there is a decrease in the glomerular filtration rate and creatinine clearance, slowing the metabolism of any drug that requires renal biotransformation. There is also a decreased ability to clear fluid and sodium loads, making fluid overload and hypernatremia potential hazards of fluid administration.

Skeletal system

Infants have a relatively immature skeletal system, epiphyses are not yet fused, and fontanelles remain open. The nurse must be careful when carrying and positioning these patients. Protection from falls is imperative.

Integumentary system

Infants possess extremely sensitive skin, which requires care when placing and removing tape, ECG leads, and automatic blood pressure cuffs. In addition, infants have little subcutaneous fat and a relatively large surface area. Heat loss may be profound in even a short period of time. Neonates, in particular, are at risk because compensatory heat generation is achieved by nonshivering thermogenesis or the metabolism of brown fat. Use of this mechanism increases oxygen demands and may contribute to acidosis.

Developmental issues related to surgery and hospitalization

For pediatric patients hospitalization evokes feelings of separation, loss of control, and fear of injury and pain. Clearly, the response of the patient to hospitalization and surgery will vary with the patient's level of intellectual and verbal functioning. The infant who is unable to verbalize or understand explanations may react strongly to separation by crying, and he or she may be difficult to comfort. The toddler may respond with physical aggression and verbal uncooperativeness. The school-aged child may passively withdraw, but children in this age group are generally able to understand that family members are waiting to see them. Adolescents, likewise, understand separation.

Preoperative assessment

Despite the observation that by the age of 2 years the pediatric patient may be viewed as physiologically similar to the adult, it is still important to obtain a preoperative baseline. Most pediatric patients are hospitalized for surgical correction of anatomic deviations (congenital or acquired); physiologic derangements are usually minimal or absent. However, a history and physical examination, including laboratory values, should be included as part of the preoperative assessment. Gestational age as well as chronologic age should be recorded, as should any history of birth trauma or distress in infancy.

Ideally, the preoperative assessment should be done in the presence of family members, for this allows for a more reliable history, facilitates the development of a relationship between the family and members of the health care team, and allows for the beginning of patient and family teaching. Observing family and child interactions may also provide clues about family strengths and potential postoperative problems.

Preoperative medications

Preoperative medications may be administered to decrease the anxiety felt by children about the operating room and about separation from parents. In addition, preoperative medications may be used to increase patient safety and to decrease the anesthetic requirement intraoperatively.

Anticholinergics, specifically atropine and scopolamine, are used to minimize the cholinergic effects of halothane and succinylcholine, to offset vagal bradycardia at intubation, and to decrease secretions, which might, if unchecked, result in laryngospasm.

Sedatives (benzodiazepines and barbiturates) and opioids may be administered to decrease apprehension, to cause the child to fall asleep while the parent is present and before entering the operating room, and to decrease the anesthetic requirement.

Antiemetics may be given, but the lower gastric pH (2.5) and the increased residual gastric volume in children must be taken into consideration. The antiemetic is useful in decreasing the risk of aspiration and in reducing the incidence of postoperative nausea and vomiting.

Preoperative medications may be administered orally, intravenously, intramuscularly, or rectally. Oral medications are well tolerated by children, but they may have a delayed onset of action. Intravenous and intramuscular administrations require a needle stick, but these forms of administration increase the predictability of absorption. Rectal administration may be useful when intravenous access is difficult to attain. Absorption and onset of action are slowed and may be unpredictable.

Pharmacologic differences

The administration of anesthetic agents to infants and children requires knowledge not only about the physiologic differences in these patients but also about the pharmacologic differences. Although the drugs selected to provide anesthesia are not different than those used in adults, the delivery of the drugs will be different because of age-related differences in uptake, extravascular fluid volume, and receptor maturity.

Inhalation anesthesia. Induction of anesthesia by mask is likely to be well tolerated in infants and school-aged children, but it may be met with resistance by toddlers and preschoolers. However, inhalation induction is often preferred to a "shot." Halothane provides a more rapid and smooth induction than does enflurane or isoflurane. Enflurane and isoflurane are pungent and are associated with a higher incidence of airway irritation, specifically laryngospasm.

Inhalation induction in neonates and infants is extremely rapid because of a lower functional residual capacity for body weight and a greater blood flow to vessel-rich tissues, including the brain, heart, liver, and kidneys. Vessel-rich tissues make up 22% of the total body weight in neonates, as compared with only 10% in adults.

The incidence of hypotension and bradycardia during an inhalation induction is higher in neonates and infants than in adults; this is another result of the more rapid uptake of the anesthetic by vessel-rich tissues, in this case the myocardium. Cardiac monitoring (ECG and blood pressure) and oximetry are essential; and the presence of an intravenous line is strongly recommended.

Intravenous anesthetics. Because of an immature blood-brain barrier and a decreased ability to metabolize drugs, neonates are extremely sensitive to barbiturates and opioids. Because of an immature respiratory center, infant apnea is often an expected consequence of opioid administration.

Muscle relaxants. Infants are significantly more sensitive to nondepolarizing muscle relaxants than are adults; and infants require a lower plasma concentration to achieve neuromuscular blockade. Initial doses, however, are similar to adult doses. Infants have an increased extracellular volume, which dilutionally lowers plasma concentrations of the muscle relaxant.

In addition, because neonates experience decreased renal clearance of drugs, *d*-tubocurarine, metocurine, and pancuronium may have a prolonged duration of action. The immature hepatic system will delay clearance of vecuronium, prolonging the neuromuscular blockade.

Compared with adults, infants require increased doses of succinylcholine, probably because of the dilutional effect of a high-extravascular volume.

General anesthesia is the technique of choice for the pediatric patient because it provides a rapid, smooth induction. In some centers, to ease the induction even more, a parent may be present for the mask induction.

Regional anesthesia. In the pediatric patient, regional anesthesia may be used as an adjunct to general anesthesia, as the sole anesthetic, or for postoperative pain management. Although the option to use regional anesthesia is available, its use may be limited by patient cooperation factors and the anesthesiologist's level of comfort and proficiency in performing the procedures. The child may refuse to cooperate for the procedure because of fear of needles and apprehension about the operating room.

Axillary blocks may be used for procedures on the forearm, outer arm, and hand. Combination ilioinguinal and iliohypogastric blocks are useful for postoperative pain management after herniorrhaphy. The block is performed intraoperatively in the anesthetized child. Penile ring blocks are extremely effective for minimizing postoperative discomfort after a circumcision.

Caudal anesthesia is increasing in popularity in infants for perineal and lower abdominal surgery because of the ease of locating landmarks. Spinal anesthesia, injected at the level of L4-5 or L5-S1, is used for procedures below the level of the diaphragm. The use of intramuscular or intravenous ketamine may be beneficial in increasing the older child's cooperation in regional anesthesia.

Postoperative priorities

In addition to recovering from surgery and anesthesia, pediatric patients have unique needs and concerns specific to their physiologic and psychologic level of functioning. Concerns lie in the areas of altered ventilation, hypothermia, fluid balance, emergence, and comfort.

Alterations in ventilation. When we remember the anatomic and physiologic differences in the pediatric population, it becomes possible to identify two goals specific to alterations in ventilation. First, it is important to *promote oxygenation*. The demand for oxygen is high in the pediatric patient, and as anesthetic agents depress respirations, it is important for the PACU nurse to ensure airway patency, to provide oxygen (particularly for sleeping patients), and to institute pulse oximetry monitoring for any sleeping or critically ill patient.

Second, it is important to *monitor for compromised function*. Unless contraindicated, many pediatric patients scheduled for short procedures will be maintained intraoperatively by mask, as opposed to endotracheal, anesthesia. As a result, few patients will be admitted to the PACU with an endotracheal tube in place. There are, however, several potential airway alterations that may be seen in the postoperative pediatric surgical patient.

Infant apnea. Anesthetic agents that directly depress respiratory function may act on the immature respiratory center of the infant to cause periods of protracted apnea. This is especially problematic in infants with a history of respiratory distress, prematurity, or bronchopulmonary dysplasia. Hypothermia may also contribute to apneic episodes. Treatment includes administration of oxygen, stimulation to breathe, and initiation of pulse oximetry and/or apnea monitoring. Infants who are younger than a hospital-defined standard gestational age (usually 48 weeks) are usually kept hospitalized overnight for apnea monitoring after even the most minor procedure.

Postextubation croup. Postextubation croup is the name given to the hoarse, barking cough that may be seen in children after extubation. It is most commonly seen in children between 1 and 4 years of age, particularly when accompanied with intubation trauma, prolonged intubation, or movement of the endotracheal tube in patients who are awake. It is diagnosed by its characteristic cough. Treatment includes the administration of cool, humidified oxygen, and, if stridorous, racemic epinephrine.

Obstruction. To prevent airway obstruction, children are usually transported to the PACU in the lateral decubitus position (tonsillar), which results in the tongue falling away from the pharynx and allows for any secretions to drain away from the oropharynx. The PACU nurse should maintain children in this position until they awaken.

Hypothermia. Because of the infant's large body size, decreased subcutaneous fat, decreased catecholamine stores, and increased need for oxygen, it is important to restore normothermia. Hypothermia may result in apnea, bradycardia, hypotension, and metabolic acidosis. Therefore the best treatment is intraoperative prevention of hypothermia. If the patient is admitted to the PACU with a decreased temperature, the PACU nurse should initiate rewarming immediately.

Fluid balance. Because of the pediatric patient's alterations in renal function, including the decreased ability to handle fluid and sodium loads, restoration of circulating volume and fluid maintenance is critical. Ideally, to prevent iatrogenic dehydration, infants and toddlers should be scheduled as the first cases of the day.

Fluid therapy is designed *to meet normal physiologic needs, to restore deficits, and to replace losses*. It may be difficult to maintain an intravenous line in an infant or toddler. However, if fluid therapy is indicated, the PACU nurse must protect and secure the intravenous line. Maintenance fluid needs and urine outputs of the pediatric patient are identified in Table 9-2.

As an additional note, given that the pediatric patient is susceptible to fluid overload, fluid therapy is usually administered with a buretrol via a volumetric infusion pump. Documentation of intake and output is essential, as fluid replacement may be based on ml/ml replacement.

Table 9-2.   **Maintenance fluids in pediatric patients and normal urine output**

Electrolytes	Daily amount (mEq/kg)
Na	3
K	2
Cl	2

Body weight and age	24-hour fluid requirement
Premature and full-term newborn less than 5 days of age	50-70 ml/kg
Premature and full-term newborn over 5 days of age (5 days to 1 month of age)	150 ml/kg
3-10 kg (over 1 month of age)	100 ml/kg
10-20 kg	1000 ml plus 50 ml/kg over 10 kg
20 kg to adult	1500 ml plus 20 ml/kg over 20 kg

Normal urine output	
Age	**ml/kg/hr**
1 to 4 days	0.3-0.7
4 to 7 days	1.0-2.7
Over 7 days	3
Over 2 years	2
5 years to adult	1
Insensible loss	28

From Dripps R, Eckenhoff J, and Vandam L: Introduction to anesthesia, Philadelphia, 1988, WB Saunders Co.

Emergence. Most pediatric patients will awaken with some degree of disorientation and awareness of unfamiliarity with the environment. It is generally possible for the PACU nurse to quickly reorient these children to person and place. However, emergence delirium—as evidenced by persistent confusion, unruliness, and disorientation—may occur in up to 15% of young children and adolescents. It is important to immediately evaluate respiratory adequacy to rule out hypoxemia as the cause. If pain is the cause, pharmacologic intervention may be required. The need for patient safety must be attended to and may include the use of restraints or padded side rails. Sedation is not usually required. The nonpharmacologic interventions of touch, reassurance, parental visitation, and time may be the only intervention necessary.

Comfort. A number of myths exist about pediatric pain. Perhaps the most damaging is the belief that children do not have pain. Research has provided evidence of a pain response in all ages, including infancy. The goals in providing comfort for the pediatric patient include *preventing or minimizing separation, minimizing loss of control, and minimizing pain.*

Parental or care-giver reunion should be instituted as soon as possible. Some hospitals have gone as far as to allow parents to accompany their children into the operating room for induction and to be present on admission to the PACU for emergence.

To minimize loss of control, explanations and reorientation should begin postoperatively as soon as the child coherently awakens. Choices may be allowed when feasible. Restoration of control is particularly important in the adolescent patient.

Pain management may include the use of nonpharmacologic interventions such as touch (holding), rewarming, parental visitation, and feeding (for example, a bottle). Often nonpharmacologic interventions are tried first, particularly in nonverbal patients. Pharmacologic intervention may include small, titrated doses of intravenous narcotics (with subsequent apnea monitoring). Acetaminophen (Tylenol), liquid or tablets, usually 10 to 15 mg/kg by mouth, is an effective analgesic.

Discomfort from nausea and vomiting rarely requires intervention. Children usually report feeling better immediately after an emesis. Antiemetics are rarely necessary.

Summary

The pediatric patient does have unique needs that require attention, especially during infancy. By recognizing that physiologic differences exist, it becomes important for the PACU nurse to take the time to obtain a preoperative assessment and to set postoperative priorities for all pediatric patients.

AMBULATORY SURGICAL PATIENTS

Providing quality care for the ambulatory surgical patient requires a patient capable of accepting this type of surgery and a system capable of supporting this type of patient. It is the purpose of this section to discuss the concept of and rationale behind ambulatory surgery and to discuss patient selection factors. Issues related to the types of procedures being performed and to preoperative and postoperative concerns shall also be presented.

Rationale behind ambulatory surgery

Ambulatory surgery has been defined as "surgery of an uncomplicated nature that traditionally has been done on an inpatient basis, but which can be done with equal efficiency and safety without a hospital admission."[49]

It is the concept of efficiency that has fostered the growth of ambulatory surgery, specifically financial efficiency. Ambulatory surgical procedures performed in a physician's office save approximately 70% of costs of the same procedure performed in a traditional inpatient setting. The same procedure performed in a free-standing ambulatory center saves an average of 60% of outpatient costs. If the procedure is performed on an outpatient basis in a hospital-integrated system, savings average 50% of costs. Much of the savings are seen in the areas of bed costs, pharmacy, and laboratory testing.[61]

Cost savings are felt by patients, insurance companies, and other third-party payers.

Health-care cost containment is a national priority. Ambulatory surgery began its surge with full consumer support.

An additional advantage of ambulatory surgery is that it allows better use of inpatient beds. When ambulatory surgery is accepted as a viable alternative to inpatient hospitalization, bed congestion can be reduced, and inpatient beds can be used most efficiently. While some hospitals, particularly those with high occupancy rates, welcome this as a form of traffic control, smaller hospitals may experience this as a loss of revenue, and not as economic efficiency. Empty beds do not generate revenue.

Ambulatory surgery has been advantageous to patients as well. There is a lower incidence of nosocomial (hospital-acquired) infections and decreased morbidity associated with surgical procedures. Psychologically, ambulatory surgery promotes the concept of wellness, early ambulation, and restoration of functioning.

Types of ambulatory surgical facilities

The *free-standing ambulatory surgical center* is usually owned and operated by a physician. The centers are often located in densely populated areas, and they are designed to meet the needs of a targeted patient population. Access to the center is facilitated by public transportation, or the center will be conveniently located near interstate exits. These centers tend to be efficient and not highly bureaucratic operations, and they report high levels of patient and staff satisfaction.

Disadvantages of this type of center include high start-up and operating costs. Because these centers are usually independent, revenue generated must cover and exceed costs. In addition, independence from the bureaucracy of a large medical center also means independence from inpatient resources. If more complex procedures or extensive surgery are needed, referrals must be made. An affiliation must be made with an inpatient facility for transfer of the patient and continued care in an emergency.

The second type of ambulatory surgical facility is the *hospital-separated, or satellite center*. These centers exist as branches of a hospital or medical center and are designed to meet the needs of a geographic area, for example, a suburban or downtown commuter population. Operating costs are often subsidized by the hospital or medical center. Marketing is usually done by the main facility. A separate ambulatory facility decreases competition for operating rooms and eases scheduling demands. If additional surgery is needed or a complication arises, admission to the inpatient facility is facilitated.

The major disadvantage of this type of arrangement is the start-up costs associated with its development. Although the satellite center is initially subsidized by the inpatient facility, it is required to generate revenue by its caseload. An additional disadvantage may be the distance between the satellite center and the main hospital. Surgeons who operate on both inpatients and outpatients may not want to travel between two facilities.

The most common type of ambulatory surgical facility is the *hospital-integrated facility*. In some medical centers, no distinction other than a title (Ambulatory Surgical Unit) is given to the facility. With a hospital-integrated facility, existing resources (operating rooms, laboratories, billing) can be used, and existing personnel (physicians, anesthesiologists, nurses, central supply) can staff both the ambulatory center and the inpatient facility. Although this creates an increase in workload, it maximizes the productivity of the staff and the facility. With the resources of the inpatient facility readily available, it is possible to schedule an outpatient procedure that has the potential to become a major invasive surgery, for example, a diagnostic laparoscopy that has a probability of becoming a laparotomy, or a cystoscopy that may become a prostatectomy. In addition, because of the availability of inpatient resources, it is possible to schedule borderline, or "sicker," patients for outpatient surgery, with the awareness that the inpatient facility is available as a back-up if necessary.

Disadvantages of this type of arrangement reflect the increased costs associated with operating an inpatient facility. There is no question that it is more expensive to operate an inpatient facility than a free-standing facility. Many more resources and personnel must be supported. In addition, ambulatory surgical patients may be displaced on the operating schedule in favor of inpatients, particularly emergency cases. This disruption in schedules may result in ambulatory patients entering the operating room at late times and, as a result, being discharged to home at very late hours, which is often undesirable when patient safety is a priority.

In hospital-integrated facilities, ambulatory surgical patients are often side-by-side with inpatients, increasing the potential for nosocomial infections. Ideally, inpatients and outpatients should be separated, particularly as the ambulatory patient progresses into the secondary recovery phase of progressive ambulation, taking fluids, voiding, and discharge teaching.

Patient selection

Appropriate patient selection is imperative if the goals of ambulatory surgery centers—specifically, financial efficiency and patient safety—are to be met. Traditionally, ambulatory surgery has been an option only for physical status 1 and 2 patients (defined in Chapter 2). However, because of demands from patients, third-party payers, and physicians, the number of physical status 3 patients being scheduled for ambulatory procedures is increasing. With appropriate screening and care, this may prove acceptable, but the change in selection variables has been associated with an increase in unplanned, postoperative hospitalization (or transfers, in the case of free-standing units).[61]

Regardless of the physical status classification assigned to the patient, it is possible to identify ideal characteristics of an ambulatory surgical patient. First and foremost, the patient must be in good health. For the physical status 1 and 2 patient, this is not usually a problem. For the physical status 3 patient with severe systemic disease that is not incapacitating (for example, insulin-dependent diabetes mellitus, obesity, and hypertension), the system disorder should be well-controlled. Medical consults might be recommended, with patients receiving documented clearance for surgery from their internist or cardiologist. The anesthesiologist should also see the patient for a preoperative evaluation and clearance.

The patient should also be physically and intellectually capable of complying with preoperative, and ultimately, postoperative instruction. If the patient has physical or intellectual limitations because of age, impaired mobility, or diminished intellectual ability, a care-giver must be willing to accept responsibility for the patient; the care-giver may be the parent of a minor child or an adult child of an elderly parent.

As previously mentioned, patients should be willing to participate in the procedure preoperatively and postoperatively. Responsibilities of patients should be clearly identified, and their willingness to participate ascertained and documented.

Elderly patients present a special challenge in ambulatory surgery. As outpatients, elderly patients are able to return to a familiar home environment without the disruption of hospitalization. Because many elderly people live alone and might need help on the night of surgery, it is important to ensure the presence of a competent care-giver in the home environment. In addition, because of the normal physiologic changes associated with aging, combined with pathophysiologic conditions that may exist, it is important to assess the elderly patient's physiologic age, rather than chronologic age, in determining acceptability for ambulatory surgery. The requirement of accepting patients only if they are in good health is especially true with the elderly population.

The pediatric patient in ambulatory surgery also presents unique concerns. A parent or care-giver must participate in the experience by giving consent and by ensuring compliance with preoperative and postoperative instructions.

Infants of less than 46 weeks' gestational age and those with a history of prematurity, apnea, feeding aspiration, or anemia are not candidates for ambulatory surgery. Because of the higher incidence of postoperative apnea and sudden infant death among these infants, they are admitted to an inpatient facility for overnight apnea monitoring. If no respiratory distress is noted, the infant will generally be discharged to home the following morning.

Procedural selection

Ideally, the selection of a specific procedure as being acceptable for ambulatory surgery should be based on a mutual agreement among the physicians (surgeon and anesthesiologist) and the patient. Unfortunately, many procedures have been determined to be ambulatory in nature by the third-party payers as a result of diagnostic-related groups (DRGs) and reimbursement issues.

The goals in electing to perform a procedure on an ambulatory basis should be patient safety and quality care. Financial consideration may be the outcome in a procedure being done on an outpatient basis, but it should not be the goal in determining procedural suitability.

It is possible to identify six specifications that are usually adhered to in determining whether it is acceptable to perform a procedure on an ambulatory basis. Although summarized in the box on p. 237, each will be specifically addressed.

The first specification is that there will be no invasion of a major body cavity or cranial vault. Penetration of a body cavity reflects the invasiveness of the procedure, a greater potential for postoperative complications, including infection, the likelihood of pain requiring parenteral narcotics, and the need for continued monitoring (including laboratory data, x-ray, hemodynamic) or follow-up (with physical therapy or respiratory therapy).

SPECIFICATIONS FOR AMBULATORY SURGERY

There will be no invasion of a major body cavity or the cranial vault.
Minimum physiologic derangement is expected.
Transfusion of blood bank blood is not expected.
The procedure will take a relatively short time (<4 hours).
Postoperative complications are unlikely.
Professional nursing care is not needed.

The second specification is that the procedure is associated with minimum physiologic derangement. Electrolyte imbalance, dehydration, hemorrhage, pneumonia, and sepsis should not be expected outcomes of an ambulatory procedure, because all are associated with an increased morbidity and mortality and the need for medical and nursing intervention and monitoring.

The third specification is that transfusion of blood bank blood should not be required by the procedure. Ideally, patients with severe anemia will not be candidates for ambulatory surgery. Low hemoglobin values are associated with a higher incidence of oxygenation problems, including desaturation and hypoxemia. In addition, patients are not usually given transfusions unless blood loss exceeds 500 to 1000 ml, dropping a patient's hemoglobin to less than 10 g/dl.

The fourth specification is that the procedure will take less than 4 hours of anesthesia time. This specification has been so challenged that it is possible it will be eliminated altogether. Initially, ambulatory procedures were limited to 60 to 90 minutes in duration. More than 4 hours of anesthesia time has been associated with a higher incidence of postoperative respiratory depression (decreased tidal volume and negative inspiratory force) and generalized fatigue and malaise. However, the relationship between anesthesia time and recovery time appears weak.

The fifth specification is that the procedure be associated with a minimal probability of postoperative complications, including pain, nausea and vomiting, bleeding, and surgery-specific complications.

The sixth specification—that professional nursing care should not be needed after recovery from anesthesia is complete—is perhaps one of the most important. If professional nursing care is required to assist the patient in regaining, maintaining, or attaining an optimum level of physiologic functioning, the patient should be admitted to an inpatient facility.

Although these six specifications exist as guidelines for selecting patients for ambulatory surgery, the decision also depends on the type of ambulatory surgical facility in which the procedure will be performed. The procedure may be performed in a physician's office, a free-standing facility, or a hospital-integrated facility, depending on the likelihood of needing an inpatient bed after surgery. If the need for postoperative medical and nursing care does exist, the procedure should be performed strictly on an inpatient basis. The overlap in the categories for this determination is illustrated in Fig. 9-1. The most commonly performed ambulatory surgical procedures are identified in the box on p. 239.

Despite the recommendations that exist for determining the suitability of ambulatory surgical procedures, a number of surgeons have begun trials with procedures traditionally thought to be inpatient procedures, including vaginal hysterectomy, tonsillectomy, cholecystectomy, mastoidectomy, and mastectomy. The rationale behind this trend came from monitoring patients postoperatively and determining that care priorities and patient needs centered on rest and sleep and pain management, all of which can be provided in the ambulatory setting.

Obviously, not all patients undergoing these types of surgeries are candidates for having them performed in an ambulatory setting. Ambulatory surgery requires healthy patients who are capable and willing to follow a preoperative and postoperative routine. It also requires surgeons who are innovative and willing to operate in this manner.

Preoperative evaluation. Although it is the surgeon who first proposes ambulatory surgery to a patient, the ultimate clearance for the procedure is usually given by an anesthesiologist in a preoperative visit. It is the anesthesiologist who sees the patient preoperatively, obtaining a medical, surgical, and anesthesia history. The anesthesiologist orders preoperative laboratory tests based on individual patient findings. This preoperative visit is usually scheduled anywhere from 30 days in advance of the surgery to the day of surgery. It is advantageous to see the patient prior to the day of surgery to maximize patient safety, minimize cancellations, and help decrease patient anxiety by answering questions about the anesthesia and surgery.

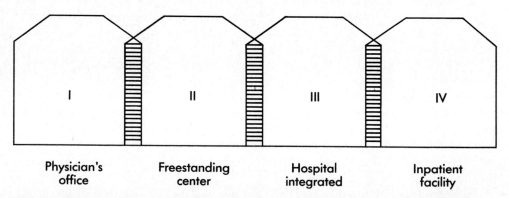

I	II	III	IV
Physician's office	Freestanding center	Hospital integrated	Inpatient facility

FIG. 9-1. Surgical classifications. *I,* Procedures requiring only local anesthesia. *II,* Procedures requiring anesthesia with no expectation of prolonged recovery or hospitalization. *III,* Procedures requiring anesthesia with minimal expectation of the need for hospitalization, *IV,* Patients who are receiving anesthesia and who may require postoperative medical and surgical care.

COMMON AMBULATORY PROCEDURES

Gynecologic

*Dilation and curettage
Tubal ligation
Diagnostic laparoscopy
Examination under
    anesthesia
Biopsy

Urologic

*Cystoscopy
Circumcision
Vasectomy
Lithotripsy
Biopsy

Orthopedic

*Arthroscopy
Carpal tunnel release
Bunionectomy
Fracture repair
Joint manipulation

General

*Biopsy
Breast biopsy
Hemorrhoidectomy
Herniorrhaphy
A-V fistula placement
Central line placement
Excision of lesions

Opthalmology

*Cataract extraction
Lens implant
Lacrimal duct probing
Examination under
    anesthesia

Dental

*Multiple extractions

Otolaryngoscopy

*Myringotomy (tubes)
Adenoidectomy
Laryngoscopy
Submucous resection
Septorhinoplasty
Tonsillectomy

Plastic surgery

*Rhinoplasty
Mammoplasty
Basal cell carcinoma
    excision
Scar revision
Dermabrasion
Blepharoplasty
Liposuction

Thoracic surgery

*Bronchoscopy
Tracheal dilation
Esophageal dilation
Pacemaker battery
    change

---

*Represents most common procedure in each specialty.

Laboratory testing. The use of laboratory testing to screen patients preoperatively has been extremely controversial, especially in the ambulatory surgical population. Physicians have been criticized for ordering "routine" laboratory tests without considering individual patient specifics. Roizen[57] advocates ordering laboratory tests only for recognizable indications, finding that 60% of currently ordered tests are unnecessary. Ideally, laboratory tests should be ordered in consideration of the patient's medical history, age, medications, and type of scheduled procedure. Commonly ordered laboratory tests for the ambulatory surgical patient are identified in Table 9-3.

Nursing assessment. Nurses play a vital role in the preoperative preparation of patients. In fact, it is often a nurse who fulfills the role of preoperative coordinator. The preoperative nurse will ensure that the patient is seen and cleared medically by an anesthesiologist, laboratory tests are performed, results are obtained, and a chart is com-

Table 9-3. **Laboratory testing in ambulatory surgery**

Test	Males	Females	Miscellaneous information
Hematocrit or hemoglobin	Over age 60	All	—
Urinalysis (BUN/glucose)	Over age 40	Over age 40	In all diabetic patients
Electrocardiogram	Over age 40	Over age 40	Younger if indicated by history
Chest roentgenogram	Over age 60	Over age 60	Younger if indicated by history
Coagulation profile	Only if indicated by history or surgery		
Electrolytes	Only if indicated by history or surgery		

piled. A nursing history and physical examination will also be obtained. Each interviewer should complement the others, documenting findings.

A nursing history and physical examination is obtained for a number of reasons. Initially, it is a means to determine the patient's understanding of the ambulatory surgical procedure and process. More important, it is a means to identify and clarify any misunderstandings the patient may have about the procedure, anesthesia, and the preoperative and postoperative routines. By obtaining a history and physical examination targeted toward activities of daily living (mobility, nutrition, toileting, life-style), it is possible to identify potential alterations in patient functioning that may have an impact on a successful recovery. Perhaps the most important underlying reason for obtaining a nursing history and physical examination is that it provides the opportunity for preoperative teaching. Planning for discharge begins on admission into the ambulatory process, not on completion of the procedure.

Preoperative teaching will include logistic instructions for the day of surgery. The nurse should instruct the patient as to where and when to arrive for surgery, including any necessary details about parking. The patient should be instructed about NPO (no oral intake) status. For adults, nothing should be taken by mouth, including water, after midnight of the night before surgery. For children ages 6 months to 3 years, clear liquids may be given up to 6 hours before induction. For infants less than 6 months of age, clear liquids may be given up to 4 hours before induction. It is important for the nurse to clarify the definition of clear liquids; it does not include milk or juices such as orange or tomato. Clear liquids are liquids that one can "see through," including water, apple juice, and cranberry juice.

Preoperative teaching should also emphasize the desirability of patients not smoking prior to surgery, especially the day of surgery, but ideally for as long as possible before surgery. The nurse should also instruct the patient as to any preoperative medications that should be taken, whether the medication is ordered as a single-dose preoperative medication or is taken routinely for a preexisting medical disorder.

Preoperative teaching should also include arrangements for discharge, including arranging for transportation, emphasizing the need for a responsible adult to accompany the patient home, and making any necessary arrangements for follow-up care.

Time should be allowed for questions by both the patient and the patient's family member or significant other. Frequently, in addition to answering questions during the preoperative visit, many centers call the patient (or parent) the night before surgery to reinforce teaching and to answer any last minute questions. The nurse should document all teaching that is done in the patient's chart.

Day of surgery. Prior to entering the operating room, the patient will once again be screened by an anesthesiologist and by a nurse. The anesthesiologist will review all documentation, will determine if any acute changes have occurred, and will grant final clearance for the procedure. The nurse will screen the patient to confirm adherence to preoperative routines and to confirm that a responsible adult will be available postoperatively to accompany home any patient having general, regional, or sedation anesthesia.

Anesthesia for ambulatory surgery. General anesthesia has traditionally been the anesthetic technique of choice for ambulatory surgery, and it remains so, especially with the advent of newer anesthetic agents such as isoflurane, fentanyl, and alfentanil. General anesthesia provides a rapid and smooth induction, intraoperative amnesia and analgesia, good surgical conditions, and a relatively short recovery with minimal side effects.

Regional anesthesia in ambulatory surgery has traditionally been limited to peripheral nerve blocks. Increasingly, however, epidural, spinal, and caudal anesthesia have been used successfully with ambulatory patients. Regional anesthesia does not cause the secondary side effects of general anesthesia, which include nausea, malaise, headache, and fatigue. In addition, regional anesthesia may decrease the need for postoperative analgesics. The use of regional anesthesia will have an impact on discharge because additional criteria must be included in assessment; for example, the patient must be able to ambulate without hypotension or dizziness after an epidural, spinal, or caudal anesthetic.

Local anesthesia is perhaps the safest anesthetic technique; it is associated with few complications or side effects and has the most rapid recovery. It also has the benefit of allowing the patient to return to home or work without being accompanied by a family member or friend. Unfortunately, many procedures cannot be performed under local anesthesia, and so its usefulness is limited.

Local anesthesia may be used in conjunction with the intravenous sedation of a narcotic and a benzodiazepine, for example, fentanyl and midazolam. The addition of intravenous sedation helps to increase both the effectiveness of the local anesthetic and patient comfort and to decrease pain and anxiety.

The choice of anesthetic technique depends on (1) the surgical procedure; (2) the patient's health, history, and emotional state; and (3) the anesthesiologist's judgment as to the ideal anesthetic.

Postoperative priorities. The ambulatory patient who has undergone a surgical procedure has postanesthetic and postsurgical needs. The assessment by the PACU nurse must be directed toward both areas. Postoperative priorities are established on the basis of this assessment, and the ultimate goal is discharge of the patient to home. The components of the postanesthetic and postoperative assessment are described in Chapter 5. It is the purpose of this section to identify unique considerations for the ambulatory surgical patient.

The most important goal postoperatively is to maintain patient safety while maintaining the patient's ambulatory status. There are a number of intraoperative and postoperative events that may compromise patient safety if the patient is discharged to home. These events may be categorized as medical, surgical, anesthesia-related, or social. Examples from each category are provided in the box below.

Medical conditions that result in admission generally necessitate continued monitoring and laboratory testing, which cannot be performed on an outpatient basis. The most common surgical reason for admission is the need for more extensive surgery. The surgeon may have had to perform a mastectomy instead of a biopsy. A cystoscopy may need to be rescheduled as a lithotripsy. Surgical complications (for example, a uterine perforation during a laparoscopy) may necessitate admission for monitoring of bleeding or monitoring for infection.

Aspiration is considered to be an anesthesia-related reason for admission—the result, perhaps, when an outpatient does not consider two cups of coffee the morning of surgery "eating breakfast." Nausea and vomiting may result in admission, particularly if continued emesis is likely to result in dehydration. Pain requiring management with parenteral narcotics may also be cause for admission.

Social reasons for admission include a patient's request for hospitalization, which may be made because of concerns about mobility, transportation, or care-giver capabilities. A family member may request patient hospitalization for similar reasons. A physician may request that a patient be hospitalized because of uncertainty about the patient's or family's reliability, ability to manage postoperatively, or compliance. Hospital administration may mandate hospitalization if no care-giver is available to take home the patient who has had anesthesia and surgery. This type of admission stems from medi-

---

OUTPATIENT → INPATIENT: REASONS FOR HOSPITALIZATION

Medical

Chest pain
ECG changes/dysrhythmias
Exacerbation of a chronic condition
   (diabetes/hypertension)
Electrolyte abnormalities

Surgical
Need for more intensive surgery
Need for drainage system monitoring
Bleeding—actual or high potential
Surgical misadventures

Anesthesia

Aspiration
Nausea and vomiting
Pain

Social
Patient request
Family request
Physician request
Hospital directive

BASELINE DISCHARGE CRITERIA
——————— **FOR THE AMBULATORY SURGICAL PATIENT** ———————

1. Stable vital signs for 30 minutes that are consistent with the preoperative baseline
2. No respiratory distress
3. Minimal nausea, vomiting, and dizziness
4. Alert and oriented to surroundings
5. Able to ambulate unless inappropriate for age
6. No signs or symptoms that may jeopardize the safety of recovery (e.g., bleeding, swelling, extreme pain)
7. Void as indicated by surgery (gynecologic, urologic)

Additional discharge criteria following regional anesthesia (epidural and spinal)

1. Presence of normal sensation
2. Able to ambulate (indicates strength and balance)
3. Able to void (return of sympathetic nervous function)

colegal concerns about the level of functioning of patients after anesthesia and the safety in discharging them to home alone.

As the patient begins to stabilize from both the anesthesia and the surgery, oxygen therapy and ECG monitoring will be discontinued. The PACU nurse will then assist the patient into the second phase of post anesthesia recovery. In this phase, the patient will move from the PACU cart to a chair, usually a recliner. Fluids will be offered. If the fluids are tolerated without nausea and vomiting, the intravenous line will be discontinued. The PACU nurse will assist the patient to the bathroom as necessary.

As previously stated, the most important goal in ambulatory surgery is to maintain patient safety. It is imperative, therefore, for practitioners within ambulatory surgical centers to establish written discharge criteria that are consistently applied when determining patient readiness for discharge to home. Discharge criteria used to assess patient readiness, including criteria for the patient who has received regional anesthesia, are listed in the box above.

After the discharge criteria are met and documented by the PACU nurse, the patient should ultimately be assessed for discharge by the anesthesiologist as well. Medical clearance for discharge is the final criterion that must be met.

Inherent in planning for discharge is that patients receive post anesthesia and postsurgical teaching. Postanesthesia teaching includes recommendations not to drive or to make major decisions until the day after surgery. If the patient complains of a sore throat after intubation, instruction is given about warm salt-water gargles and acetaminophen. If the patient has had a spinal anesthetic, instruction is given about the possibility of developing a postdural puncture headache. Patients should be instructed to call their anesthesiologist if they have a headache that is unrelieved by analgesics or one that is accompanied by a stiff neck. For patients who have had spinal anesthetics, bedrest with bathroom privileges is usually recommended for the evening of surgery to decrease the potential for developing a headache.

Postsurgical instruction should include procedure-specific information, including expected complications. Patients should be instructed to notify their surgeon in the event of unanticipated complications. Activity recommendations or limitations will be reviewed. Finally, follow-up instructions should be given.

All discharge teaching should be documented in the patient's chart. In addition, because of the amnesiac effects of anesthetic medications, patients should be given written copies of their post anesthesia and postoperative instructions. A family member might also be included in the teaching.

Future of ambulatory surgery. As ambulatory surgery becomes increasingly more liberal in patient and procedure selection, new alternatives for care delivery have been developed, with a goal of maintaining patient safety.

One interesting alternative is a 23-hour postoperative observation unit, which is being used for extended recovery of ambulatory patients. As long as the patient occupies the unit for less than 24 hours, outpatient status is maintained.

Some hospitals use a hotel for continued availability of medical care. The ambulatory medical hotel encourages patient independence, but it provides the reassurance of available medical personnel in the event of an emergency.

Surgeons are utilizing nurse clinicians or home health nursing care to provide postoperative follow-up for patients. Home visits may be required for pain management, fluid administration, or in the event of complications.

Patient-controlled analgesia is being tried in the ambulatory patient population for continuing parenteral pain medication in the home setting. Single-patient use infusion devices have been made portable to allow for easier mobility.

Summary. The concept of ambulatory surgery is well accepted by physicians, nurses, third-party payers, and, most important, by patients. In selecting patients, procedures, or anesthetic techniques in ambulatory surgery, the primary goal is the maintenance of patient safety. Vigilance and attention to detail by the surgeon, anesthesiologist, and nurse will help to ensure this goal.

REFERENCES
Elderly Patients
1. Bentley J, Borel J, Nenad R, and Gillespie T: Age and fentanyl pharmacokinetics, Anesth Analg 61:968-971, 1982.
2. Brocklehurst JC and Hanley T: Geriatric medicine for students, London, 1978, Churchill Livingstone, Inc.
3. Cassel C and Walsh J (editor): Geriatric medicine, vol II, New York, 1984, Springer-Verlag, Inc.
4. Crawford F: Ambulatory surgery: the geriatric patient, Am Assoc OR Nurs 2:356-359, 1985.
5. Davenport H: Anesthesia in the elderly, New York, 1986, Elsevier Science Publishing Co, Inc.

6. Del Guercio L and Cohn J: Monitoring operative risk in the elderly, JAMA 243(13):1350-1355, 1980.
7. Ellison N: Problems in geriatric anesthesia, Surg Clin North Am 55:929, 1975.
8. Evans T: The physiologic basis of geriatric general anesthesia, Anaesth Intensive Care 1:319, 1973.
9. Farrow S et al: Epidemiology in anaesthesia II: factors affecting mortality in hospital, Br J Anaesth 54:811, 1982.
10. Gambert S (editor): Contemporary geriatric medicine, vol II, New York, 1986, Plenum Publishing Corp.
11. Gibson J, Mendelhall M, and Axel N: Geriatric anesthesia: minimizing the risk. In Brindly G (editor): Clinics in geriatric medicine, Philadelphia, 1985, WB Saunders Co, p 313.
12. Gordon JL: Planning a safe anesthesia for the elderly patient, Geriatrics 32:69-72, 1977.
13. Halbrecht T, Garrison R, and Fry D: Role of infection in increased mortality associated with age in laparotomy, Am Surg 49:173-178, 1983.
14. Johnson J: The medical evaluation and management of the elderly surgical patient, J Am Geriatr Soc 31:621, 1983.
15. Katz R (editor): Anesthesia and the elderly. In Seminars in anesthesia 5(1), Orlando, March 1986, Grune & Stratton.
16. Krechel S (editor): Anesthesia and the geriatric patient, New York, 1984, Grune & Stratton.
17. Linn BS, Linn MW, and Wallen N: Evaluation of results of surgical procedures in the elderly, Ann Surg 195:90-96, 1982.
18. Mohr DN: Estimation of surgical risk in the elderly: a correlative review, J Am Geriatr Soc 31:99-102, 1983.
19. Masunuru V: The geriatric patient, Curr Rev Recov Room Nurses 8(7):58-63, 1985.
20. Pathy MS (editor): Principles and practice of geriatric medicine, New York, 1985, John Wiley & Sons, Inc.
21. Rowe J et al: The effect of age on creatinine clearance in man: a cross-sectional and longitudinal study, J Gerontol 31:155, 1976.
22. Roy R: General vs regional anesthesia in the elderly patient—does it matter? American Society of Anesthesiologists annual meeting, Chicago, ASA Annual Refresher Course Lectures 431:1-6, 1986.
23. Rupp S, Caotagnoli K, Fisher D, and Miller R: Pancuronium and vecuronium pharmacokinetics and pharmacodynamics in young and elderly adults, Anesthesiology 67:45-49, 1987.
24. Sear J, Cooper G, and Kumar V: The effect of age on recovery, Anaesthesia 38:1158, 1983.
25. Stephen C and Assaf R (editors): Geriatric anesthesia: principles and practice, Boston, 1986, Butterworth Publishers.
26. White DG: Anesthesia in old age, Br J Hosp Med 24:145-150, 1980.

Pediatric Patients

27. Berry F: Anesthetic management of difficult and routine pediatric patients, New York, 1986, Churchill Livingstone, Inc.
28. Berry F: Pediatric outpatient anesthesia. In Hershey SG (editor): ASA Refresher Courses in Anesthesiology 10:17-26, 1982.
29. Berry F: Pediatric anesthesia. Otolaryngol Clin North Am 14(3):533-556, 1981.
30. D'Apolito K: The neonate's response to pain, Am J Maternal-Child Nurs 9(4):256-257, 1984.
31. Dorn L: Children's concepts of illness: clinical applications, Pediatr Nurse 10(5):325-327, 1984.
32. Dripps R, Eckenhoff J, and Vandam L: Introduction to Anesthesia, Philadelphia, 1988, WB Saunders Co.
33. Eger E, Bahlman S, and Munson E: The effect of age on the rate of increase of alveolar anesthetic concentration, Anesthesiol 35:365-372, 1971.
34. Gotch G: Caring for children needing anesthesia, AORN 35(2):218-226, 1982.

35. Gregory G: Pediatric anesthesia, New York, 1985, Churchill Livingstone, Inc.
36. Hannallah R and Rosales J: Experience with parent's presence during anaesthesia induction in children, Can Anaesth Soc J 30:286-289, 1983.
37. Johnson, G: Day care surgery for infants and children, Can Anaesth Soc J 30:553-557, 1983.
38. Koka B et al: Postintubation croup in children, Anesth Analg 56:501, 1977.
39. Korberly B: Pharmacologic treatment of children's pain, Pediatr Nurse 11(4):292-294, 1985.
40. Liu L et al: Life-threatening apnea in infants recovering from anesthesia, Anesthesiology 59:506-510, 1983.
41. Nelson M: Identifying the emotional needs of the hospitalized child, Am J Maternal-Child Nurs 6(3):181-183, 1981.
42. Rowe P (editor): The Harriet Lane handbook: a manual for pediatric house officers, ed 11, Chicago, 1987, Year Book Medical Publishers, Inc.
43. Smith R: Anesthesia for infants and children, ed 4, St Louis, 1980, The CV Mosby Co.
44. Whaley P and Wong D: Nursing care of infants and children, ed 3, St Louis, 1987, The CV Mosby Co.

The Ambulatory Surgical Patient

45. Ashcraft K, Guinee W, and Golladay E: Clinical assessment of hematocrit and hemoglobin, Anesthesiol Rev 9(2):37, 1982.
46. Boyle W and White P: Preoperative assessments and management of adults with pre-existing problems, Ambulatory Anesthesia: Newsletter of the Society for Ambulatory Anesthesia 2(4):4, December 1987.
47. Carson J and Eisenberg J: The preoperative screening examination. In Goldmann D et al (editors): Medical care of the surgical patient: a problem-oriented approach to management, Philadelphia, 1982, JB Lippincott Co, pp 16-30.
48. Comprehensive preop telephone interviews are smoothing ways for ambulatory patients, Anesthesiol News, June 25, 1987.
49. Davis JE and Detmer DE: The ambulatory surgical unit, Ann Surg 175:856, 1972.
50. Detmer DE and Buchanan-Davidson DJ: Ambulatory surgery, Surg Clin North Am 62:685, 1982.
51. Egdahl R: Should we shrink the health care system? Harvard Bus Rev 61(1):125, 1984.
52. Faculty expert explains steps to low hospital admission rates, Same Day Surg 6(11):136, 1982.
53. Jensen S and Wetchler B: The obese patient: an acceptable candidate for outpatient anesthesia, JAANA 50:369, 1982.
54. Kitz D et al: Discharging outpatients: factors nurses consider to determine readiness, AORN 48(1):87-91, 1988.
55. Liv L et al: Life-threatening apnea in infants recoverying from anesthesia, Anesthesiol 59:506, 1983.
56. Meridy HW: Criteria for selection of ambulatory surgical patients and guidelines for anesthetic management: a retrospective study of 1553 cases, Anesth Analg 61:921-926, 1982.
57. Roizen M: Routine preoperative evaluation. In Miller R (editor): Anesthesia, ed 2, Chicago, 1989, Churchill Livingstone, Inc, pp 225-254.
58. Schneider A: Assessment of risk factors and surgical outcome, Surg Clin North Am 63:1113, 1983.
59. Squibb C: Outpatient surgical evaluations, Nurs Manage 19(1):32L-32P, 1988.
60. Wetchler B: Outpatient anesthesia. In Barash P, Cullen B, and Stoelting R (editors): Clinical anesthesia, Philadelphia, 1989, JB Lippincott Co, pp 1339-1364.
61. Wetchler B: Anesthesia for ambulatory surgery, Philadelphia, 1985, JB Lippincott Co.
62. Wetchler B: Anesthesiologists serve as watchdogs in ambulatory surgical settings, Same Day Surgb 8(7):83, 1984.
63. White P: Anesthetic considerations for the adult outpatient, Am Soc Anesthesiol Rev Course Lectures 273:1-7, 1986.

Review Questions

1. *The loss of large artery elasticity seen in the elderly person* ——————————.
   a. Contributes to increased vascular resistance
   b. Compromises organ perfusion in all body systems
   c. Increases circulation speed
   d. Increases cardiac output

2. *The oxygen content of blood (Pao$_2$) in the elderly person* ——————————.
   a. Increases with age
   b. Is unaffected by age
   c. Is equal to the carbon dioxide content of blood (Paco$_2$)
   d. Decreases with age

3. *In the elderly patient, sympathetic responsiveness* ——————————.
   a. Increases with age
   b. Decreases with age
   c. Remains equal to that of a younger adult
   d. No longer occurs

4. *Medications should be administered cautiously to elderly patients because* ——————————.
   a. Large doses are required to achieve desired effects
   b. Renal and hepatic metabolism of drugs is slower
   c. The elderly have a decreased sensitivity to drugs
   d. The elderly have rapid circulation times

5. *Medications taken routinely by elderly persons for pathophysiologic alterations may adversely affect the patient intraoperatively. For example, beta-adrenergic antagonists may decrease autonomic functioning, causing* ——————————.
   a. Bronchodilation and tachycardia
   b. Bronchospasm and bradycardia
   c. Acidosis and hypotension
   d. Alkalosis and hypertension

6. *Anesthetic agents administered to the elderly should be given* ——————————.
   a. In higher doses because of a decreased sensitivity
   b. In higher doses because of slowed renal and hepatic clearance
   c. In decreased doses because of declining hepatorenal function
   d. In decreased doses because of increased renal clearance

7. *Inhalation induction in children* ——————————.
   a. Should be attempted only after intravenous sedation is given
   b. Is slower than in adults
   c. Causes no cardiac alterations as seen in adults
   d. Is extremely rapid because of rapid tissue uptake

8. *Narcotic administration in infants* ——————————.
   a. Is absolutely contraindicated
   b. Is associated with episodic apnea
   c. Requires intensive care hospitalization
   d. Is not associated with any problems that do not also occur in adults

9. *Hypothermia in infants and children may result in* _____.
   a. Apnea, bradycardia, hypotension, and metabolic acidosis
   b. Bleeding, hypotension, and cardiac arrest
   c. Tachycardia, hypertension, and respiratory alkalosis
   d. Myocardial protection and stability

10. *An unexpected decrease in a child's heart rate is assumed to be caused by* _____ *until proven otherwise.*
   a. Pain
   b. Hypotension
   c. Hypoxemia
   d. Fluid overload

11. *At birth, the* _____ *nervous system is underdeveloped.*
   a. Parasympathetic
   b. Sympathetic

12. *Which of the following statements is true in describing the infant's respiratory system?*
   a. The infant's tidal volume is the same as that of an adult
   b. The infant's respiratory rate is equal to that of an adult
   c. In an infant, hypoxemia produces tachycardia
   d. An infant's tidal volume is 3 ml/kg

13. *Nonshivering thermogenesis* _____.
   a. Is an efficient mechanism to generate heat
   b. Increases oxygen demand and may contribute to acidosis
   c. Is a mechanism to promote heat loss
   d. Conserves oxygen and decreases neonatal stress

14. *Antiemetics may be given to children preoperatively* _____.
   a. To lower gastric pH
   b. Because children are allowed to eat before surgery
   c. To slow gastric motility
   d. To decrease the risk of aspiration

15. *The overriding goal of ambulatory surgery is* _____.
   a. Financial efficiency
   b. Patient safety
   c. Creativity
   d. Increased patient satisfaction

16. *A hospital-integrated ambulatory center is* _____ *cost effective to operate than a free-standing center.*
   a. More
   b. Less

17. *A physical status* _____ *should not be selected for ambulatory surgery.*
   a. I patient
   b. II patient
   c. III patient
   d. IV patient

18. *Infants of less than 46 weeks' gestational age should not be discharged to home after ambulatory surgery because of the risk of* _____.
    a. Pain requiring intravenous narcotics
    b. Hypothermia
    c. Apnea
    d. Feeding aspiration

19. *Spinal anesthesia in ambulatory surgery* _____.
    a. Is contraindicated because of the need to keep patients flat for 24 hours
    b. Is contraindicated because of the risk of postdural puncture headache
    c. Is only an option in the pediatric patient
    d. Avoids the secondary side effects of general anesthesia

20. *Assessment of patient readiness for discharge to home is best achieved by* _____.
    a. Nursing judgment
    b. Patient opinion
    c. Consistently applied discharge criteria
    d. Family readiness

21. *Phase II recovery is designed* _____.
    a. To help the patient progress toward home readiness
    b. As a back-up mechanism if an outpatient requires hospitalization
    c. To occur if the patient is returned to the operating room for bleeding
    d. Only for patients receiving local anesthesia

Answers

21. a	14. d	7. d
20. c	13. b	6. c
19. d	12. a	5. b
18. c	11. b	4. b
17. d	10. c	3. b
16. b	9. a	2. d
15. b	8. b	1. b

CHAPTER 10

At any given time, the patient in the PACU is under the care of a surgeon, an anesthesiologist, and a nurse. If the hospital is a teaching hospital, residents for the surgical service and for anesthesia and perhaps a medical or nursing student are also involved in the patient's care. The patient is at risk for numerous postanesthetic and postoperative problems and complications. When one considers the number of patients who pass through the PACU on any given day, it becomes easy to recognize the potential for injury that exists.

Initially, the patient has just been moved from a highly controlled setting (the operating room) into the PACU. At no time is the potential for physiologic instability as high. Monitoring must be initiated, assessments performed, and priorities set, often simultaneously. As more and more PACUs are caring for intensive care patients, patient acuity is increasing, as is the use of more sophisticated technologies.

In addition, the anesthesiologist's priorities may differ from those of the surgeons. In no other area of the hospital is the chain of command so unclear. Each physician may feel his or her priorities and demands deserve preference. Verbal orders are the norm rather than the exception.

With the extremely rapid pace of the PACU, there is little control over admissions or the daily schedule. The average length of stay in most PACUs is an hour to an hour and a half.

Perhaps in no other area in the hospital is the patient at greater risk of injury. It is the unique nature of the PACU that contributes to this level of risk. As a result, no text on PACU nursing would be complete without a chapter on legal implications of PACU nursing practice.

LEGAL IMPLICATIONS
OF PACU PRACTICE

Chapter Objectives

After reading this chapter, the reader should be able to:

1. Define the four criteria that determine professional liability.
2. Identify the major allegations being brought against nurses.
3. Identify the components of informed consent.
4. Identify the *only* condition that may override the need to obtain informed consent.
5. Describe techniques to improve documentation.
6. Identify mechanisms to minimize legal risks within the PACU.

STANDARDS OF CARE

Fundamental to any discussion of professional liability is the need to discuss the concept of standards of care. Standards of care are defined as the level of skill and diligence that would be used by the majority of members of a professional discipline in the same or similar circumstances. Standards of care are defined by the members of the profession as accepted practice. If care that is delivered falls below these standards, the practitioner may be held liable.

The American Society of Post Anesthesia Nurses (ASPAN) has developed Standards of Nursing Practice for the immediate preanesthesia period and for post anesthesia care (Appendix A).[3] The American Society of Anesthesiologists also approved Standards for Postanesthesia Care (Appendix B).[2] Both sets of standards will influence practice within the PACU.

LIABILITY

For professional liability to exist, four separate but related criteria must be met. First, *there must be a relationship between the health care provider and the health care recipient* (patient). This relationship implies that a certain duty is owed by one person to another. This relationship may be professional, implied, contractual, or written.

A professional relationship is exemplified by the traditional nurse-patient or doctor-patient relationship and implies a duty to care. An implied relationship is not expressed or written, but is inferred by an act or behavior. A contractual relationship is an agreement to do or not do a particular act. An example of a contractual relationship would be a verbal agreement by a patient to allow a particular surgeon to perform a total hip replacement. A written relationship contains the terms and conditions of a contractual agreement. The signing of an operative consent form is an example of a written relationship. In signing an operative consent, a patient gives permission for the surgeon to perform a specified operation and for the anesthesiologist to administer an anesthetic.

Second, *there must be damages.* If the patient is not injured physically or mentally, there is no liability, no matter how negligent or careless a care-giver might have been. Usually damages are obvious, including loss of life or limb. Damages in the form of pain and mental suffering are more difficult to quantify and evaluate. In short, damages may be physical, financial, or emotional.

Third, *the damages must be caused by negligence or substandard care.* Negligence is defined as conduct that falls below the standard established by law for the protection of others against unreasonable risk of harm and may involve acts of commission (performance of an improper or unsafe act) or omission (failure to act). In the determination of professional negligence, the standard of care is determined by the degree and skill customary to that profession in similar circumstances or communities.

The injured person (through legal representation) must prove beyond a reasonable doubt that the injuries suffered were caused by negligence by a member of the health care team. The relationship between the damages and the negligent act must be determined.

Clearly, untoward events or poor outcomes can occur in patient care, often for idiosyncratic or unexplainable reasons. If, however, the untoward event or poor outcome was caused by an act of negligence of a health care provider, liability may exist.

Fourth, *damages must be the direct and proximate cause of the negligent act.* This criterion is best explained by the case of *Fayson v. Saginaw General Hospital et al.*[35]

In this case, a patient was scheduled for electroconvulsive therapy. During his fourth treatment, the patient vomited and aspirated. The anesthesiologist had not determined whether the patient had eaten prior to initiating anesthesia for the procedure. As a result of the aspiration, the patient developed adult respiratory distress syndrome and required intubation and ventilation in the intensive care unit.

The patient continued to improve over the next 10 days. On the eleventh day, while under the care of an inexperienced licensed practical nurse, the patient became disconnected from the ventilator. The disconnection went undetected, and the patient suffered severe, hypoxic brain damage; thereafter the patient required total care.

When the case was filed, the anesthesiologist, psychiatrist, and the hospital were sued. Although the anesthesiologist had been negligent in failing to determine whether the patient had eaten, his negligent act was neither the direct nor proximate cause of the patient's adverse outcome. The undetected disconnection was the cause, as was the nurse's failure to recognize and correct the disconnection. The complaints against the anesthesiologist and the psychiatrist were dismissed. The hospital (as the employer of the nurse) settled the case out of court.

NURSING LIABILITY

Increasingly, nurses are being held liable for their patient care activities. Nursing negligence may be based on a failure to act or on the performance of an improper or unsafe act.

Case examples

In the discussion that follows, the most common allegations brought against nurses are presented; when possible, each allegation is illustrated by a case example specific to PACU practice or PACU nursing.[15,23] Although some of the case examples are from actual legal case files, others are drawn from anecdotal reporting by PACU personnel. Patient, nurse, and institutional confidentiality has been maintained in the citing of anecdotal data.

Failure to administer medications promptly and properly. PL was taking care of a 67-year-old male who had had a femoral-popliteal bypass graft. The operating room course was unremarkable. In the PACU, the patient's leg dressing repeatedly became saturated with blood. PL notified the surgeon and "20 of protamine" was ordered to be given intravenously; 20 ml of protamine was drawn up and administered. Shortly thereafter, PL was unable to palpate or Doppler the dorsalis pedis or posterior tibial pulses. The surgeon was notified and the patient was returned to the operating room for surgical reexploration. In reviewing the events leading up to the loss of pulses, it was determined that the "20 of protamine" order was meant as 20 mg of protamine. Instead, 20 *ml* (25 mg/ml or 500 mg) was administered. PL, unfortunately, was a new nurse in the PACU and was unfamiliar with the medication and the usual doses.

Failure to administer medications promptly and properly includes such actions as incorrectly administering a medication, administering a medication to a patient with a known allergy to the drug, mixing incompatible medications, missing scheduled doses of medications, and not having knowledge of the drugs being administered (for example, not knowing usual dose, contraindications, adverse effects).

Failure to take correct phone orders. The previous example involving protamine administration illustrates the importance of taking correct phone orders. In that example, the surgeon gave a telephone order for "20 of protamine" to be given intravenously. Unfortunately, the nurse gave 20 ml (25 mg/ml or 500 mg), instead of 20 mg, which was the intention of the surgeon.

In the PACU, nurses take phone orders on a daily basis, commonly for intravenous fluids or pain medications. Phone orders are usually sought out and obtained as a matter of convenience. The nurse obtains the desired order, and the anesthesiologist or surgeon, who may be back in the operating room, is spared the necessity of returning to the

PACU to write the order. It is interesting to note that most hospitals have policies concerning verbal or telephone orders. Verbal and telephone orders are usually permissible only in the event of an emergency or if the physician is out of the hospital. Many hospital units, including PACUs, have expanded this policy (unofficially) to include situations in which the physician (surgeon or anesthesiologist) is physically out of the unit (back in the operating room).

Although routinely taking telephone orders for medications is not recommended, if telephone orders for medications are taken, it is imperative for the nurse to verify the five "rights" of medication safety: the right patient, the right medication, in the right dose, delivered by the right route of administration, at the right time. It has been recommended by some that whenever verbal or telephone orders are taken, the nurse repeat the order back to the physician for verification. This step will minimize or eliminate medication errors caused by miscommunication or misunderstanding.

Additional methods used by some hospitals to prevent problems with verbal orders, caused by either miscommunication or misunderstanding, include requiring two registered nurses to listen when a verbal order is being given, with both nurses signing the order in the chart, or using an answering machine to record all telephone orders. The physician is ultimately responsible for signing off the verbal order in the medical record.

Failure to adequately monitor patients. NR was caring for a 59-year-old woman who had undergone bronchoscopy. Her history was remarkable for a chronic cough and progressive dyspnea. Intraoperatively, the patient received 4 ml (200 μg) of fentanyl and 2.5 mg of midazolam. In the PACU, the patient was lethargic, but arousable with stimulation. The ECG showed sinus rhythm with an average rate of 74. Blood pressures were within the patient's preoperative range, averaging 140/90. High-humidity oxygen at 28% FiO_2 was administered by face tent. Twenty minutes after admission the nurse noted premature ventricular contractions (PVCs) on the ECG monitor, averaging 4 to 6 per minute. Suddenly, the patient was noted to be cyanotic and apneic. The nurse manually ventilated the patient. Anesthesia personnel were notified, and the patient was reintubated. In reviewing the events leading up to the reintubation, it was noted that, despite its availability, pulse oximetry monitoring was never initiated. Given the patient's history, surgery, and the anesthetic agents received, pulse oximetry monitoring should have been initiated. The patient had become progressively hypoxemic. Unfortunately, the hypoxemia was not detected. It was not until the patient was found to be cyanotic and apneic that intervention was initiated. (Anecdotal report.)

Failure to follow physicians' orders promptly and properly. BD was a 72-year-old man who had had an aortic bifurcation graft. Postoperative orders included an order for low-molecular weight dextran to be given as a continuous infusion at 20 ml/hour. The admitting PACU nurse failed to initiate the order. Four hours later, patient report was given to another nurse, who also failed to initiate the order. At 8 AM, 12 hours after surgery, the patient was returned to the operating room for exploration of the graft site for a suspected occlusion. In reviewing documentation, it was noted that all postoperative orders, with the exception of the dextran, had been signed off and initiated. The dextran order was missed by both the admitting nurse and receiving nurse and as a result was never initiated.[33] (Anecdotal report.)

Failure to report significant changes in a patient's condition. MP was a 37-year-old woman admitted to the PACU after a partial hysterectomy. Her past medical history was unremarkable; however, the patient weighed 350 pounds (159 kilograms). In the PACU, the patient complained of being cold. Warm blankets were applied. The PACU record included documentation of hypotension (blood pressure 94/60), cyanosis, and dilated pupils. The patient was also noted to be lying flat in bed. Within 5 minutes of admission and the chart notation, the patient became unresponsive and apneic. Despite resuscitation, the patient remained comatose for 2 years before dying. In reviewing the case, it was noted that although documentation of clinical signs of hypoxemia were made in the PACU chart, the PACU nurse failed to notify either the patient's anesthesiologist or surgeon about the changes in patient status. In addition, no interventions (oxygen therapy, elevating the head of the patient's bed) were instituted, despite the patient's status and physical condition (obesity). This particular case resulted in a *$52 million* wrongful death judgment and is currently under appeal.[29,37]

Failure to protect the patient from falls. DK was a 37-year-old man who was admitted as an outpatient for an arthroscopy. The procedure was performed with the patient having received general anesthesia. At the end of the case, just as the anesthesiologist was preparing to extubate the patient, the patient suddenly "bucked" on the endotracheal tube, became combative, and fell off of the operating room table. X-ray examination revealed no fracture damage. In reviewing the events leading up to the fall, it was noted that the patient restraints, normally in place during any operative procedure, had been removed prematurely. Restraints are normally removed at the end of the procedure just before the patient is transferred from the operating table to the PACU cart. (Anecdotal report.)

The patient in the PACU is at risk for injury because of alteration in consciousness and judgment. The PACU nurse must recognize the patient's potential for injury and institute appropriate interventions as necessary to ensure patient safety.[11]

Failure to follow established nursing protocol. In *Goldsby v. Evangelical Deaconness Hospital,* failure to follow established nursing protocol resulted in a patient's death.[36] In this case, the patient was admitted to the PACU after an open reduction and internal fixation of a mandibular fracture. Although the patient's jaws were wired shut, the patient was extubated in the operating room and brought to the PACU with a patent airway. Postoperative orders specified how the patient was to be positioned and that wire cutters were to be placed at the patient's bedside. Shortly after admission, the PACU nurses left the unit to attend an inservice meeting. An operating room nurse was called to care for the patient. Although not oriented to the PACU, the operating room nurse followed PACU protocol and went to obtain vital signs 15 minutes after taking report. Unfortunately, by this time, the patient had developed an obstructed airway and suffocated, and he could not be resuscitated. In review of the case, not only was nursing care found to be negligent, but the patient had not been positioned as ordered and the wire cutters were not at the bedside. The anesthesiologist, surgeon, and hospital were sued. The cases against the anesthesiologist and surgeon were ultimately dismissed, but the hospital was held liable for damages as employer of the nurses.

This case is useful not only in representing a common allegation against nurses (failure to follow established nursing protocol) but also in presenting the doctrine of *respondeat superior*. Under the doctrine of respondeat superior, a hospital may be held liable for the negligent action of its employees if the negligent act occurred at the place of employment and the employee was acting within the scope of his or her employment. As a result, negligent actions on the part of the PACU nurses (in leaving a postoperative patient with an inexperienced nurse) and the operating room nurse (for failing to initiate postoperative orders and to recognize airway obstruction) resulted in the hospital being held liable for the actions and failure to act of its employees. Damages against the hospital were in excess of $600,000.

Other areas of professional liability

Although uncommon, nurses are also being held liable for assault and battery, breach of promise, fraud, and abandonment.

Assault and battery. *Assault* is defined as a threat to inflict bodily harm. Threatening someone with a weapon (gun, knife, or other instrument) is referred to as *aggravated assault*. Battery is defined as the actual physical act of violence against another person. *Aggravated battery* is defined as the commission of an act of violence against someone using a weapon.

The allegation of assault or battery, or both, may be raised whenever a nurse intervenes or acts in a way that affects a patient without having obtained consent from the patient to do so. This is based on the premise that the individual has the right to control what may or may not be done to his or her body. To quote Justice Cardozo,

Every human being of adult years and sound mind has a right to determine what shall be done with his own body and a surgeon who performs an operation without his patient's consent commits an assault for which he is liable in damages.[38,39]

The right to self-determination also includes the right to refuse medical intervention or treatment (for example, blood transfusions or resuscitation).

The process of determining whether a procedure will or will not be performed is based on the concept of *informed consent*. Informed consent is an active, shared decision-making between the provider and the recipient of care. For informed consent to be valid, three conditions must be met.

First, there must be *adequate disclosure* by the provider of the diagnosis, the nature and purpose of the proposed treatment, the risks and consequences of the proposed treatment, the probability of a successful outcome, the availability, benefits, and risks of alternative therapies, and the prognosis if treatment is not instituted. The person performing the treatment is usually responsible for obtaining the consent. Therefore, the physician is usually responsible for obtaining patient consent.[12]

The explanation of the diagnosis and proposed treatment should be presented in nontechnical terms directed toward the patient's level of understanding. The discussion of *risks* associated with an intervention includes presenting outcomes that have a probability of occurring or that might occur. *Consequences* of an intervention are those outcomes generally expected to occur.

Second, the recipient of the care must demonstrate *sufficient comprehension* of the information provided. Ideally, the patient should be able to demonstrate comprehension by being able to explain to the health care provider his or her understanding of the information provided. Unfortunately, research has shown that the vast majority of patients do not comprehend that to which they have consented.[30]

Third, the recipient of care must give consent *voluntarily,* free from coercion or undue influence. Under this provision, patients are also free to withdraw from treatment at any time. The health care provider should identify the risks and consequences associated with withdrawal, leaving the ultimate decision up to the individual patient.

There are a number of special situations pertaining to the concept of informed consent that warrant additional discussion.

Emancipated minors. In most cases, consent for treatment of or surgery on a child of less than 18 years of age must be given by the child's parent or legal guardian. Emancipated minors, including those so declared by a court of law or as a result of marriage, may give their own consent.

Emergency care. A true medical emergency may override the need to obtain consent. When *immediate* medical treatment is required to preserve life or to prevent serious impairment to life, the individual patient is incapable of giving consent, and reaching the next of kin is impossible or would result in unnecessary delay of treatment, the physician may institute treatment without liability for battery.

In these instances, the essential focus is the patient's need for immediate care and the delay of treatment to obtain consent would further threaten the individual's life.

In *Jackovich v. Yocum,* a 17-year-old boy was brought to an emergency room after having been injured jumping from a freight train.[34] The emergency room physician, in providing emergency care, concluded that the boy's arm had to be amputated above the elbow because it had been crushed beyond repair. Two other physicians examined the boy and confirmed the necessity for surgery to protect the boy's life. The boy was unconscious. The boy's parents could not be reached. The surgery was begun without consent. After the boy's recovery, the boy's parents brought suit against the physician, charging that the amputation was unnecessary and was performed without authorization. The jury ruled in favor of the defendant (the physician), stating,

If a surgeon is confronted with an emergency which endangers the life or health of the patient, it is his duty to do that which the occasion demands, within the usual and customary practice among physicians and surgeons in the same or similar localities, without consent of the patient.[34]

Inability to reach next of kin. In any instance in which the patient is unable to give his or her consent and it is impossible to reach the next of kin to obtain proxy consent, the physician should document the existence of a medical emergency. If possible, consultation should be sought by another physician who also agrees with the opinion of medical necessity. It is also suggested that all attempts to notify the next of kin be documented, to show that all reasonable attempts were made. Documentation protects the physician and the hospital from liability.[27]

Operative consent after preoperative medication. It is generally the policy of most hospitals that an operative consent cannot be obtained after a preoperative medication has been given. This is based on the premise that the preoperative medication has the potential to alter the patient's comprehension ability and therefore to compromise informed consent.

If the consent is not signed, many hospitals have refused to allow the surgery to proceed. However, risk managers have begun to question the practice of cancelling surgery. Cancelling the surgery is not recommended, particularly if the patient has been admitted to the hospital specifically for the surgery. The ambulatory surgical patient who arrives the morning of surgery is specifically showing up for the scheduled procedure.

Another alternative is to permit the surgery to proceed as scheduled after the surgeon documents in the progress notes that the procedure has been explained to the patient and that patient has consented to the procedure. In addition, if the patient is still seen as mentally competent, the consent should still be obtained, even though the preoperative medication has been given. An "unusual occurrence report" should also be completed in situations in which signed consent forms are obtained after premedication.

Breach of promise. The allegation of breach of promise is usually made when a patient has been promised a specific outcome that, for whatever reason, does not occur. This allegation is usually made against physicians who promise that surgery will ensure a cure or a complete recovery from an illness or disease. However, as nurses increase their role in patient care delivery, their ability to influence and predict patient outcomes increases.

Breach of promise may also become an issue when patient confidentiality is violated. Every nurse, beginning in nursing school, has been told never to discuss a patient's case with anyone not involved in the direct care of that patient. Stories of cases overheard as a result of elevator and cafeteria conversations occur too frequently.

Every patient is due the right and courtesy of privacy and confidentiality. The patient's chart is considered an extension of the patient and is therefore due the same right of privacy and confidentiality.

Fraud. The allegation of fraud is raised when it is believed that unnecessary procedures have been performed. Again, this allegation has been traditionally brought against surgeons for performing unnecessary surgical procedures. An anecdotal report specific to the PACU provides an example of how this charge might be applied to a PACU nurse.

RM, a night nurse in the PACU, was caring for a patient after repair of an esophageal rupture. The patient was stable and intubated. The care plan was to have him remain ventilated, without weaning, for 3 days to promote healing along the suture lines. At 5 AM, RM obtained all of the physician-ordered morning laboratory tests, including arterial blood gases, electrolytes, red blood counts, and coagulation profiles. At 7:15

AM, RM reported on her patient to FJ, the day shift nurse in the PACU. At 9 AM, FJ obtained another full set of blood tests. In making rounds, the PACU head nurse inquired about the rationale for the repeated laboratory tests. Laboratory tests had been ordered daily; they had been obtained 4 hours earlier. No ventilator changes had been made. No change in patient status had occurred. The additional laboratory charges would have added $390 to the patient's bill unnecessarily. As a result, the laboratory billing office was instructed to take the charges off of the patient's bill and to post the charges to the PACU. In this age of utilization review, external agencies are replacing the unit head nurse in monitoring for cost containment.

Abandonment. Once a physician-patient or nurse-patient relationship is established, the patient develops the expectation that the physician or nurse will be available to provide continued, ongoing care. If the physician or nurse is not available to perform any necessary or expected services, and a substitute care-giver has not been designated, the allegation of *abandonment* may be raised.

Although no anesthesiologist, surgeon, or primary nurse will be available 24 hours a day, arrangements must be made for a substitute care-giver to assume patient care responsibilities. The PACU nurse reports to another PACU nurse at the end of the shift, relating any actual or potential patient problems. Any significant patient variables or medical history should also be shared. Reporting and the accepting of a report should be documented in the patient's PACU record. Likewise, if the attending surgeon or anesthesiologist is going home while the patient is still in the PACU, arrangements should be made to identify the physician who is responsible for medical care of the patient, for example, an on-call physician or PACU medical director.

CHARGES OF MALPRACTICE AND NEGLIGENCE

Because adverse outcomes do occur and charges of malpractice are made, the PACU nurse should have an understanding of the process through which the allegation will proceed.

Initially, the injured person or a family member of the injured person (the plaintiff), through legal representation, will present a complaint against a practitioner (the defendant). A *complaint* outlines the alleged negligence, states the outcome injury, and indicates the amount of compensation demanded. At this point, the defendant (on the advice of legal counsel) may choose to acknowledge and respond to the complaint by providing the compensation specified, or the defendant may choose to refuse to accept the allegation of negligence and may refuse to provide compensation.

If this occurs, the legal representatives for both the plaintiff and the defendant will begin the process of pretrial *discovery*, which includes the gathering of facts and of clarifying issues. This may include the use of interrogatories, expert witnesses, and depositions.

An *interrogatory* is a detailed, information-seeking questionnaire designed to produce information that supports or refutes the complaint. *Expert witnesses* are persons whose expertise in a given area is designed to support or refute the complaint; they are solicited by either the plaintiff or the defendant. *Depositions* are legal testimonies given by witnesses in the presence of legal counsel. The deposition is a legal document, with all testimony recorded. Depositions may be introduced into court during the trial.

As information is gathered, the relative strength of the complaint will be realized. At this time, the plaintiff may terminate the proceedings by withdrawing the suit; the defendant may choose to negotiate a settlement with the goal of avoiding a trial and minimizing the costs associated with the settlement; or the case may proceed to trial. It should be noted that only one in twenty cases ever reach trial.

If the case goes to trial, it will be the responsibility of the plaintiff's attorney to prove beyond a reasonable doubt to a jury that the four elements of negligence (professional liability) against the defendant exist. If negligence is determined, the jury will find in favor of the plaintiff and will determine the amount of damages to be paid. If negligence cannot be proved, the judge will dismiss the suit. Both the plaintiff and the defendant may appeal the verdict.

WHAT TO DO IF YOU ARE SUED

Given the high-risk nature of post anesthesia care, it is not out of the realm of possibility that the PACU nurse will at some time be served with a notice of complaint in which she or he has been named as a defendant.

If this occurs, the PACU nurse is encouraged to work closely and to cooperate with the hospital's legal counsel. Chances are excellent that if a nurse has been named as a defendant in a case, the hospital has also been named. Cooperation is essential in maintaining a united front.

The PACU nurse is reminded to never discuss the case with anyone, particularly colleagues. Any concerns, questions, or speculations should be shared only with legal counsel.

Finally, it is important to never alter existing medical (hospital) records. Because complaints may be raised some time after patient care has been provided, details specific to the case may have been forgotten. Medical records may be reviewed as a means to familiarize oneself with the case. In reviewing the records, the PACU nurse may recognize deficiencies in charting, either omissions or incomplete notations. Despite the temptation to correct the deficiency, the PACU nurse is reminded to *never alter existing records*. Even if it was well intended, altering a record may be seen as an attempt to cover up, to hide, or to alter facts. The PACU nurse should remember that while the original patient record may be available to him or her through medical records, the legal representatives of the plaintiff and the defendants have copies of the chart.

REDUCING THE RISKS

Although the PACU is a high-risk patient care area, it is possible for PACU practitioners to decrease the risk of liability. It has been speculated that 90% of the liability issues could be eliminated with better documentation and the remaining 10% with better communication.

Good communication

The importance of establishing good doctor-patient and nurse-patient relationships cannot be overemphasized. Although adverse outcomes do occur in patient care, it is the patient who receives no explanation, no information, and no support who is the most likely to sue. Good communication is essential for maintaining patient satisfaction and for minimizing the liability of health care practitioners. Primary care has done much to foster doctor-patient and nurse-patient relationships. Patients are able to identify "my doctor" and "my nurse" as the individuals responsible for coordinating their medical and nursing care.

Guidelines for documentation

If 90% of the liability issues could be eliminated with better documentation, then it is essential to review guidelines designed to improve documentation. It is important for the PACU nurse to remember that every part of the patient's chart may be introduced into a court of law as evidence. Completeness and accuracy are essential.

The PACU record is initiated on the patient's arrival to the PACU. Initial documentation will include a summary of the anesthetic management of the patient (ideally obtained from a verbal report from the anesthesiologist), documentation of admission vital signs and of the admission assessment. Documentation will then continue per the PACU routine (for example, vital signs every 15 minutes) and for any interventions initiated (medications administered, treatments applied). The PACU nurse should document not only the intervention but also the patient's response to the intervention. If, for example, a patient complains of pain at the surgical incision site, the PACU nurse might document, "Patient complaining of pain at surgical site. Medicated with 2 mg MSO4 (morphine sulphate) IV (intravenously), with good relief."

It is important that the patient's name appear on every page of the PACU record. Stamping the patient's record with his or her identification plate ensures that the patient's name and number are both on the record, preventing errors.

Every entry should be timed and, if appropriate, dated. Most patients admitted to the PACU will remain for an average length of stay of 1 to 2 hours on one given day. However, as PACUs are frequently being used to provide ongoing intensive care to patients when surgical intensive care units are full, patients may remain in the PACU overnight, or even longer. One PACU in a tertiary medical center kept a patient for three and a half days before a bed became available in the intensive care unit! When a patient stay overlaps days, entries should be dated to avoid confusion.

Every entry should be written legibly in permanent ink. Illegible entries leave much to speculation. Entries should never be written in pencil. Every entry should be specific, complete, and accurate. If an error is made in charting, the error should never be obliterated. A line should be drawn through the error with the nurse's initials and any other documentation required by hospital policy (for example, writing "error" or "void").[20]

Entries should be made in formats consistent with unit protocol. If it is routine to chart in narrative format, then charting should be in narrative form. If it is routine to chart in care plan format (SOAP charting), then documentation should be in care plan format.

Entries should be made promptly and continuously, avoiding gaps in time. No blank spaces should be left on a record. If a notation finishes in the middle of a line, then a line should be drawn through any space not used. If data requested are not applicable to a specific patient, then a notation of "N/A" (not applicable) should be made, rather than leaving blank spaces.

The PACU record should be objective. Personal comments, opinions, and criticisms should be avoided. The record should be a transcription of facts only.

It is also important that the PACU nurse use only hospital-approved abbreviations in charting. This is done to ensure that the abbreviation is well accepted and will not be subject to misunderstanding. Many abbreviations have more than one meaning, and documentation may be misinterpreted if the wrong meaning is applied. For example, MS may refer to morphine sulfate, multiple sclerosis, or mental status. MD may refer to medical doctor, muscular dystrophy, or manic-depressive. D/C may refer to discharge or discontinue. The symbol ↑ may refer to increasing, elevated, or high. When only hospital-approved abbreviations are used, the clarity and accuracy of charting is increased. (Commonly used hospital abbreviations are identified in Appendix C).

Every entry should be initialled or signed by the nurse making the notation. No nurse should ever make or sign an entry for someone else.

Although these guidelines for documentation are not exhaustive, implementing them can assist the PACU nurse in documenting care and will provide the PACU nurse with clear evidence in the defense of allegations of malpractice. The cardinal rule, "if you didn't document it, you didn't do it" is an adage under which to practice.

Defining nursing practice

In an effort to reduce liability, it is recommended that the practice of nursing in the PACU be defined by clear practice roles, standards of care, and written policies and procedures.

Staff should be adequately trained under supervision to work in the PACU. Orientation expectations should be clearly defined. Sufficiently trained personnel should be available to provide patient care according to predetermined staffing ratios (usually 1:2 or 1:3).

Resources should be available to meet the needs of the physiologically unstable patient, including equipment (reintubation supplies, cardiac monitors, pulse oximetry, and suction), medications (emergency and routine), and medical personnel (anesthesiologists, surgeons, respiratory therapists).

Most important, deviations from accepted practice should be avoided, and situations that may result in deviations from accepted practice should be corrected. The risks of both are far too great.

SUMMARY

The high-risk, unique nature of the PACU must be recognized and acknowledged. Just as defensive driving can help to reduce the risks of highway travel, delivery of defensively planned nursing care will help to reduce the risk of liability associated with PACU practice.

REFERENCES

1. Abreiter J: A buyer's guide to malpractice insurance, RN 49(5):65-66, 1986.
2. American Society of Anesthesiologists: Standard for postanesthesia care, Chicago, 1988, The Society.
3. American Society of Post Anesthesia Nursing: Standards of nursing practice, Richmond, 1986, The Society.
4. Appelbaum P, Lidz C, and Melsel A: Informed consent: legal theory and clinical practice, New York, 1987, Oxford University Press.
5. Bernsweig E: Don't cut corners on informed consent, RN 47(12):15-16, 1984.
6. Brent N: Avoiding legal risks in the ICU, Nurs Life 5(4):48-51, 1985.
7. Creighton H: Recovery room nurses: legal implications, Nurs Manage 18(1):22-23, 1987.
8. Creighton H: Informed consent, Nurs Manage 17(10):11-12, 1986.
9. Creighton H: Patient teaching, Nurs Manage 16(1):12-18, 1985.
10. Creighton H: Law every nurse should know, ed 4, Philadelphia, 1981, WB Saunders Co.
11. Cushing M: First anticipate the harm . . . patient safety, Am J Nurs 85(2):137-138, 1985.
12. Cushing M: Informed consent: an MD responsibility? Am J Nurs 84(4):437-440, 1984.
13. Dean K: Nursing judgement . . . narcotics in the postoperative patient, Focus Crit Care 11(5):24-25, 1984.
14. DeKornfeld T: Medico-legal implications of recovery room care, Curr Rev Recov Room Nurse 4(1):27-31, 1979.
15. Frost E: Recovery room practice, Boston, 1985, Blackwell Scientific Publications, Inc.
16. Gosfield A: Health law handbook, New York, 1989, Clark Boardman.
17. Heher J: Nursing malpractice in the postoperative recovery room, Curr Rev Recov Room Nurse 13(2):99-103, 1980.
18. Kapp M: If you question your patient's competence, RN 48(10):59-60, 1985.
19. Kiely D: Ethical considerations in critical care nursing, Crit Care Nurse 5(2):61-63, 1985.
20. Missing Progress Notes: Nurses' "whiteouts" x-rayed, Regan Rep Nurs Law 25(10):1, 1985.
21. Murphy E: The professional status of nursing: a view from the courts, Nurs Outlook 35(1):12-15, 1987.
22. Patient's word v. nurse's word: documentation, Regan Rep Nurs Law 25(6):4, 1984.
23. Putkowski S: Liabilities of the recovery room team. In Frost E (editor): Recovery room practice, Boston, 1985, Blackwell Scientific Publications, Inc.
24. Quimby C and Bailey M: Anesthesia recovery care, New York, 1986, Igaku-Shoin, Medical Publishers, Inc.
25. Rabinow J: Avoiding legal risks in the O.R., Nurs Life 5(6):24-26, 1985.
26. Rahn J: I was negligent: will I lose my nursing license? Focus Crit Care 13(1):38-39, 1986.
27. Rosoff A: Informed consent: a guide for health care providers, Rockville, MD, 1981, Aspen Systems.
28. Rozovsky F: Consent to treatment: a practical guide, Boston, 1984, Little, Brown & Co, Inc.
29. Sella M: More big bucks in jury verdicts, ABA J July 1989, pp 69-72.

30. Silva M and Zeccolo P: Informed consent: the right to know and the right to choose, Nurs Manage 17(8):18-19, 1986.
31. Totton T: Legal issues in nursing practice, Kentucky Nurse 33(4):10, 1985.
32. Veatch R and Fry S: Case studies in nursing ethics, New York, 1987, JB Lippincott Co.
33. When nurses fail to follow doctor's orders: disaster, Regan Rep Nurs Law 26(7):1, 1985.

Legal References

34. *Jackovich v Yocum,* 212 Iowa 914, 237 NW 444 (1931).
35. *Fayson v Saginaw General Hospital et al,* Saginaw County Circuit Court, 1978.
36. *Goldsby v Evangelical Deaconess Hospital,* Wayne County Circuit Court, 74-004-754 NM, 1978.
37. *Palacios v Medical Arts Hospital of Houston, Texas,* 1985.
38. *Canterbury v Spence* 464 F. 2d 772 (DC Cir 1972).
39. *Schloendorff v Society of New York Hospital,* 211 NY 125, 105 NE, 92,93 (1914).

Review Questions

1. *The PACU is considered a high-risk patient care area because of* _____.
   a. Unclear administrative roles
   b. High patient acuity
   c. Rapid turnover of patients
   d. All of the above
2. *Standards of care are* _____.
   a. Defined by the profession as accepted practice
   b. Defined by the courts as legal precedent
   c. Defined by the courts as required practice
   d. Defined by the profession as required practice
3. *Negligence may involve* _____.
   a. An act of omission
   b. An act of commission
   c. Substandard care
   d. All of the above
4. *The four criteria that must exist for liability to be claimed are:*
   a.
   b.
   c.
   d.
5. *Which of the following is a complete medication order?*
   a. M.S. 2-4 IV
   b. Demerol 25-50 mg IM
   c. Zantac 50 mg IV rider q 8 hours
   d. Tylenol 10 mg/kg now
6. *Respondeat superior means* _____.
   a. Physicians are responsible for the nurses caring for their patients
   b. The hospital may be held liable for its employees
   c. Patients will sue the person (institution) with the most money
   d. The patient is always right
7. *Assault is defined as* _____.
   a. A threat to do harm to an individual
   b. The act of physical violence against an individual
8. *If a care-giver violates a patient's right to self-determination, the care-giver may be charged with* _____.
   a. Breach of promise
   b. Fraud
   c. Abandonment
   d. Assault and battery

9. *List the three criteria that must be met for true informed consent to be given.*
   a.

   b.

   c.

10. *Informed consent is not required if* _____.
    a. The patient is an emancipated minor
    b. Next of kin are unavailable
    c. Immediate medical intervention is required to sustain life
    d. The patient has been premedicated

11. *If the patient's right to confidentiality is violated, the care-giver may be charged with* ____.
    a. Assault and battery
    b. Breach of promise
    c. Abandonment
    d. Fraud

12. *In documenting a situation, you remember several items you forgot to include. You should*
    _____.
    a. Add the omitted items at the end of your note with the date and time
    b. Forget adding it altogether
    c. White out your notes and make the needed correction
    d. Tear out the page and start over

13. *Your patient has had a cystoscopy. In documenting on your PACU record the condition of the patient's dressing you write* _____.
    a. Internal
    b. Invisible
    c. Dry and intact
    d. Not applicable or N/A

14. *In using abbreviations in charting* _____.
    a. Any initials used verbally may be used
    b. Only hospital-approved abbreviations should be used
    c. The nurse becomes liable for any misunderstandings that result
    d. Abbreviations with more than one meaning are acceptable

15. *Reducing nursing liability in the PACU* _____.
    a. Is beyond the scope of nursing practice
    b. Requires medical supervision of all nursing care delivered in the PACU
    c. May be accomplished with communication, documentation, and defined nursing practice
    d. Is pointless because patients will sue anyway

Answers

1. d
2. a
3. d
4. a. A professional relationship must exist.
   b. There must be damages.
   c. Damages must be caused by negligence.
   d. Damages must be the direct and proximate result of negligence.
5. c
6. b
7. a
8. d
9. a. Adequate disclosure
   b. Sufficient comprehension
   c. Voluntarily given
10. c
11. b
12. a
13. d
14. b
15. c

CHAPTER 11

Unfortunately, when the term *quality assurance* is mentioned, it is met with reactions of resistance ("Why do we have to?"), frustration ("I don't know what to do or how to do it"), resentment ("I'm a staff nurse, my job is patient care"), and general dislike by PACU practitioners and managers. Quality assurance and quality assurance activities are often seen as busywork, mandated by nursing administration or by an external agency. Quality assurance is seen as time consuming (because it involves organization and documentation), as threatening (because the data may be reviewed or the unit itself may be visited by an internal or external surveyor), and as another activity that pulls often overworked (their perception) staff members away from the bedside. Almost every article, book chapter, or reference on quality assurance acknowledges—usually in the opening paragraphs—the generally negative perceptions held by practitioners about quality assurance.

Quality assurance is usually viewed as a way to identify problems and to concretely define areas for improvement. Quality assurance may also and should also be used as a way to identify strengths of individuals, of units, and of organizations. It can be a way to recognize excellence in a care-giver. It can be a way for a unit to recognize that in providing care to many thousands of patients the incidence of untoward events is less than 1%. It can be the way for an ambulatory surgical unit to recognize that as a result of carefully conceived patient prescreening, their rate of outpatients requiring unplanned hospitalizations is almost nonexistent.

Quality assurance may be an avenue to identify areas for improvement, but it should also be recognized as a means to identify strengths.

QUALITY ASSURANCE IN THE PACU

Chapter Objectives

After reading this chapter, the reader should be able to:

1. Define quality assurance.
2. Identify why quality assurance is important.
3. Identify the essential components of quality assurance.
4. Discuss the three types of quality assurance indicators.
5. I｡ tify examples of quality assurance that may be implemented in the PACU.

DEFINING QUALITY ASSURANCE

The Joint Commission for the Accreditation of Healthcare Organizations (JCAHO) defines quality assurance as an ongoing process designed to objectively and systematically monitor and evaluate the quality and appropriateness of patient care and as a means to pursue opportunities to improve patient care and to resolve identified problems.[18]

The American Nurses' Association defines quality assurance as a sum of all of the activities that ensure that patients receive the best possible nursing care.[3,4] Quality assurance has also been defined as the examination and analysis of a product.[15] Specific to the PACU, it is an inspection and analysis of post anesthesia care (the product).

Quality assurance is a means for the nursing profession to assure the patient of a specialized degree of excellence of nursing care by continuously and objectively measuring the structural, procedural, and outcome components of nursing against preestablished criteria of nursing standards.[31]

Although the words used in each of these definitions vary, a number of commonalities exist, forming the basis of quality assurance. Quality assurance is a *process*. A process implies an activity that moves in a direction over time. It is not static. Quality assurance is a *purposeful monitoring of care*. Some define purposeful monitoring as systematic, planned, or structured. Purposeful monitoring of care implies a focused assessment of a product; in this instance, the product is the nursing care in the post anesthesia care unit.

Finally, quality assurance involves the *evaluation* of nursing care. The care provided may be evaluated against a standard defined by a professional organization, or it may be evaluated by comparing data against predetermined criteria. The evaluation of care involves making a judgment about the *effectiveness* and *efficiency* of care delivery.

Simply stated, effectiveness is a measure of our doing the "right" things. Effectiveness implies outcomes—being able to determine what the "right" things or ideal outcomes might be. Efficiency is a measure of our doing things "right." Efficiency implies an evaluation of the likelihood of a successful outcome. If care is delivered in a prescribed manner, what is the likelihood or probability of a successful outcome?

WHY IS QUALITY ASSURANCE IMPORTANT?

Ideally the impetus for quality assurance would have come from within the profession. Quality assurance within business and industry was internal in its origin, in recognition of competition. Unfortunately, quality assurance activities in health care had to be encouraged, and in some cases mandated, by external agencies.

In an effort to ensure that federal dollars were being optimally used, the United States Congress called on the Department of Health, Education and Welfare in 1972 to determine the necessity of health care services provided, that these services met standards of care, and that these services contained costs. Third-party payers, also in an effort to evaluate care delivery and to control the exorbitant costs of health care, formed professional standards review organizations (PSROs).

PSROs were developed to review patient care activities financed by the federal government; specifically, they were established to determine the necessity of services performed. The PSROs were also given the task of evaluating whether or not services performed met standards of care and that services were being maximally used. In 1982, findings from the PSROs led to the development of the concept of diagnosis-related groups (DRGs). DRGs (initially identifying 467 categories) were developed as a means to mandate cost containment in health care, ideally without sacrificing quality care. PSROs were ultimately replaced with peer review organizations (PROs), whose task remains essentially that of the PSROs, now targeted to the state level.

Health care consumers also began to pressure health care providers and organizations to be accountable for care delivery. This pressure arose from recognition of the ever-increasing costs of health care in combination with a perceived lack of quality.

The professional organizations whose members provide health care services also recognized their responsibility to society to provide quality health care. In 1973, the American Nurses' Association developed initial Standards of Practice. The American Society of Post Anesthesia Nurses approved Standards of Care for the immediate post anesthesia phase in 1984, expanding the Standards of Care in 1986 to include the preanesthesia phase, phase one post anesthesia care, phase two post anesthesia care, and management standards (Appendix A). The American Society of Anesthesiologists first developed a practice advisory for recovery room care in 1973. In 1988, the most recent Standards for Post Anesthesia Care were approved (Appendix B).

The accrediting agencies, specifically the Joint Commission for the Accreditation of Healthcare Organizations (JCAHO) also identified standards, including standards of practice, standards of performance, and standards of care. *Standards of practice* focus on the provider of care, describing what the practitioner (the PACU nurse) does and how the practitioner provides care. *Standards of performance* focus on quality, specifying how well the practitioner (the PACU nurse) should carry out patient care. *Standards of care* focus on the patient and outcomes of care that can be expected by the patient and family.

Standards are defined as "accepted practice" by professionals who provide direct care or who evaluate care to patients. Although standards were developed to serve as practice guidelines, they have been interpreted as mandatory or obligatory by members of society and the legal profession. If care that is delivered is seen as falling below these standards, the practitioner may be held liable (see Chapter 10). Evaluation of care through quality assurance activities may reduce personal and organizational exposure to liability.

THE ESSENTIAL COMPONENTS OF QUALITY ASSURANCE

Quality assurance has been defined as a process, thereby implying a directional flow of activities. As outlined by the Joint Commission for the Accreditation of Healthcare Organizations (JCAHO), the process involves identifying the most important aspects of care within an organization, formulating measurable indicators to monitor the care in an ongoing manner, evaluating the care to identify opportunities for improvement or problems in delivery, implementing actions to address identified problem areas, and evaluating the effectiveness of the actions.

This process has been further detailed by the JCAHO into a ten-step quality assurance process, identified in the box on p. 272.[18]

Several terms identified in the ten-step process deserve clarification or further definition. *Aspects of care* are activities that affect a large number of patients. If these care activities are not performed correctly or when indicated, patients are at risk for increased morbidity. *Thresholds* are identified as desired levels of compliance for a particular indicator, often defined as a percentage rate. The frequency of *data collection* will be directly related to the frequency of occurrence of the aspect of care and the significance of the care activities.

FOCUS OF QUALITY ASSURANCE

Three types of quality assurance indicators may be applied to the practice of nursing within the PACU. These indicators are characterized as structural, process, or outcome oriented.

TEN-STEP PROCESS FOR QUALITY ASSSURANCE

1. Assign responsibility for monitoring and evaluation activities.
2. Delineate the scope of care provided by the organization.
3. Identify the most important aspects of care provided by the organization.
4. Identify indicators (and appropriate clinical criteria) for monitoring the important aspects of care.
5. Establish thresholds (levels, patterns, trends) for the indicators that trigger evaluation of care.
6. Monitor the important aspects of care by collecting and organizing the data for each indicator.
7. Identify problems or opportunities to improve care, evaluate care when thresholds are reached.
8. Take action to improve care or correct identified problems.
9. Assess the effectiveness of the actions, and document the improvement in care.
10. Communicate the results of the monitoring and evaluation process to relevant individuals or departments and to the organization-wide quality assurance program.

Structural indicators are used to evaluate the environment in which postanesthetic care is delivered. A structural indicator may be used to evaluate the adequacy of the size of and space within the PACU. Because much postanesthetic care delivery depends on monitoring equipment and supplies, a structural indicator might be used to evaluate product safety, product evaluation, orientation of staff to equipment, and prepurchase evaluations. The box on p. 273 provides an example of a prepurchase evaluation form used to evaluate and determine the type of pulse oximeter to be purchased by a PACU.

Process indicators are used to evaluate the application of the nursing process in the PACU. The implementation of the nursing process (assessment, planning, implementation, and evaluation) results in nursing practice. Within the PACU, when a nurse admits a patient, vital signs are obtained, monitoring and oxygen therapy are initiated, and a postanesthetic and postoperative assessment is performed (step one of the nursing process). On the basis of data obtained in the admission assessment, the PACU nurse identifies the existence of actual and potential problems, individualized to the newly admitted patient. The PACU nurse develops a plan of care for the patient, designed to address and resolve actual problems and to prevent potential problems (step two of the nursing process). The plan is then put into action (step three of the nursing process). The patient's response to interventions is evaluated (step four of the nursing process). Because the patient's status may change or a response to the interventions may be noted, the PACU nurse will continue to assess the patient, revising the nursing care plan, initiating actions, and evaluating the patient until the patient is deemed ready for discharge from the PACU.[22]

Outcome indicators focus on the end-point in care delivery or the patient's condition at a predetermined point in time. For example, the patient who is ready for discharge

```
┌──────────────── PREPURCHASE EVALUATION FORM ────────────────┐
│                                                             │
│   Oximeter used        Circle all that apply                │
│                        Nellcor                              │
│                        PhysioControl                        │
│                        Ohmeda                               │
│                        Criticare                            │
│                        Other (specify)_____      │
│   Type of patient      Circle all that apply                │
│                        Pediatric    Child    Adult    Elderly│
│                        Light skin color    Dark skin color  │
│                        Less than 95°    Greater than 95.1°  │
│                        Quiet in bed    Moving about in bed   │
│   Problems             Circle all that apply                │
│                        Did not read oxygen saturation consistently│
│                        Probe difficult to use               │
│                        Probe had to be taped on             │
│                        Did not pick up pulse                │
│                        Required much time to establish good site for pulse│
│                        Did not read until patient warmed up │
│                        Other (specify)_____      │
│   Benefits of unit used  Circle all that apply              │
│                        Size                                 │
│                        Portability                          │
│                        Easy to use                          │
│                        Easy to set/reset alarms             │
│                        Did not need to change probes for different patients│
│                        Aesthetics                           │
│                        No problems encountered during this use│
│                        Other (specify)_____      │
│                                                             │
└─────────────────────────────────────────────────────────────┘
```

from the PACU can be expected to be adequately ventilating and perfusing, maintaining an adequate cardiac output, responsive and responding appropriately, normothermic, and physically comfortable. The use of a PACU care plan (Chapter 5), discharge checklist (Fig. 11-1), or direct observation may facilitate outcome audit data collection.

APPLYING QUALITY ASSURANCE TO THE PACU

The previous discussion of quality assurance has been theoretic and historical. In an effort to make quality assurance relevant to the PACU and PACU practitioner, a number of quality assurance projects specific to post anesthesia care will be presented and discussed. The list of projects is not meant to be exhaustive. It is designed to provide examples of quality assurance projects that may be implemented by PACU staff and management.

RUSH-PRESBYTERIAN-ST. LUKE'S MEDICAL CENTER
CHICAGO, ILLINOIS 60612

POST ANESTHESIA ORDER AND DISCHARGE SHEET

SIGNATURE AND TITLE REQUIRED WITH EACH ORDER

DATE & TIME		DEPARTMENT OF ANESTHESIOLOGY	CRITERIA FOR DISCHARGE	
			TICK	✓ APPROPRIATE BOX
		(PLEASE CIRCLE ORDERS TO BE IMPLEMENTED AND COMPLETE BLANKS WHERE APPROPRIATE)		Patient awake
		1. Admit to P.A.R.		Vital signs stable
		2. V.S. per P.A.R routine.		No excess bleeding, Drainage
		3. Medicate for pain as follows:		Minimal nausea, vomiting
				No Respiratory Depression
				Extubated more than 1 hour
				Discharge to Floor
		4. IV Fluids: a. Per surgical service		Discharge to Special Care Area
		b. As follows:		Signed _____ MD
				Signed _____ RN
		5. Face tent / T-Piece		
		6. Ventilator–Initial Setting		
		Mode FIO$_2$ V / T		
		Respiratory Rate Other		
		7. ABG's in _____ min. from A - line, then		

Signed _____ M.D.   Date _____

FORM NO. 7867   REV 11/89

FIG. 11-1. Post anesthesia order and discharge sheet. (Reprinted with permission of Rush-Presbyterian-St. Luke's Medical Center, Chicago.)

Morbidity and mortality reports

Although the compiling of morbidity and mortality reports has been traditionally associated with departments of medicine, surgery, and anesthesia, the collection of morbidity and mortality data may be useful in the PACU as well.

The collection of morbidity and mortality data involves recording a brief synopsis of untoward or unusual events that occur in the PACU. An example of a report form is provided in the box below. This may include such events as reintubation, patients who were taken back to the operating room because they were bleeding, acute cardiac emergencies, and patient injury.

Ideally, the data will be recorded as soon after the unusual event as possible, that is, once the emergency is reconciled. At the end of each month, the morbidity and mortality reports can be compiled into categories, for example, respiratory (reintubations, respiratory arrests), cardiovascular (dysrhythmias, myocardial infarctions), surgical (bleeding, dehiscence, error), or procedural (medication or policy error) (Table 11-1).

The documentation of unusual events is important, but review of the data is even more important. Review of the data may identify the need for in-service training, for a change in policy, or for ongoing monitoring. For example, in one PACU, it was noted that in a 1-month period, a significant number of patients required emergency reintubation within minutes of arrival in the PACU. Each was attributed to inadequate assessment of the patient's neuromuscular status in the operating room. As a result of the review, an in-service training seminar was provided in the department of anesthesia about neuromuscular blockade and reversal. In addition, the PACU nurses developed an ad-

---

SAMPLE MORBIDITY AND MORTALITY REPORT FORM

Date _____

(Addressograph plate)

Surgeon _____
Anesthesia team _____
Surgical procedure _____

Description of event:

Patient outcome:

Addendum:

For quality assurance purposes only

Table 11–1. PACU morbidity and mortality report (month of March 1990)

	Date	Patient	Procedure	Reason/complication
Respiratory	3/4/90	R.V.	Drainage of empyema	Reintubation
	3/19/90	T.K.	Herniorraphy	Pulmonary edema
	3/25/90	B.R.	Diagnostic laparotomy	Pseudocholinesterase deficiency—prolonged intubation
Cardiovascular	3/5/90	C.Z.	Exploratory laparotomy	Intraoperative MI
	3/7/90	V.M.	CABG	Tamponade
	3/18/90	H.N.	CABG	Postoperative CVA
Surgical	3/4/90	P.B.	TURP	Return to OR—bleeding
Procedure	3/12/90	W.T.	Exploratory laparotomy	Dopamine infiltration
Miscellaneous	72 patients (7%) admitted with temperature of <93° F; overnight stay patients (no beds in SICU) 55			

mission protocol that included an assessment of respiratory and neurologic functioning.

Also as a result of the incidents and further review, it was noted that the reintubations did not occur smoothly. Resuscitation equipment was either poorly organized or not immediately available. Again, as a result, the PACU nurses placed Ambu-bags and masks at every bedside, and the emergency carts were reorganized into adult and pediatric carts.

It should be noted that morbidity and mortality reports may identify problems within departments or across departments. It is suggested, therefore, that a copy of the PACU monthly morbidity and mortality report be given to and discussed with the quality assurance committee of the department of anesthesia and with any department whose actions may have contributed to an untoward event in the PACU.

The morbidity and mortality report may be used as a structural, process, or outcome indicator. A presentation or discussion of an untoward event can clarify what occurred and what actions or lack of actions on the part of a practitioner may have contributed to the event (process). It is possible to discuss the patient's actual status as a result of the event (outcome). It is also possible to evaluate or discuss the circumstances under which the event occurred (structure).

It is important to recognize that morbidity and mortality reports should be viewed as a monitoring tool. Determination of blame is not what is important. It is important to identify the action or failure to act that contributed to the event and to initiate plans to correct deficiencies to prevent the event from recurring.

Chart audits

Chart audits are designed as a mechanism to evaluate adequacy of documentation or as an outcome or process indicator. Charts are reviewed for completeness, conformity to standards, and legibility. Charts are selected randomly from the entire day's schedule to ensure variability of cases reviewed and of nurses doing the charting (see the box below). For example, if only the first five cases out of the operating room in the morning are reviewed, it is likely that the cases will be short procedures, including cystoscopies and tubal ligations, and that the patients will be ambulatory surgical patients who are relatively healthy. In addition, only the nurses who are scheduled to work in the morning will have their documentation of care evaluated. Random chart selection increases the reliability of data collection across cases, patient types, and nurses.

Evaluation of documentation is designed not only to identify deficiencies in a nurse's charting but also to evaluate the deficiencies in the records used. The nurses may be charting per unit standards, but the PACU record or flow sheet may prove cumbersome or inadequate, or it may not be conducive to the patient population being served.

PACU CHART AUDIT

STANDARD: ALL AREAS ON THE PACU RECORD ARE COMPLETE

THRESHOLD: 100%

	Yes	Not complete	Not applicable
I. *Anesthesia report of preoperative and intraoperative events*			
A. Surgical procedure	☐	☐	☐
B. Name of surgeon	☐	☐	☐
C. Name of anesthesiologists	☐	☐	☐
D. Patient history (indication for surgery)	☐	☐	☐
E. Anesthetic agents used	☐	☐	☐
F. Intraoperative medications given (antiemetics/antibiotics)	☐	☐	☐
G. IV fluid totals (includes blood products)	☐	☐	☐
H. Estimated blood loss	☐	☐	☐
I. Only hospital-approved abbreviations used	☐	☐	☐
II. *PACU admission assessment*			
A. Are breath sounds assessed bilaterally?	☐	☐	☐
B. Are admission vital signs documented?	☐	☐	☐
C. Has an admission ECG strip been obtained?	☐	☐	☐
D. Has the patient's neurologic status been evaluated?	☐	☐	☐
E. Has the patient's position been noted?	☐	☐	☐

This last problem is clearly evident with the changing acuity and status of patients in some PACUs. With an increase in patient acuity, demand for surgical intensive care beds has increased tremendously. Unfortunately, the supply of intensive care beds is not always sufficient to meet the demand, and postsurgical patients who need intensive care beds are remaining overnight (or even longer) in the PACU. Most PACU records are not designed, either in size or space, for extended stay patients. Charting, particularly of medications and intake/output, may become confusing as the PACU record grows to several pages. In an attempt to increase clarity, many PACUs have been forced to develop new records to better document the status of overnight or extended recovery patients.

Identification of problems in the format of a chart or in the way in which it is filled out should be addressed, and plans should be made to correct the problem. Ongoing and periodic monitoring will help to ensure that charting deficits that have been identified have been corrected and that no new deficits have arisen.

In performing chart audits, it is also desirable to evaluate problem identification and problem resolution when evaluating documentation. If, for example, a PACU nurse documents that the patient has "a respiratory rate of 36-40 with wheezing heard throughout all lung fields bilaterally, and a saturation of 86% on 50% FIO_2 high humidity face mask," subsequent documentation might include, "head of the cart elevated 30 degrees, anesthesiologist notified and present. Alupent treatment given. After treatment, breath sounds clear, respiratory rate 24-26, oxygen saturation 95% on 50% FIO_2 high humidity mask." In this example, the PACU nurse has identified the presence of a problem (respiratory distress) and its resolution (anesthesiologist involvement, interventions provided, patient response). With this type of chart audit, process and outcome indicators may be identified and evaluated.

Joint Commission for Accreditation of Healthcare Organizations (JCAHO) visits

The purpose of a JCAHO accreditation survey visit is to assess the extent of a hospital's compliance with defined standards. Compliance with the standards is assessed either by documentation of compliance by hospital personnel, by examples of the implementation of a standard as evidence of compliance, or by on-site observation by JCAHO surveyors. Currently, the JCAHO has defined standards in twenty-three areas (identified in the box on p. 279).[18]

The rating scale used by the JCAHO to assess compliance has six rankings, the numbers 1 through 5 and NA (not applicable). The scale may also be applied by the hospital staff in self-assessment. An explanation of the scale follows:[18]

1. *Substantial Compliance* indicates that the hospital consistently meets all major provisions of the standard or required characteristic.
2. *Significant Compliance* indicates that the hospital meets most provisions of the standard or required characteristic.
3. *Partial Compliance* indicates that the hospital meets some provisions of the standard or required characteristic.

STANDARDS OF THE JOINT COMMISSION FOR THE ACCREDITATION OF
HEALTHCARE ORGANIZATIONS

Alcoholism and other drug dependency services
Diagnostic radiology services
Dietetic services
Emergency services
Governing body
Hospital-sponsored ambulatory care services
Infection control
Management and administrative services
Medical records services
Medical staff
Nuclear medicine services
Nursing services
Pathology and medical laboratory services
Pharmaceutical services
Physical rehabilitation services
Plant, technology, and safety management
Professional library services
Quality assurance
Radiation oncology services
Respiratory care services
Social work services
Special care units
Surgical and anesthesia services

4. *Minimal Compliance* indicates that the hospital meets few provisions of the standard or required characteristic.
5. *Noncompliance* indicates that the hospital fails to meet the provisions of the standard or required characteristic.
NA. *Not applicable* indicates that the standard or required characteristic does not apply to the hospital.

To be accredited a hospital must demonstrate that it is in *substantial compliance* with the standards. Accreditation is then awarded for 3 years, with or without recommendations. At the end of 3 years, the hospital must reapply for reaccreditation. Recommendations are identified areas of concern that should receive the highest priority in a hospital's plans for improvement. A hospital that receives a recommendation is expected to direct attention toward the recommendations within the time schedule established by the JCAHO Accreditation Committee. Monitoring of progress toward compliance may occur through written progress reports at identified intervals or through focused, on-site survey visits. During a focused survey visit, generally only those areas identified in the recommendations are addressed.

Although the JCAHO does not identify a set of standards specific to the PACU, standards that have an impact on the operation, care delivery, and practice of nursing within the PACU may be found in the sections on Surgical and Anesthesia Services, Special Care Units, Hospital-Sponsored Ambulatory Care Services, and Nursing Services.

In these sections, either standards or characteristics specific to the PACU may be found. For example, under Surgical and Anesthesia Services is the standard, "Surgical and anesthesia services, as appropriate for the hospital, are available to meet the needs of patients." Characteristics that apply to the PACU under this standard include:

●The postoperative status of the patient is evaluated on admission to and discharge from the post anesthesia recovery area.

●Documentation includes a record of vital signs and level of consciousness, intravenous fluids administered, including blood products, all drugs administered, post anesthesia visits and any unusual events or postoperative complications and the management of those events.[18]

Under Special Care Units is the standard, "Special care units, as appropriate for the hospital, are established for patients requiring extraordinary care on a concentrated and continuous basis." Characteristics that apply to the PACU under this standard include:

●Each special care unit is well organized and integrated with other units and departments/services of the hospital, and the scope of services provided is specified.

●The relationship of each special care unit to other units and departments/services of the hospital is specified within the overall hospital plan.

●Written criteria for patient admission and discharge from a special care unit, including priority determination, are developed by the medical staff, with participation of the nursing department/service.[18]

It is interesting to note that the following statement may be found within the introductory definition of special care units, "A special care unit is ordinarily not combined with a post anesthesia recovery unit."[18]

Standards applicable to PACU practice are also found under Hospital-Sponsored Ambulatory Care Services. For example, in this section is the standard, "The hospital implements structures, systems, policies, and procedures for safety management, life safety, equipment management, and utilities management in all areas where ambulatory care patients are provided services."[18] Within this standard several specifications apply to the PACU, including characteristics defining the need for patient privacy, the provision of anesthesia and post anesthesia services, communication systems in an emergency situation, equipment and supplies appropriate to the sizes of patients treated, and verification of emergency equipment, drugs, and supplies.

Standards and characteristics applicable to PACU practice found under Nursing Services include specifications concerning organization, administration, standards of practice, staffing, care delivery, in-service education, policies and procedures, and quality assurance.

Practitioners and managers of post anesthesia care units would be advised to peruse all of these sections when preparing for JCAHO visits, as well as when preparing for JCAHO accreditation. Use of the standards and characteristics for ongoing monitoring will help to increase staff familiarity with the standards, will provide a mechanism for prompt detection of discrepancies, and will, ideally, increase the unit's compliance with the standards.

Workload monitoring and staffing patterns

Establishment of staffing patterns in the PACU is difficult at best. Recommendations have been made about staffing by the numbers (one nurse for every two patients in primary recovery), staffing by acuity (one nurse for every intubated, ventilated patient), and staffing by staff experience (one orientee for one simple postoperative patient). Clearly, the use of one method, without consideration of any of the others, presents problems.

Staffing by the numbers, or by patient census, is calculated by recording the time that patients enter and exit the PACU. The hours worked by nurses are also recorded. The data are then tabulated and compared. Unfortunately, this method can only provide retrospective data. By obtaining census data on a daily or weekly basis, trends and days of heavier patient loads can be determined. The data can be used to determine scheduling needs, days off, days requiring additional nurses, and schedules of part-time nurses. Census data can also be used to assist in the scheduling of support service personnel, including clerks, transporters, and unit assistants.

Staffing by acuity is difficult, at best, for it is difficult to predict with any certainty the acuity of patients on any given day. A number of patient classification systems have been developed for use in critical care units, including the APACHE (acute physiology and chronic health evaluation), the TISS (therapeutic interventions scoring system), and the Medicus System (Rush-Presbyterian-St. Luke's Medical Center, Chicago).[11,20] Unfortunately, the unique variables of PACU care prevent reliable prediction or evaluation of staffing requirements in the PACU. To date, there is no workload tool that accurately predicts staffing requirements of the post anesthesia unit.

The development of a workload tool is another example of a quality assurance activity that can be individualized to the unique considerations of the PACU. A PACU that provides care only to ambulatory surgical patients may have a high volume of low-acuity cases. A PACU that provides 24-hour care to inpatient, outpatient, and intensive care patients will be faced with a high-acuity and high-volume census.

An example of a PACU workload tool may be found in the box on p. 282. This tool, currently being piloted, attempts to correlate physiologic alterations with length of stay, ASA physical status rating, surgical procedure, and type of anesthesia. The tool was developed by the PACU nurses and was designed to identify variables that increased patient acuity, workload, and staffing needs.

Others have attempted to identify surgical procedures as an indicator of acuity and staffing requirements. Bodenstein and DeLozier classified procedures as type one, two, three, and four.[8] This system is based on the premise that the more complicated or invasive the surgery, the greater the demand on PACU nurses.

PACU WORKLOAD CRITERIA LOG

Patient ID number _____   *Type of anesthesia:*
        1   9   General _____ (24)

Admission time _____   Epidural _____ (25)
       10   14   Spinal _____ (26)

Surgical procedure _____ (_____)   IV sedation _____ (27)
            15   Local _____ (28)

ASA class _____
           16

Age _____   Discharge time _____
    17   18   19   23

CARE CATEGORIES
Check all that apply

1. *ISOLATION* _____ (29)
2. *HYPOTHERMIA* _____ (30)
3. *OUTPATIENT* _____ *(31)*
4. *SENSORIUM*
    a. Emergence delirium _____ (32)
    b. Prolonged somnolence
       _____ (33)
    c. Sensory deficit _____ (34)
5. *RESPIRATORY*
    a. Respiratory arrest/obstruction
       _____ (35)
    b. Pneumothroax _____ (36)
    c. Apnea/hypoventilation _____ (37)
    d. Hyperventilation _____ (38)
    e. Bronchospasm/laryngospasm/wheezing
       _____ (39)
    f. Pulmonary emboli _____ (40)
    g. Pulmonary edema _____ (41)
    h. Artificial airway _____ (42)
    i. Frequent suctioning _____ (43)
    j. Reintubation _____ (44)
    k. Ventilator _____ (45)
6. *CARDIOVASCULAR*
    a. Arrhythmias _____ (46)
    b. CHF _____ (47)
    c. Hypotension _____ (48)
    d. Hypertension _____ (49)
    e. Angina _____ (50)
    f. MI _____ (51)
    g. Cardiac arrest _____ (52)
7. *HEMORRHAGE* _____ (53)
8. *SPECIAL PROCEDURES*
    a. Blood administration _____ (54)
    b. Swan-Ganz _____ (55)
    c. CVP/A-line/multiple IV
       _____ (56)
    d. ECT _____ (57)
    e. Minor surgery _____ (58)
    f. ICU patient _____ (59)
    g. Insertion of tubes _____ (60)
    h. Specimen of
       collection _____ (61)
    i. Epidural drip _____ (62)
9. *MISCELLANEOUS*
    a. Blood reaction _____ (63)
    b. Return to OR _____ (64)
    c. Requires assistance of another RN $> \frac{1}{2}$ hour _____(65)

Type one patients were identified as patients who have had minor surgery and who require minimal care for less than one and a half hours of PACU time. Examples of type one surgeries include arthroscopies, diagnostic laparoscopies, biopsies, and vasectomies.

Type two patients were identified as patients who have had minor surgery, but who require slightly more care than type one patients, including more observation or treatments. Examples of type two surgeries include amputations, appendectomies, vaginal hysterectomies, and ventral herniorrhaphies.

Type three patients were identified as patients who have had major surgery and who will require time to stabilize (2 to 3 hours), more medications, more treatments, and closer observations. Examples of type three surgeries include cholecystectomies, colon resections, nephrectomies, and joint replacements.

Type four patients were identified as patients who have had major surgery and who will require prolonged observation (more than 3 hours) in the PACU before returning to a surgical unit or who will require continued care in an intensive care unit. Examples of type four surgeries include craniotomies, bypass grafts, transplants, and thoracic surgeries.[8] It should be remembered that none of these workload tools have undergone the rigors of intensive, multisite clinical validation studies. They serve as examples only.

Staffing for patient acuity matches care delivery to the unique needs of individual patients. Unfortunately, because acuity varies on a daily basis, it is difficult to use acuity data in scheduling. Acuity data is useful, however, in justifying decisions to refuse additional PACU admissions, in justifying the need to call in an on-call nurse, or in justifying the need for additional staff to provide care for ICU overflow patients.

Staffing by staff experience should be a variable in any staffing decisions. New orientees and new graduates cannot be expected to carry the same patient load (by number or acuity) as an experienced practitioner. As a result, many managers will not count orientees in their staffing numbers when preparing monthly schedules.

SUMMARY

Whether mandated by external agencies or internal administration, quality assurance activities should be the responsibility of every practitioner within the PACU. Quality assurance activities are a way for the individual practitioner to evaluate self-performance, care delivery, and patient outcomes. Quality assurance activities are a way for the individual practitioner to contribute to the overall functioning and evaluation of the PACU.

It is no longer acceptable to simply "do the job." The demand is now for high-quality, cost-effective care. Health care is a business, mandating effective and efficient care delivery. Quality assurance activities can help to conform effective and efficient performance and can help serve as a means to identify areas for individual or unit improvement.

Quality assurance data can help to assure individual PACU practitioners, unit managers, hospital administrators, and departmental managers that we are providing high-quality post anesthesia care.

REFERENCES

1. Aduddell P and Weeks L: A cost-effective approach to quality assurance, Nurs Economics 1:279-282, 1984.
2. American Nurses Association: Standards of nursing practice, Kansas City, MO, 1973, The Association.
3. American Nurses' Association: Nursing quality assurance management/learning system: guide for nursing quality assurance coordinators and administrators, Kansas City, MO, 1982, The Association.
4. American Society of Anesthesiologists: Standards for postanesthesia care, Park Ridge, 1988, The Society.
5. American Society of Association Executives: Assess your strengths and weaknesses: a workbook for evaluating your association, Washington, DC, 1988, The Society.
6. American Society of Post Anesthesia Nurses: Standards of nursing practice, Richmond, 1986, The Society.
7. Bodenstein J and DeLozier A: Staffing the recovery room, Nurs Manage 14(10):34C-E, 1983.
8. Brown E: Quality assurance in anesthesiology: the problem-oriented audit, Anesth Analg 63:611-615, 1984.
9. Coyne W: Nurses are the key to quality health care, RN 53(2):69-74, 1990.
10. Cullen D et al: Therapeutic intervention scoring system: a method for quantitative comparison of patient care, Crit Care Med 2:57, 1974.
11. Decker C: Quality assurance: accent on monitoring, Nurs Manage 16(11):20-24, 1985.
12. Donabedian A: The quality of care: How can it be assessed? JAMA 260:1743-1748, 1988.
13. Duberman S: Quality assurance in the practice of anesthesiology 1986, Park Ridge, IL, 1986, American Society of Anesthesiologists.
14. Eichhorn J: Quality assurance, Curr Rev Post Anesth Care Nurse 11(17):133-140, 1989.
15. Ennis H: Staffing of the recovery room: a view of systems, Curr Rev Recov Room Nurse 1(15):115-119, 1979.
16. Green E and Katz J: A quality-assurance tool that works overtime, RN 9:30-31, 1989.
17. Joint Commission on Accreditation of Hospitals: Accreditation manual for hospitals, Chicago, 1987, The Commission.
18. Joint Commission: First indicators set for pilot tests, Agenda for Change 2(1):1-8, 1988.
19. Knaus W et al: APACHE-acute physiology and chronic health evaluation: a physiologically based classification system, Crit Care Med 9(8):591-597, 1981.
20. Kovner C: Using computerized databases for nursing research and quality assurance, Comput Nurs 7(5):228-231, 1989.
21. McConnell E: Quality assurance in recovery room nursing: objectives of nursing service recruitment, Curr Rev Recov Room Nurse 2(4):27-31, 1980.
22. Meisentheimer C: Incorporating JCAH standards into a quality assurance program, Nurs Adm QA Update 7:1-8, 1983.
23. Meisentheimer C: Quality assurance, Rockville, MD, 1985, Aspen Systems.
24. Miciorowski L, Larson E, and Keane A: Quality assurance evaluate thyself, J Nurs Adm 15:38-42, 1985.
25. Miller T and Rantz M: Quality assurance: guaranteeing a high level of care, J Gerontol Nurs 15(11):10-15, 1989.
26. Miller T and Rantz M: Management structures to facilitate practice changes subsequent to QA activities, J Nurs Assur 3(4):21-27, 1989.
27. New N and New J: Quality assurance that works, Nurs Manage 20(6):21-24, 1989.
28. Robinson M: Sneak preview: JCAHO's quality indicators, Hospitals 62(13):38-43, 1986.
29. Schroeder P and Maibusch R: Nursing quality assurance, Rockville, 1984, Aspen Systems.
30. Smeltzer C: Organizing the search for excellence, Nurs Manage 14(6):19-21, 1983.

Review Questions

1. *Quality assurance may be used as a means to identify* _____.
   a. Strengths
   b. Areas for improvement
   c. Problems
   d. All of the above

2. *Effectiveness is a measure of* _____.
   a. Doing the "right" things
   b. Doing things "right"

3. *Efficiency is a measure of* _____.
   a. Doing the "right" things
   b. Doing things "right"

4. *Standards of practice focus on* _____.
   a. The quality of care
   b. The patient
   c. The provider of care
   d. Outcomes of care

5. *Standards of care focus on* _____.
   a. The providers of care
   b. The environment of care delivery
   c. Quality of care
   d. Patient outcomes

6. *A structural indicator addresses all of the following EXCEPT* _____.
   a. Unit space
   b. Patient response to intervention
   c. Monitoring equipment
   d. Safety inspections

7. *The four components of the nursing process are* _____.
   a. Assessment, planning, implementation, and evaluation
   b. Problem identification, problem evaluation, problem resolution, and follow-up monitoring
   c. Effectiveness, efficiency, compliance, and successful outcome
   d. Process, implement, evaluate, and change

8. *Making a judgment about patient status is an example of* _____.
   a. Assessment
   b. Evaluation
   c. Monitoring
   d. Problem resolution

9. *An outcome audit determines whether which group meets preestablished criteria at a point in time?*
   a. Anesthesiologists
   b. PACU nurses
   c. Surgeons
   d. Patients

10. *The use of a discharge checklist is useful for which type of audit?*
    a. Structural
    b. Process
    c. Outcome
    d. Nursing care

11. *Morbidity and mortality reports* ⸻⸻⸻⸻.
    a. Identify untoward patient events
    b. Are given to lawyers to identify professional liability
    c. Are compiled with the goal of assigning blame
    d. May be done by physicians only

12. *The purpose of a JCAHO survey is to* ⸻⸻⸻⸻.
    a. Find fault with hospital personnel and organization
    b. Assess organizational compliance with defined standards
    c. Compare one hospital with another
    d. Compare patient care costs within geographic areas

13. *As JCAHO does not have a category of standards specific to the PACU, the PACU*
    ⸻⸻⸻⸻.
    a. Will not be evaluated
    b. Must define its own standards
    c. Should identify relevant standards from related categories
    d. Will be evaluated against the standards applied to anesthesiologists

14. *To be accredited by JCAHO, a hospital must demonstrate* ⸻⸻⸻⸻ *compliance
    with defined standards*
    a. Total
    b. Significant
    c. Minimal
    d. Substantial

15. *Staffing by census data is limited because* ⸻⸻⸻⸻.
    a. Patient acuity is not considered
    b. Trends in use of the PACU cannot be determined
    c. Scheduling of staff is not facilitated
    d. The need for support service personnel cannot be determined

Answers

15. a	10. c	5. d
14. d	9. d	4. c
13. c	8. b	3. b
12. b	7. a	2. a
11. a	6. b	1. d

APPENDIX A

ASPAN STANDARDS OF PRACTICE

PART I: STANDARDS OF NURSING PRACTICE: AMBULATORY CARE, PREANESTHESIA OR PREPROCEDURAL PHASE.

I. Assessment

Health status data is collected. This data is recorded, retrievable, continuous and communicated. Data is obtained by interviewing the patient and/or significant other, physical exam, review of records, and consultation.

A. Assessment factors include but are not limited to:
1. Relevant preoperative physical status including: electrocardiogram, radiology findings, laboratory values, allergies, disabilities, drug use, physical impairments, mobility limitations, prostheses (including hearing aids), and cardiac, respiratory and diabetic history
2. Relevant preoperative, emotional, safety, and psychosocial needs
3. Previous anesthetic (patient and family, with or without complications)
4. Length of fasting (NPO)
5. Understanding of anesthesia (local, local with sedation, regional block, general)
6. Understanding of procedure
7. Understanding of preoperative teaching to include for both short stay and same day admit patients: pain and nausea control, length of stay in PACU Phase I and II as appropriate, use of oxygen, need for coughing and deep breathing post anesthesia
8. Understanding of preoperative teaching for short stay patients to also include discharge criteria, home care instructions and an understanding of the need to have a responsible adult drive the patient home and provide support
9. Need for home care services.

From American Society of Post Anesthesia Nurses: Standards of Practice, Richmond, VA.

B. Initial physical assessment to include the documentation of:
1. Temperature, blood pressure, pulse, and respirations
2. Review of systems as indicated per type of anesthesia and patient status
3. Assessment of potential complicating factors.

II. Nursing Diagnosis

Nursing diagnosis is a concise statement and represents a decision based upon analysis of the data collected during the assessment phase.

A. Nursing diagnosis is consistent with current scientific knowledge.

B. Nursing diagnoses are based on identifiable data as compared with established norms or previous conditions.

C. Nursing diagnoses include but are not limited to:
1. Anxiety
2. Alterations in fluid volume (deficit)
3. Potential for physical injury
4. Potential for respiratory dysfunction
5. Knowledge deficit.

III. Care Plan

The plan for nursing care describes a systematic method for achieving the preanesthesia or preprocedural goal of adequately preparing the patient physically, emotionally, and psychologically.

A. The plan includes setting priorities for appropriate nursing actions.

B. The plan is based on current scientific knowledge.

C. The plan is developed with and communicated to the patient, family and/or significant others and appropriate health care team personnel.

D. The plan is formulated in conjunction with preanesthesia health status data and assessments.

E. The plan includes but is not limited to the following nursing actions:
1. Identification of the patient
2. Adequate physical and emotional preparation for surgery
3. Interpretation and documentation of data obtained during assessment
4. Documentation of nursing plan, action or interventions with outcomes
5. Discharge planning and home care instructions with patient and significant others
6. Appropriate transportation after discharge.

IV. Implementation

The plan for nursing care is implemented to achieve the goal as stated under care plan.

A. Nursing actions remain consistent with the written plan to provide continuity of care in accordance with established policy and procedure.

B. Comfort, safety, efficiency, skill, and effectiveness are reflected in nursing action.

C. Nursing decisions and actions regarding patient care reflect upholding the dignity of the patient and family.

D. The plan may be added to meet the changing needs of the patient in each phase.

V. Evaluation

The plan for nursing care is evaluated.

A. Current assessment data is collected and recorded to evaluate the patient's readiness for transfer to the operating room:
   1. All required radiology findings, laboratory values, and electrocardiogram results documented
   2. Vital signs documented
   3. Consent forms signed and witnessed as required by the individual institution
   4. Ordered shave preps or scrubs completed
   5. Preoperative teaching complete
   6. Preoperative medication administered and documented, if ordered
   7. Patient properly attired
   8. Intravenous started, if applicable
   9. Allergies documented
   10. Dentures, contact lenses, hearing aides, and prostheses removed if indicated.

PART II: STANDARDS OF NURSING PRACTICE: POST ANESTHESIA CARE, PHASE ONE

I. Assessment

Health status data is collected. This data is recorded, retrievable, continuous and communicated. Data is obtained by physical exam, review of records and consultation.

A. Assessment factors include but are not limited to:
1. Relevant preoperative status, including: electrocardiogram, vital signs, radiology findings, laboratory values, allergies, disabilities, drug use, physical or mental impairments, mobility limitations, prostheses (including hearing aids)
2. Anesthesia technique (general, regional, local), effect of pre-op medications
3. Anesthestic agents, muscle relaxants, narcotics and reversal agents used
4. Length of time anesthesia administered
5. Type of surgical procedure
6. Estimated fluid/blood loss and replacement
7. Complications occurring during anesthetic course, treatment initiated, response.

B. Initial physical assessment to include the documentation of:
1. Vital signs
    a. Respiratory rate and competency, airway patency, breath sounds, type of artificial airway, mechanical ventilator and settings
    b. Blood pressure—cuff or arterial line
    c. Pulse—apical—peripheral—cardiac monitor pattern
    d. Temperature—oral—rectal—axillary—digital through dermal sensors
2. Pressure readings—central venous—arterial blood—pulmonary artery wedge and intracranial pressure if indicated
3. Position of patient
4. Condition and color of skin
5. Circulation—peripheral pulses and sensation of extremity(ies) as applicable
6. Condition of dressings
7. Condition of suture line, if dressings are absent
8. Type and patency of drainage tubes, catheters and receptacle
9. Amount and type of drainage
10. Muscular response and strength
11. Pupillary response as indicated
12. Fluid therapy, location of lines, type and amount of solution infusing (including blood)
13. Level of consciousness
14. Level of physical and emotional comfort
15. Numerical score if used.

II. Nursing Diagnosis

Nursing diagnosis is a concise statement and represents a decision based upon analysis of the data collected during the assessment phase.

A. Nursing diagnosis is consistent with current scientific knowledge.

B. Nursing diagnoses are based on identifiable data as compared with established norms or previous conditions.

C. Nursing diagnoses include but are not limited to:
1. Altered level of consciousness
2. Alterations in comfort
3. Anxiety
4. Alterations in cardiac output
5. Alterations in fluid volume (both excess and deficit)
6. Impairment of mobility (including decrease in muscle strength)
7. Potential for physical injury
8. Respiratory dysfunction
9. Impairment in skin integrity
10. Abnormal tissue perfusion
11. Alterations in urinary elimination
12. Alterations in body temperature.

III. Care Plan

The plan for nursing care describes a systematic method for achieving the goal of post anesthesia nursing care—to assist the patient in returning to a safe physiological level after an anesthetic by providing safe, knowledgeable, individualized nursing care to patients and their families in the immediate post anesthetic phase.

A. The plan includes setting priorities for appropriate nursing actions.

B. The plan is based on current scientific knowledge.

C. The plan is developed with and communicated to the patient, family and/or significant others and appropriate health care team personnel.

D. The plan is formulated in conjunction with preoperative, intraoperative, and current post anesthetic health status assessments.

E. The plan is developed to maintain patient's privacy, dignity and safety.

F. The plan includes but is not limited to the following nursing actions:
1. Identify the patient
2. Monitor, maintain, and/or improve respiratory function
3. Monitor, maintain, and/or improve circulatory function
4. Promote and maintain physical and emotional comfort
5. Receive report from operating room nurse, anesthesiologist, and/or anesthetist
6. Monitor surgical site
7. Interpret and document data obtained during assessment
8. Document nursing plan, action, and/or interventions with outcome
9. Notify family and/or significant others of patient's arrival and discharge from PACU
10. Notify patient care unit of any needed equipment
11. Notify patient care unit when patient is ready for discharge from PACU.

IV. Implementation

The plan for nursing care is implemented to achieve the goal as stated under care plan.

A. Nursing actions remain consistent with the written plan to provide continuity of care in accordance with established policy and procedure.

B. Nursing actions are performed with safety, skill, efficiency, effectiveness and knowledge.

C. Nursing decisions and actions regarding patient care reflect upholding the dignity of the patient and family.

D. The plan may be altered to meet the changing needs of the patient.

V. Evaluation

The plan for nursing care is evaluated.

A. Current assessment data are collected and recorded to evaluate the patient's status for discharge:
1. Airway patency and respiratory function
2. Stability of vital signs, including temperature
3. Level of consciousness and muscular strength
4. Mobility
5. Patency of tubes, catheters, drains, intravenous lines
6. Skin color and condition
7. Condition of dressing and/or surgical site
8. Intake and output
9. Comfort.

VI. Discharge

The post anesthesia nurse shall discharge the patient in accordance with written policies set forth by the Department of Anesthesia and also in accordance with the criteria and data collected through use of the nursing process. A final nursing assessment and evaluation of the patient's condition will be performed and documented. If a numerical scoring system is used, the discharge score will be recorded to reflect the patient's status. The post anesthesia nurse arranges for the safe transport of the patient from the PACU.

PART III: STANDARDS OF NURSING PRACTICE: POST ANESTHESIA CARE, PHASE TWO

I. Assessment

Health status data is collected. This data is recorded, retrievable, continuous and communicated. Data is obtained by interviewing the patient, and/or significant other, physical exam, review of records and consultation.

A. Assessment factors include but are not limited to:
1. Relevant preoperative or preprocedural data
2. Relevant anesthesia and surgical data
3. Relevant post anesthesia phase I data.
B. Initial post anesthesia phase II physical assessment to include the documentation of:
1. Vital signs
   a. Respiratory rate and competency
   b. Blood pressure
   c. Pulse
   d. Temperature
2. Position of patient
3. Condition and color of skin
4. Neurovascular assessment as applicable
5. Condition of dressings, drains, tubes as applicable
6. Muscular response and strength
7. Fluid therapy, location of lines, type and amount of fluid infusing
8. Level of consciousness
9. Level of physical and emotional comfort
10. Numerical score, if used.

II. Nursing Diagnosis

Nursing diagnosis is a concise statement and represents analyses of the data collected during the assessment phase to prepare the patient for discharge.

A. Nursing diagnosis is consistent with current scientific knowledge.

B. Nursing diagnoses are based on identifiable data as compared to established norms or previous conditions.

C. Nursing diagnoses include but are not limited to:
1. Altered level of consciousness
2. Alterations in comfort
3. Alterations in fluid volume (both excess and deficit)
4. Impairment of mobility (including decrease in muscle strength)
5. Respiratory dysfunction
6. Impairment in skin integrity
7. Abnormal tissue perfusion
8. Alterations in urinary elimination
9. Alterations in body temperature
10. Knowledge deficit.

III. Care Plan

The plan for nursing care describes a systematic means for achieving the post anesthesia phase II goal—to assist the patient in returning to a safe physiological level after enabling discharge with an appropriate knowledge base for home care.

A. The plan includes setting priorities for appropriate nursing action.

B. The plan is based on current scientific knowledge.

C. The plan is developed with and communicated to the patient, significant other, and appropriate health care team personnel.

D. The plan is formulated in conjunction with preoperative, intraoperative, and current post anesthetic health status assessments.

E. The plan includes but is not limited to the following nursing actions:
   1. Identification of the patient
   2. Receiving report from post anesthesia phase I nurse
   3. Provide for maximum degree of privacy
   4. Provide for confidentiality of information and records
   5. Provide for safety/security of patients belongings
   6. Administer pain medication as necessary, record results
   7. Administer other medication as ordered, record results
   8. Complete ordered tests and treatments
   9. Monitor, maintain, and/or improve respiratory function
   10. Monitor, maintain, and/or improve circulatory function
   11. Promote and maintain physical and emotional comfort
   12. Monitor surgical site
   13. Interpret and document data obtained during assessment
   14. Document plan, action, and/or intervention and outcome
   15. Position patient gradually from supine to Fowler's position
   16. Offer fluids by mouth
   17. Ambulate with assistance
   18. Ask patient to urinate prior to discharge
   19. Review discharge planning, provide written home care instructions to patient and significant other
   20. Provide home care if needed for extended care or evaluation of home per social service. Next day follow up phone call is recommended to evaluate status.

IV. Implementation

The plan for nursing care is implemented to achieve the goal as stated under care plan.

A. Nursing actions remain consistent with the written plan to provide continuity of care in accordance with established policy and procedure.

B. Nursing actions are performed with safety, skill, efficiency, effectiveness and knowledge.

C. Nursing decisions and actions regarding patient care reflect upholding the dignity of the patient and family.

D. The plan may be altered to meet the changing needs of the patient.

V. Evaluation

The plan for nursing care is evaluated.

A. Current assessment data are collected and recorded to evaluate the patient's status for discharge to home:
   1. Adequate respiratory function
   2. Stability of vital signs, including temperature
   3. Level of consciousness and muscular strength
   4. Ability to ambulate consistent with developmental age level
   5. Ability to swallow oral fluids, cough or demonstrate gag reflex
   6. Ability to retain oral fluid
   7. Skin color and condition
   8. Pain minimal
   9. Adequate neurovascular status of operative extremity
   10. Able to demonstrate proper use of crutches
   11. Able to demonstrate proper care of drains and catheters
   12. Able to describe care of and changing of dressings
   13. Able to demonstrate proper method of administering eye and ear drops
   14. Able to describe the "proper" taking of prescribed medications
   15. Patient and home care provider understands all home care instructions
   16. Written discharge instruction given to patient/family
   17. Concur with prearrangements for safe transportation home.

VI. Discharge

The post anesthesia (Phase II) nurse shall prepare to discharge the patient in accordance with approved written policy and also in accordance with criteria and data collected through the use of the nursing process. A final nursing assessment and evaluation of the patient's condition will be performed and documented. If a numerical scoring system is used, the discharge score will be recorded to reflect the patient's status and meet the facility's written policy. The post anesthesia (Phase II) nurse ensures availability of safe transport of the patient to his or her home.

PART IV: ASPAN'S STANDARDS OF NURSING PRACTICE: MANAGEMENT STANDARDS

I. Personnel

A. Head Nurse

The head nurse must be a registered nurse with appropriate education, experience and ability to demonstrate proficiency in nursing practice and management. Plans, coordinates, directs, evaluates, and delegates nursing activities for the PACU, twenty-four hours a day. The head nurse is administratively responsible to a designee of the Department of Nursing and medically responsible to the Chairperson of the Department of Anesthesia. The head nurse has the responsibility and authority to take those actions needed to assure that optimal care is given in the PACU.

B. Staff Nurse

The staff nurse must be currently registered and complete a formal orientation program that is specific to the PACU. The staff nurse must be able to function in emergency situations and possess the skills required for the use of the Nursing Process.

C. Ancillary Staff

Ancillary staff shall meet requirements set by the individual facility's policy, position descriptions and be familiar with written protocols and procedures.

II. Education

Education preparation for the RN in the PACU will include but is not limited to:

1. Airway management
2. Management of the patient during altered states of consciousness
3. Management of monitoring and respiratory equipment
4. Management of fluid lines
5. Management of tubes, drains, and catheters
6. Cardiopulmonary resuscitation
7. Administration of drugs and drug related problems
8. Knowledge of anesthetic agents, techniques, actions, and interactions
9. Arrhythmia recognition and treatment
10. Assessing learning needs and patient education as appropriate per unit.

An educational curriculum will be developed to promote clinical experience and professional growth. Programs will be on-going to reflect new developments in patient care and offer continued opportunity for self-fulfillment. Individual educational records will be maintained with documentation of participation in educational programs.

III. Patient-Staff Ratio

Patient-staff ratio will vary according to patient classification and is recommended as follows:

Class 1-1:3—One nurse to three patients who are awake and stable, uncomplicated patients.

Class II-1:2—One nurse to two patients; a) any stable, unconscious patient, b) any uncomplicated pediatric patient, c) patients who have undergone major surgery and whose systems have stabilized.

Class III-1:1—One nurse to one patient at the time of admission to the PACU for any patient requiring life support care. A second care nurse must be available to assist as needed.

It is recommended that two licensed staff nurses, one of whom is an R.N., be present whenever a single patient is recovering from anesthesia. It is also recommended that increased staff be available when difficult patient educational needs are evident.

Physical Aspects

A. The Post Anesthesia Care Units, Phase I and Phase II will be in close proximity to the area in which anesthesia is to be administered.

B. It is recommended that Phase I PACU and Phase II PACU be two separate rooms or areas. It is also recommended that preoperative patients not be present when patients are recovering from anesthesia.

C. One and one half beds will be available in the PACU for every one operating room. Two beds will be available in the PACU for every one operating room when dealing with short, simple procedures on relatively healthy patients.

D. Each patient care unit will be equipped to provide various means of oxygen delivery, constant and intermittent suction, a means to monitor blood pressure, adjustable lighting, and the capacity to ensure patient privacy.

E. In Phase I PACU there will be one EKG monitor for every two patient care units minimally. When dealing with more acute patients, one monitor for every patient care unit is recommended. Monitors for arterial, central venous, and/or pulmonary artery pressures, for those patients requiring these measures, will be available. In Phase II PACU one EKG monitor should be available for emergency situations. Emergency carts should be available in both Phase I and Phase II PACUs.

F. One ventilator will be maintained in the Phase I PACU at all times. A sufficient number of ventilators will be available to care for any post anesthesia patient who requires one.

G. Portable oxygen, suction, and cardiac monitoring equipment will be available for those patients requiring such equipment during transport.

H. Patients requiring isolation (as detailed by the Infection Control Committee of Department) will be cared for in a designated area in the PACU (preferably a separate room), apart from other patients. If such is not available, continuous post anesthesia care will be provided elsewhere in the facility. The quality of care in this situation will be equal to that available in the PACU.

I. Those patients requiring strict or respiratory isolation must be housed in a private room.

J. A method of calling for assistance in emergency situations shall be provided in all areas.

K. A plan for transport of patients from a free standing facility to a full service hospital setting must be in place for emergency situations.

APPENDIX B

STANDARDS
FOR POSTANESTHESIA CARE
(Approved by House of Delegates on October 12, 1988)

These Standards apply to postanesthesia care in all locations. These Standards may be exceeded based on the judgment of the responsible anesthesiologist. They are intended to encourage high quality patient care, but cannot guarantee any specific patient outcome. They are subject to revision from time to time as warranted by the evolution of technology and practice.

STANDARD I

ALL PATIENTS WHO HAVE RECEIVED GENERAL ANESTHESIA, REGIONAL ANESTHESIA, OR MONITORED ANESTHESIA CARE SHALL RECEIVE APPROPRIATE POSTANESTHESIA MANAGEMENT.

1. A Postanesthesia Care Unit (PACU) or an area which provides equivalent postanesthesia care shall be available to receive patients after surgery and anesthesia. All patients who receive anesthesia shall be admitted to the PACU except by specific order of the anesthesiologist responsible for the patient's care.
2. The medical aspects of care in the PACU shall be governed by policies and procedures which have been reviewed and approved by the Department of Anesthesiology.
3. The design, equipment and staffing of the PACU shall meet requirements of the facility's accrediting and licensing bodies.
4. The nursing standards of practice shall be consistent with those approved in 1986 by the American Society of Post Anesthesia Nurses (ASPAN).

From American Society of Anesthesiology: ASA Standards for post anesthesia care, Park Ridge, IL.

STANDARD II

A PATIENT TRANSPORTED TO THE PACU SHALL BE ACCOMPANIED BY A MEMBER OF THE ANESTHESIA CARE TEAM WHO IS KNOWLEDGEABLE ABOUT THE PATIENT'S CONDITION. THE PATIENT SHALL BE CONTINUALLY EVALUATED AND TREATED DURING TRANSPORT WITH MONITORING AND SUPPORT APPROPRIATE TO THE PATIENT'S CONDITION.

STANDARD III

UPON ARRIVAL IN THE PACU, THE PATIENT SHALL BE RE-EVALUATED AND A VERBAL REPORT PROVIDED TO THE RESPONSIBLE PACU NURSE BY THE MEMBER OF THE ANESTHESIA CARE TEAM WHO ACCOMPANIES THE PATIENT.

1. The patient's status on arrival in the PACU shall be documented.
2. Information concerning the preoperative condition and the surgical/anesthetic course shall be transmitted to the PACU nurse.
3. The member of the Anesthesia Care Team shall remain in the PACU until the PACU nurse accepts responsibility for the nursing care of the patient.

STANDARD IV

THE PATIENT'S CONDITION SHALL BE EVALUATED CONTINUALLY IN THE PACU.

1. The patient shall be observed and monitored by methods appropriate to the patient's medical condition. Particular attention should be given to monitoring oxygenation, ventilation and circulation. While qualitative clinical signs may be adequate, quantitative methods are encouraged.
2. An accurate written report of the PACU period shall be maintained. Use of an appropriate PACU scoring system is encouraged for each patient on admission, at appropriate intervals prior to discharge, and at the time of discharge.
3. General medical supervision and coordination of patient care in the PACU should be the responsibility of an anesthesiologist.
4. There shall be a policy to assure the availability in the facility of a physician capable of managing complications and providing cardiopulmonary resuscitation for patients in the PACU.

STANDARD V

A PHYSICIAN IS RESPONSIBLE FOR THE DISCHARGE OF THE PATIENT FROM THE POSTANESTHESIA CARE UNIT.

1. When discharge criteria are used, they must be approved by the Department of Anesthesiology and the medical staff. They may vary depending upon whether the patient is discharged to a hospital room, to the ICU, to a short stay unit, or home.
2. In the absence of the physician responsible for the discharge, the PACU nurse shall determine that the patient meets the discharge criteria. The name of the physician accepting responsibility for discharge shall be noted on the record.

APPENDIX C

COMMONLY USED ABBREVIATIONS IN THE PACU

A

ā	before
A2	aortic second sound
AAA	abdominal aortic aneurysm
AB	abortion
ABGs	arterial blood gases
abd	abdomen
ac	before meals
ACF	anterior cervical fusion
ACL	anterior cruciate ligament
ACLS	advanced cardiac life support
ACTH	adrenocorticotropic hormone
acid phos	acid phosphatase
ADA	American Diabetes Association
ADD	adduction
ADH	antidiuretic hormone
ADL	activities of daily living
ad lib	as much as desired
adm	admission
admin	administer or administration
A/E or AE	above-elbow amputation
AF	atrial fibrillation
AGA	appropriate for gestational age
AI	aortic innsufficiency
AICD	automatic implantable cardioverter defibrillator
AIDS	acquired immunodeficiency syndrome
A/K amputation or AKA or AKamp	above-knee amputation
alb	albumin
alk phos	alkaline phosphatase
ALS	amyotrophic lateral sclerosis

AM, am, or a.m.	morning before noon
AMA	against medical advice
AMP	amputation
amt	amount
Anes	anesthesiology
Ant	anterior
AODM	adult onset diabetes mellitus
A-P	anteroposterior
A-P & Lat	anteroposterior and lateral
approx	approximately
ARC	AIDS related complex
ARDS	adult respiratory distress syndrome
ARF	acute renal failure
AS	aortic stenosis
ASAP	as soon as possible
ASD	atrial septal defect
ASF	Anterior spinal fusion
ASHD	arteriosclerotic heart disease
Asst	assistance
AVM	arteriovenous malformation
AVR	aortic valve replacement
A & W	alive and well
ax	axillary

B

B	both/bilateral
BBB	bundle-branch block
B/E	below elbow
BID, b.i.d. or bid	two times a day
BKA	below-knee amputation
bl cult	blood culture
BM	bowel movement
BMA	bone marrow aspirate

BMR	basal metabolic rate	CSF	cerebrospinal fluid
BMT	bone marrow transplant	CT or CAT	computerized axial tomography
BP	blood pressure	CV	cardiovascular
BPD	bronchopulmonary dysplasia	CVA	cerebrovascular accident
BPH	benign prostatic hypertrophy	CVN	central venous nutrition
BR	bedrest	CVP	central venous pressure
BRP	bathroom privileges	Cysto	cystoscopy
br sounds	breath sounds	cx	cervix
BS	bowel sounds	CXR	chest x-ray
BSO	bilateral salpingo-oophorectomy		
BUN	blood urea nitrogen	**D**	
Bx	biopsy		

C

		D/C	discontinue
c̄	with	D & C	dilation and curettage
C	Centigrade	decr	decreased or diminished
Ca^{++}	calcium	decub	decubitus
CABG or		Derm	dermatology
CAB	coronary artery bypass graft	D/I	dry and intact
CAD	coronary artery disease	diag, Dx,	
cath	catheter	or dx	diagnosis
CBC	complete blood count	Diff	differential
cc	cubic centimeter	DJD	degenerative joint disease
CC	chief complaint	DM	diabetes mellitus
CHD	congenital heart disease	DNR	do not resuscitate
CHF	congestive heart failure	DOA	dead on arrival
chol	cholesterol	DOB	date of birth
CI	cardiac index	DOE	dyspnea on exertion
cldy	cloudy	DP	dorsal pedis
cm	centimeter	drsgs	dressings
CMG	cystometrogram	DSA	digital subtraction angiography
CMS	circulation, motion, sensation	DTR	deep tendon reflex
CMV	cytomegalovirus	DTs	delirium tremens
CNS	central nervous system	DVT	deep vein thrombosis
C.O.	cardiac output	Dx	diagnosis
c/o	complains of		
CO_2	carbon dioxide	**E**	
cont	continued		
COPD	chronic obstructive pulmonary disease	EBL	estimated blood loss
		ECCE	extracapsular cataract extraction
		ECG or	
CP	cerebral palsy	EKG	electrocardiogram
C-PAP	continuous positive airway pressure	ECT	electroconvulsive therapy
CPB	cardiopulmonary bypass	EEG	electroencephalogram
CPK	creatinine phosphokinase	EKG or	
CPR	cardiopulmonary resuscitation	ECG	electrocardiogram
CPT	chest physical therapy	elix	elixir
CRF	chronic renal failure	EMG	electromyography
C & S	culture and sensitivity	ENT	ear, nose, and throat

EOM	extraocular movement
Eos	eosinophile
epis	episiotomy
ER	emergency room
ESWL	electroshock wave lithotripsy
ETOH	ethanol/alcohol
EVD	extraventricular drain
exp	expired
Expir	expiration or expiratory
ext	extension
ext rot	external rotation

F

F	Fahrenheit
FB	foreign body
FD	free drain
Fe	iron
Fem Pop	femoral popliteal
FEV	forced expiratory volume
FFP	fresh frozen plasma
FHT	fetal heart tones
FIV	forced inspiratory volume
FIO$_2$	fraction inspired oxygen (decimal)
flex	flexion
FRC	functional residual capacity
FSP	fibrin split products
F/U	follow up
FUO	fever of undetermined origin
FVC	forced vital capacity
Fx	fracture

G

GC	gonorrhea
gest	gestational
GFR	glomerular filtration rate
GI	gastrointestinal
GLU	glucose
Gm, g, or gm	gram
gtts	drops
GU	genitourinary
GVHD	graft vs host disease
GYN or gyne	gynecology

H

H$^+$	hydrogen ion
h or Hr	hour
HA	headache
Hb or Hgb	hemoglobin
HCO$_3$	bicarbonate
Hct or HCT	hematocrit
HEENT	head, ears, eyes, nose, throat
Hg	mercury
Hgb or Hb	hemoglobin
HHO$_2$	high humidity oxygen
HIV	human immunodeficiency virus
h/o	history of
H/P	history and physical
H$_2$O	water
HOB	head of bed
Hr or h	hour
HR	heart rate
ht	height
HTN	hypertension
HTLV III	human T-lymphotropic virus type III
Hx	history
hyperal	hyperalimentation

I

IABP	intraortic balloon pump
ICF	intracellular fluid
ICP	intracranial pressure
ICU	intensive care unit
ID	infectious disease
I & D	incision and drainage
IDDM	insulin-dependent diabetes mellitus
IHSS	idiopathic hypertrophic subaortic stenosis
I-J bypass	ileo-jejunal bypass
IM	intramuscular
IMV	intermittent mandatory ventilation
INC	incision
incr	increase or increasing
inspir	inspiration or inspiratory
int rot	internal rotation
I & O	intake and output
IOL	intraocular lens
IOP	intraocular pressure
IPPB	intermittent positive pressure breathing

irrig	irrigation	LVH	left ventricular hypertrophy
IUD	intrauterine device (contraceptive)	lytes	electrolytes
IV	intravenous		
IVP	intravenous pyelogram	**M**	
IVPB	intravenous piggyback		
IVR	intravenous rider	M	murmur
		M_1	mitral first sound
K		MAO	monoamine oxidase
		MAP	mean arterial pressure
K^+	potassium	max	maximal, maximum
KCI	potassium chloride	mcg or μg	microgram
kg	kilogram	MD	medical doctor
KUB	kidney, ureter, bladder (x-ray)	Med	medicine
KVO	keep vein open	meds	medications
		meq or	
L		mEq	milliequivalents (per liter)
		mg	milligram
L	Liter	Mg	magnesium
LA	left atrium	MI	myocardial infarction
lab	laboratory	MICU	Medical Intensive Care Unit
LAD	left anterior descending coronary	ml	milliliter or milliliters
	artery	mm	millimeter
lat	lateral	mod	moderate
lb	pound	MRI	magnetic resonance imaging
LBP	low back pain	MS	multiple sclerosis
LCE	left carotid endarterectomy	MSO_4	morphine sulfate
LCS	low continuous suction	MVA	motor vehicle accident
LCWS	low continuous wall suction	MVR	mitral valve replacement
LCX or			
LC_X	left circumflex coronary artery	**N**	
L & D	labor and delivery		
LE	lower extremity	Na^+	sodium
LGA	large for gestational age	N/A	not applicable/appropriate
LIS	low intermittent suction	NaCL	sodium chloride
LLE	left lower extremity	NAD	no acute distress
LLL	left lower lobe-lung	NCP	nursing care plan
LLQ	left lower quadrant—abdomen	Neuro	
LMP	last menstrual period	or neuro	neurology or neurological
LOC	level of consciousness	NG	nasogastric
LOS	length of stay	NGT	nasogastric tube
LP	lumbar puncture	NIDDM	non-insulin dependent diabetes mel-
LUE	left upper extremity		litus
LUL	left upper lobe—lung	NIF	negative inspiratory force
LUQ	left upper quadrant—abdomen	NKDA	no known drug allergies
LV	left ventricle	N_2O	nitrous oxide
LVEDP	left ventricular end diastolic pres-	noc	nocturnal
	sure	NPO	nothing by mouth
LVEF	left ventricular ejection fraction	NSR	normal sinus rhythm

NSVD	normal spontaneous vaginal delivery
n & v	nausea and vomiting

O

O$_2$	oxygen
OB	obstetrics or obstetrical
OBS	organic brain syndrome
O/C	on call
OD	right eye
OOB	out of bed
OP	outpatient
Ophth	ophthalmology
OR	operating room
ORIF	open reduction, internal fixation
OS	left eye
O$_2$ sat	oxygen saturation
OT	occupational therapy
OU	each eye or both eyes

P

p̄	after
PaO$_2$	partial pressure of arterial oxygen
PA	pulmonary artery
PAC	premature atrial contraction
PACU	postanesthesia care unit
PAL	posteroanterior and lateral
pap smear	Papanicolaou smear
PAR	postanesthesia recovery room
Para I, II, etc.	indicating number of children born to a woman
paracent	paracentesis
PAT	paroxysmal atrial tachycardia
PAWP	pulmonary artery wedge pressure
PCA	patient-controlled analgesia
pCO$_2$	partial pressure (p) of carbon dioxide (CO$_2$)
PCN	penicillin
PCTA	percutaneous transluminal coronary angioplasty
$\overline{PCW}$	pulmonary capillary wedge pressure mean
pcwp	pulmonary capillary wedge pressure
PD	peritoneal dialysis
PE	pulmonary embolism
Ped	Pediatrics
PEEP	positive end-expiratory pressure

PERRLA	pupils equal, reactive to light and accomodation
pH	negative logarithm of the hydrogen ion concentration
PID	pelvic inflammatory disease
PM	after noon
PMH	past medical history
PMI	point of maximum impulse
po	by mouth
PO$_2$	partial pressure of oxygen
post	posterior
post-op	postoperative
P,R	pulse, respirations
PRBC	packed red blood cells
pre-op	preoperative
p.r.n., or prn	as often as needed
procto	proctoscopy
PS	physical status
PT	posterior tibial
pt.	patient
PTA	prior to admission
PTCA	percutaneous transluminal coronary angioplasty
PTT	partial thromboplastin time
PUD	peptic ulcer disease
PVC	premature ventricular contractions
PVD	peripheral vascular disease

Q

Q or q	every
QD	every day
qid	four times a day
qns	quantity not sufficient
qod	every other day
qoh	every other hour
qs	quantity sufficient

R

R	right
RA	rheumatoid arthritis
RA	right atrium
$\overline{RA}$	right atrial mean pressure
RBC	red blood cell(s)
RCA	right coronary artery
RCE	right carotid endarterectomy
RF	rheumatic fever

rehab	rehabilitation
resp	respirations
resp distress	respiratory distress
Rh	rhesus blood factor
RLE	right lower extremity
RLL	right lower lobe — lung
RLQ	right lower quandrant abdomen
RN	registered nurse
R/O	rule out
ROM	range of motion
ROS	review of systems
RR	recovery room
r/t	related to
RUE	right upper extremity
RUL	right upper lobe — lung
RUQ	right upper quadrant — abdomen
RV	right ventricle
Rx	prescription

S

s̄	without
SA	sinoatrial (node)
SAO$_2$	arterial oxygen saturation
SBE	subacute bacterial endocarditis
sed rate	sedimentation rate
septic-A	septic AIDS
SGOT	serum glutamic-oxaloacetic tran- saminase
SGPT	serum glutamic-pyruvic transami- nase
SIADH	syndrome of inappropriate secretion of antidiuretic hormone
SIMV	synchronized intermittent manda- tory ventilation
SLE	systemic lupus erythematosus
SL	sublingual
SMR	submucous resection
SOB	shortness of breath
S/P	status post
sp gr	specific gravity
SQ	subcutaneous
s/s	signs and symptoms
staph	staphylococcus
stat	immediately and once only
STD	sexually transmitted disease
strep	streptococcus
surg	surgery or surgical

SVR	systemic vascular resistance
SVT	supraventricular tachycardia
SX	service

T

T	temperature
T & A	tonsillectomy and adenoidectomy
TAH	total abdominal hysterectomy
TB	tuberculosis
TBA	to be announced
temp	temporary
TENS	transcutaneous electrical nerve stimulator
THA	total hip arthroplasty
THR	total hip replacement
TIA	transient ischemic attack
tid	three times a day
TKA or TKR	total knee arthroplasty
TKO	to keep open
TLC	tender loving care
TMJ	temporomandibular joint
TO	telephone order
TPN	total parenteral nutrition
trach	tracheostomy
tsp	teaspoon
TUR (P)	transurethral resection of prostate
TV	tidal volume
TVR	tricuspid valve replacement
Tx	treatment, therapy

U

U/A	urinalysis
UE	upper extremity
URI	upper respiratory infection
urol	urology or urological
UTI	urinary tract infection

V

vag	vagina or vaginal
VD	venereal disease
VDRL	Veneral Disease Research Labora- tories (flocculation procedure)
v fib	ventricular fibrillation
vit cap	vital capacity
VO	verbal order

V/Q scan	ventilation perfusion lung scan	=	equals
VS	vital signs	×	times
vs	versus	°	degrees
VSD	ventricular septal defect	<	less than
VSS	vital signs stable	>	greater than
V tach	ventricular tachycardia	↑	increase
		↓	decrease
	W	2°	secondary
		1°	primary
WBAT	weight bearing as tolerated	~	approximate(ly)
WBC	white blood count	+	positive
WC or W/C	wheelchair	−	negative
WNL	within normal limits	Δ	change
W-P-W	Wolff-Parkinson-White syndrome	♂	male
wt	weight	♀	female

XYZ

y/o	year old

INDEX

Page numbers in *italics* indicate boxed material or illustrations.
Page numbers followed by *t* indicate tables.